Chemokines and Cancer

Contemporary Cancer Research

Jac A. Nickoloff, Series Editor

Chemokines and Cancer

Edited by

Barrett J. Rollins, MD, PhD

Department of Adult Oncology
Dana-Farber Cancer Institute, Boston, MA

Humana Press ✳ Totowa, New Jersey

© 1999 Humana Press Inc.
999 Riverview Drive, Suite 208
Totowa, New Jersey 07512

This publication is printed on acid-free paper. ⊚
ANSI Z39.48-1984 (American Standards Institute) Permanence of Paper for Printed Library Materials.

Cover design by Patricia F. Cleary.

For additional copies, pricing for bulk purchases, and/or information about other Humana titles, contact Humana at the above address or at any of the following numbers: Tel: 973-256-1699; Fax: 973-256-8341; E-mail: humana@humanapr.com, or visit our Website: http://humanapress.com

Printed in the United States of America. 10 9 8 7 6 5 4 3 2 1

Library of Congress Cataloging in Publication Data

Chemokines and cancer / edited by Barrett J. Rollins.
         p.   cm.—(Contemporary cancer research)
     Includes index.
     ISBN 0-89603-562-X (alk. paper)
     1. Chemokines—Therapeutic use. 2. Cancer—Chemotherapy. I. Rollins, Barrett J. II. Series.
     [DNLM: 1. Chemokines—physiology. 2. Neoplasms—physiopathology.
     QW 568 C5165 1999]
     RC271.C48C46   1999
     616.99'4061—dc21
     DNLM/DLC   98-48424
     for Library of Congress   CIP

Preface

The relationship between a malignant tumor and its host has a complexity matched only by the history of its investigation by medical scientists. Since the earliest days of histology, pathologists have noted the presence of inflammatory cells in or around a wide variety of tumors, and have inferred from these observations that the body often attempts to "reject" its tumor. As we have become more sophisticated about the physiology of leukocytes, this simple scenario has been amended to include the possibility that, in some circumstances, the host's inflammatory response may actually support rather than hinder tumor growth.

Recent advances in our understanding of inflammation and immunology are already helping to elucidate the complicated relationship between tumor and host. For example, during the past five years there has been enormous expansion in knowledge about the family of leukocyte-specific chemoattractants known as chemokines. In fact, in some instances, chemokines have been purified explicitly on the basis of their ability to attract certain leukocyte subsets into tumors. *Chemokines and Cancer* is an attempt to assess the current state of knowledge about chemokines as it applies to the cancer problem.

From a broad perspective, one can think of chemokines as acting directly on tumor cells themselves, or indirectly influencing tumor cell behavior by modulating the host's response to its tumor. So far, instances of the former are relatively rare in the literature, but examples included herein are the effects of MGSA on melanoma cell proliferation and the effects of several chemokines on tumor cell migration. Also included are examples of chemokine expression by specific tumor types (e.g., ovarian cancers) or tumor viruses, and host chemokine responses to *H. pylori*, which may be an etiologic agent in gastric carcinoma. This area will only continue to expand as more chemokine receptors are found on tumor cells and the consequences of their activation are examined.

As far as host effects are concerned, these can be subdivided into several areas. For example, chemokines can enhance tumor-specific immunity perhaps, in part, by their effects on antigen presentation. In addition, however, chemokines can enhance natural immunity through effects on macrophages and natural killer cells. Furthermore, since tumor vascularity profoundly affects growth and metastatic spread, chemokine-mediated influences on angiogenesis also have a significant effect on tumors. Finally, chapters have been included that discuss chemokine effects on stem cells, both hematopoietic and otherwise, because of their importance as a source of self-renewing tumorigenic cells and because of the adverse effects suffered by these cells as a result of cancer chemotherapy or radiation.

The chemokine field is relatively young and discoveries are occurring at a rapid pace. *Chemokines and Cancer*, therefore, can serve only as a snapshot that describes the relationship between chemokines and cancer as it is currently understood. Undoubtedly, new findings will soon expand and alter our perspectives in this area and, one hopes, provide opportunities to exploit chemokines in the treatment of malignant disease.

Barrett J. Rollins, MD, PhD

Contents

Contributors

PAOLA ALLAVENA • *Department of Immunology and Cell Biology, Istituto di Ricerche Farmacologiche, "Mario Negri," Milan, Italy*

DOUGLAS A. ARENBERG • *Division of Pulmonary and Critical Medicine, Department of Internal Medicine, The University of Michigan Medical School, Ann Arbor, MI*

FRANCES R. BALKWILL • *Biological Therapies Laboratory, Imperial Cancer Research Fund, London, UK*

HAL E. BROXMEYER • *Departments of Microbiology/Immunology, Medicine, and the Walther Oncology Center, Indiana University School of Medicine and the Walther Cancer Institute, Indianapolis, IN*

RONALD BUKOWSKI • *Department of Hematology–Oncology, Cleveland Clinic Foundation, Cleveland, OH*

MARIE BURDICK • *Department of Pulmonary Medicine, University of Michigan School of Medicine, Ann Arbor, MI*

STEPHEN W. CHENSUE • *Department of Pathology, The University of Michigan Medical School, Ann Arbor, MI*

OLEG CHERTOV • *Intramural Research Support Program, SAIC Frederick, National Cancer Institute–Frederick Cancer Research and Development Center, Frederick, MD*

JEAN E. CRABTREE • *Division of Medicine, St. James's University Hospital, Leeds, UK*

BRUNO DiGIOVINE • *Division of Pulmonary and Critical Medicine, Department of Internal Medicine, The University of Michigan Medical School, Ann Arbor, MI*

HOWARD A. FINE • *Department of Adult Oncology, Dana-Farber Cancer Institute, Harvard Medical School, Boston, MA*

JAMES FINKE • *Department of Immunology, Cleveland Clinic Foundation, Cleveland, OH*

CRAIG GERARD • *Children's Hospital and Harvard Medical School, Boston, MA*

GARARD J. GRAHAM • *The Beatson Institute for Cancer Research, Cancer Research Campaign Beatson Laboratories, Glasgow, UK*

LONG GU • *Department of Adult Oncology, Dana-Farber Cancer Institute, Harvard Medical School, Boston, MA*

HAMID HAGHNEGAHDAR • *Department of Cell Biology, Vanderbilt University, Nashville, TN*

THOMAS A. HAMILTON • *Department of Immunology, Cleveland Clinic Foundation, Cleveland, OH*

JOSEPH HESSELGESSER • *Berlex Biosciences • Division of Berlex Laboratories, Inc., Richmond, CA*

RICHARD HORUK • *Berlex Biosciences • Division of Berlex Laboratories, Inc., Richmond, CA*

CHANG H. KIM • *Departments of Microbiology/Immunology, Medicine, and the Walther Oncology Center, Indiana University School of Medicine and the Walther Cancer Institute, Indianapolis, IN*

KERSTIN KLEINE-LOWINSKI • *Universitäts-Frauenklinik, Friedrich Schiller Universität, Jena, Germany*

STEVEN L. KUNKEL • *Department of Pathology, The University of Michigan Medical School, Ann Arbor, MI*

JUN-ICHI KURATSU • *Department of Neurosurgery, Faculty of Medicine, Kagoshima University, Kagoshima, Japan*

IVAN J. D. LINDLEY • *Novartis Research Institute, Vienna, Austria*

NICHOLAS W. LUKACS • *Department of Pathology, The University of Michigan Medical School, Ann Arbor, MI*

ALBERTO MANTOVANI • *Department of Immunology and Cell Biology, Istituto di Ricerche Farmacologiche "Mario Negri," Milan, Italy and Department of Biotechnology, Section of General Pathology, University of Brescia, Italy*

RUPERT P. M. NEGUS • *Biological Therapies Laboratory, Imperial Cancer Research Fund, London, UK*

ROBERT J. B. NIBBS • *The Beatson Institute for Cancer Research, Cancer Research Campaign Beatson Laboratories, Glasgow, UK*

CHAITANYA S. NIRODI • *Department of Cell Biology, Vanderbilt University, Nashville, TN*

G. OPDENAKKER • *Laboratory of Molecular Immunology, The Rega Institute for Medical Research, University of Leuven, Leuven, Belgium*

JOOST J. OPPENHEIM • *Laboratory of Molecular Immunoregulation, Division of Basic Sciences, SAIC Frederick, National Cancer Institute–Frederick Cancer Research and Development Center, Frederick, MD*

JAMES D. OWEN • *Department of Cell Biology, Vanderbilt University, Nashville, TN*

PETER J. POLVERINI • *Laboratory of Molecular Pathology, Department of Oral Medicine, Pathology, and Surgery, The University of Michigan School of Medicine, Ann Arbor, MI*

ANN RICHMOND • *Department of Cell Biology, Vanderbilt University, and*

Department of Veterans Affairs, Nashville, TN

BARRETT J. ROLLINS • *Department of Adult Oncology, Dana-Farber Cancer Institute, Harvard Medical School, Boston, MA*

FRANK RÖSL • *Angewandte Tumorvirologie, Deutsches Krebsforschungszentrum Im Neuenheimer Feld, Heidelberg, Germany*

ARMEN SHANAFELT • *Institute of Molecular Biologicals, Bayer Corporation, West Haven, CT*

REBECCA SHATTUCK-BRANDT • *Department of Cell Biology, Vanderbilt University, Nashville, TN*

WEIPIN SHEN • *Laboratory of Molecular Immunoregulation, Division of Basic Sciences, SAIC Frederick, National Cancer Institute–Frederick Cancer Research and Development Center, Frederick, MD*

ANTONIO SICA • *Department of Immunology and Cell Biology, Istituto di Ricerche Farmacologiche, "Mario Negri," Milan, Italy*

KENZO SOEJIMA • *Department of Adult Oncology, Dana-Farber Cancer Institute, Harvard Medical School, Boston, MA*

SILVANO SOZZANI • *Department of Immunology and Cell Biology, Istituto di Ricerche Farmacologiche, "Mario Negri," Milan, Italy*

THEODORE STANDIFORD • *Department of Internal Medicine, The University of Michigan Medical School, Ann Arbor, MI*

ROBERT M. STRIETER • *Department of Internal Medicine, Division of Pulmonary and Critical Medicine, The University of Michigan Medical School, Ann Arbor, MI*

CHARLES S. TANNENBAUM • *Department of Immunology, Cleveland Clinic Foundation, Cleveland, OH*

DENNIS D. TAUB • *Clinical Immunology Section, Laboratory of Immunology, National Institute on Aging, Gerontology Research Center, National Institutes of Health, Baltimore, MD*

SUSAN TSENG • *Department of Adult Oncology, Dana-Farber Cancer Institute, Harvard Medical School, Boston, MA*

JO VAN DAMME • *Laboratory of Molecular Immunology, The Rega Institute for Medical Research, University of Leuven, Leuven, Belgium*

ANNUNCIATA VECCHI • *Department of Immunology and Cell Biology, Istituto di Ricerche Farmacologiche, "Mario Negri," Milan, Italy*

JI MING WANG • *Laboratory of Molecular Immunoregulation, Division of Basic Sciences, SAIC Frederick, National Cancer Institute–Frederick Cancer Research and Development Center, Frederick, MD*

LAUREN D. WOOD • *Department of Cell Biology, Vanderbilt University, Nashville, TN*

Teizo Yoshimura • *Immunopathology Section, Laboratory of Immunobiology, National Cancer Institute–Frederick Cancer Research and Development Center, Frederick, MD*

Harald zur Hausen • *Angewandte Tumorvirologie, Deutsches Krebsforschungszentrum Im Neuenheimer Feld, Heidelberg, Germany*

I
Chemokine Physiology

The Function of Chemokines in Health and Disease

Steven L. Kunkel, Nicholas W. Lukacs, Robert M. Strieter, Theodore Standiford, and Stephen W. Chensue

1. INTRODUCTION

The cascade of events that dictate the normal physiologic processes leading to the initiation, maintenance, and final resolution of inflammation is the result of the host responding to a variety of direct or indirect stimuli. Although these stimuli may represent either infectious agents (viruses, bacteria, and protozoans) or noninfectious processes (trauma, autoimmune disorders, and ischemia/reperfusion injury), they all result in the activation and directed migration of leukocytes into an area of tissue injury. Our current understanding of inflammation suggests that the recruitment of leukocytes from the lumen of a vessel into a localized area of injury depends on an interrelated network of events, which must occur with some fidelity in order for the cells to arrive successfully at a site of inflammation. Although many of the steps involved in leukocyte activation and elicitation have been identified, a complete understanding of these processes, including the subsequent tissue injury, are not entirely known.

Initial phases of the activation/chemotactic responses are likely to be dependent on a number of dynamic interactions that result in the expression of a variety of important inflammatory mediators. For example, the early response cytokines, interleukin-1 (IL-1) and tumor neurosis factor (TNF), have been shown to mediate leukocyte adherence to the vascular endothelium. This interaction "targets" the leukocyte to an area of inflammation and may be an important mechanism in restricting these cells to a designated area of reactivity. Interestingly, the adherence of monocytes to either endothelial or stromal cells is a strong signal for the expression of leukocyte-derived chemokines, which serves to activate further the inflammatory system. While the contact between leukocytes and endothelial cells is transient and must be reversible, it is a significant cytokine/chemokine-producing step. The transition from adherence to migration allows the activated leukocytes, first, to accumulate and then to pass through the endothelial cell and basement membrane barrier. Concomitantly, the leukocytes must recognize additional chemotactic signals that serve as homing mechanisms to "commit and direct" the cells to an area of evolving inflammation.

Studies have now shown that chemokines are not only important in recruiting cells into an area of inflammation, but that they also appear to aid in dictating the evolution of particular types of immune reactivity. For example, monocyte chemoattractant pro-

From: *Chemokines and Cancer*
Edited by: B. J. Rollins © Humana Press Inc., Totowa, NJ

tein-1 (MCP-1), which has been shown to be a potent chemotaxin for monocytes and lymphocytes, can also increase the expression of lymphocyte-derived IL-4 in response to antigen challenge and decrease the levels of IL-12. This activity may facilitate the evolution, or switch, of a Th1-type phenotypic response to a Th2-type phenotypic response. In the context of chronic inflammation, the particular cytokine/chemokine phenotype that persists at an inflammatory site may play an important role in the development of long-term disease. This may be especially true in chronic inflammation in which the continued cytokine expression pattern may predominate with characteristics of a Th2-type profile.

2. PATHOPHYSIOLOGY OF LEUKOCYTE RECRUITMENT

Historically, the pathologic assessment of various diseases and disorders has been characterized, in part, by the microscopic identification of specific leukocyte subpopulations attracted to an area of tissue injury. These *in situ* observations were important in establishing the early association between leukocytes and inflammation; however, it was not until the early 1960s and the development of the Boyden chamber that leukocyte migration could be quantitatively analyzed *(5)*. The Boyden chamber separated leukocytes from a soluble signal by a filter with a known pore size. The entire chamber could be placed in an incubator, and at specific time intervals the leukocytes that had migrated into or through the filter in response to the chemotaxin could be quantitated. One of the major scientific breakthroughs using the Boyden filters was the ability to assess the direct chemotactic activity of a given agent. A modification of the Boyden chamber has since allowed investigators to distinguish between chemotaxis, the process of directed movement of leukocytes in response to a concentration gradient, and chemokinesis, the property of random movement of activated leukocytes *(56)*.

Although these recent scientific advances were important in explaining certain aspects of leukocyte migration, credit must be given to the anatomic pathologists, who more than a century ago recognized that certain diseases were associated with specific subpopulations of leukocytes. However, these early observers could only speculate about their observations, as mechanisms responsible for the accumulation of these leukocytes were not known. One of the first investigations directed at providing a mechanism for leukocyte migration in response to a known stimulus was performed using dead microorganisms or products of human leukocytes. While descriptive, these early studies were important in providing the groundwork for a number of subsequent investigations demonstrating that bacteria products, such as *N*-formylmethionyl peptides or synthetic *N*-formylmethionyl derivatives, were potent agents for leukocyte activation and chemotaxis *(44)*. Furthermore, these subsequent investigations demonstrated that the host had developed sophisticated mechanisms to activate the chemotactic response, via specific receptor-ligand interactions, which recognize bacterial-derived products.

In addition to bacterial-derived peptides, subsequent studies demonstrated that host-derived polypeptides, such as activation products generated from the fifth component of complement (C5a) and fibrin fragments, were also chemotactic for a variety of leukocytes *(16)*. Collectively, these seminal observations provided some of the first information regarding the mechanism for the recruitment of leukocytes during infectious processes *(16,53)*. Although these investigations were important in providing insight into leukocyte recruitment, they did not address the specificity associated with the

Table 1
Some Members of the C-X-C Chemokine Family

C-X-C Chemokines
    Interleukin-8 (IL-8)
    Growth-regulated oncogene-α (GRO-α)
    Growth-regulated oncogene-β (GRO-β)
    Growth-regulated oncogene-γ (GRO-γ)
    Epithelial cell–derived neutrophil-activating Factor-78 (ENA-78)
    Neutrophil-activating peptide-2 (NAP-2)
    Granulocyte chemotactic protein-2 (GCP-2)
    Monokine induced by interferon-γ (MIG)
    Platelet factor 4 (PF4)
    Interferon-γ-inducible protein-10 (IP-10)

recruitment of leukocyte subpopulations during inflammation. The identification of other chemotactic factors such as platelet activating factor, leukotriene B_4 (LTB_4), and split products of fibronectin further complicated the issue of leukocyte movement, since these chemotactic agents also lacked any degree of specificity for the recruitment of leukocyte subpopulations *(17)*. An important aspect of these initial investigations was recognition of the redundancy in the number and types of factors that could induce leukocyte chemotaxis. The redundant nature of chemotactic factors stresses the importance of cell recruitment during an infectious/inflammatory process, as a number of systems are in place to ensure the successful elicitation of leukocytes to a site of injury.

3. THE SUPERGENE FAMILY OF CHEMOTACTIC CYTOKINES

The fact that multiple chemotactic agents possess little in the way of cell specificity remained at odds with the microscopic pathology of certain acute and chronic diseases, which are characterized by specific leukocyte populations. For example, many acute inflammatory reactions with a bacterial etiology are dominated by the presence of neutrophils, whereas many chronic immune reactions are characterized by the presence of specific mononuclear leukocyte populations. Insight into this long-standing enigma has been provided by discoveries demonstrating that a family of *chemo*tactic cyto*kines,* called *chemokines,* possess a relatively high degree of specificity for the elicitation of leukocyte subpopulations *(2,23,27,28).* These chemokines belong to related polypeptide groups, identified by the location of cysteine residues near the amino terminus that comprised the primary amino acid structure (Table 1). In one supergene family, the two amino terminal cysteines are separated by a nonconserved amino acid in a C-X-C motif, and in the other family the amino terminal cysteines are found in juxtaposition to one another in a C-C motif. The discovery of two related chemokine families of polypeptide mediators of inflammation provided a potential mechanism for the selective recruitment and activation of peripheral blood leukocytes. The chemokine field is not limited to these supergene families, as at least two additional family members have also been identified. These additional families are designated the C family, characterized by lymphotactin, and the CX_3C family, characterized by fractalkine.

Table 2
C-X-C Chemokine Family Includes Cytokines
Possessing or Lacking Glutamic Acid, Leucine,
and Arginine (ELR) Motif Near Amino Terminal End

C-X-C Chemokines Containing the ELR Amino Acid Motif
   Interleukin-8 (IL-8)
   Growth-regulated oncogene-α (GRO-α)
   Growth-regulated oncogene-β (GRO-β)
   Growth-regulated oncogene-γ (GRO-γ)
   Epithelial cell–derived neutrophil-activating Factor-78 (ENA-78)
   Neutrophil-activating peptide-2 (NAP-2)
   Granulocyte chemotactic protein-2 (GCP-2)

C-X-C Chemokines Lacking the ELR Amino Acid Motif
   Monokine induced by interferon-γ (MIG)
   Platelet factor 4 (PF4)
   Interferon-γ-inducible protein-10 (IP-10)

3.1. The C-X-C Chemokine Family

The genes encoding many of the C-X-C chemokines map to human chromosome 4(q12-q21) and their proteins possess 20–50% amino acid homology with one another *(3,35)*. Several C-X-C chemokines have been identified, including platelet factor 4 (PF4), IL-8, growth-related oncogene-α, -β, and -γ (GRO-α, -β, -γ), epithelial cell–derived neutrophil-activating factor-78 (ENA-78), granulocyte chemotactic protein-2 (GCP-2), interferon-γ-inducible protein-10 (IP-10), monokine induced by interferon (MIG), and the amino terminal processed forms of platelet basic protein: connective tissue–activating protein III, β-thromboglobulin, and neutrophil-activating peptide-2 (NAP-2) *(15,20,29,37,48,52)* (Table 1). PF4 was the first member of the C-X-C chemokine family to be described and was identified as a heparin-binding protein that could block the anticoagulation property of heparin. Many of the C-X-C chemokines were originally discovered based on their biologic activity or their ability to be expressed based on a specific stimulation. For example, the GRO family of C-X-C chemokines were originally described for their melanoma growth stimulatory activity, whereas IP-10 and MIG are specifically expressed after interferon stimulation *(1,15,20)*. IP-10 expression appears to be under the influence of interferon-α (IFN-α), IFN-β, and IFN-γ; however, MIG is expressed only by cells stimulated with IFN-γ *(15,20)*. Other C-X-C chemokines, such as IL-8, ENA-78, and GCP-2, were discovered based on their neutrophil chemotactic and activating activity, the historic biologic function that originally defined this family. Interestingly, some members of the C-X-C chemokine family do not possess neutrophil chemotactic activity, including IP-10, MIG, and PF4. Although the C-X-C amino acid motif is preserved in these proteins, they lack three important amino acids (Glu-Leu-Arg, or ELR) near the amino terminus, which is important in receptor-ligand engagement and confers neutrophil chemotactic activity to specific members of this supergene family *(3)* (Table 2).

The genomic structures for most of the C-X-C chemokine family members are highly conserved, as they have four exons and three introns (platelet basic protein and PF4 have three exons and two introns) *(26,32)*. The similarity of the exons and introns of the C-X-C family suggests that they are likely to have diverged from a common gene, as the first and second introns of the genes are highly conserved. The 5′ region of the C-X-C chemokine gene contains a variety of regulatory elements, including CCAAT and TATA boxes, as well as binding sites for known nuclear transcription factors *(33)*. Of particular interest are the binding sites for NF-κB (p65/RelA), AP-1, NF-IL-6, and octamer binding sites. Recent data support the hypothesis that more than one transcription factor is important for the activation of the IL-8 gene. The maximal induction of the IL-8 gene occurs when both the NF-IL-6 and NF-κB binding sites are occupied. Therefore, there is cooperative interaction between these two families of transcription factors in the regulation of IL-8 expression. The IL-8 promoter appears to require the binding of both transcription factors, whereas ENA-78 requires only that the NF-κB site be occupied *(8)*. These studies suggest that not all members of the C-X-C chemokine family require cooperative binding of different transcription factors for gene activation.

The mRNA of most of the C-X-C chemokines contain a short 5′ untranslated region, an open reading frame that encodes the mature polypeptide and the amino terminal sequence, and a fairly long 3′ untranslated region containing a number of AUUUA repeats. This latter characteristic is common to a number of inflammatory cytokines and has been previously shown to play a role in posttranscriptional regulation via altering mRNA stability. Using the previously cited criteria, IL-8 mRNA is 1.6 kb, with a 101 base 5′ untranslated region, a coding region containing 297 bases for the 99 amino acids, and a 1.2 kb 3′ untranslated region. The precursor polypeptide of IL-8 contains 99 amino acids plus a 20 amino acid signal sequence *(3,26,29,35)*. The secreted IL-8 polypeptide can undergo several rounds of amino terminal cleavage, resulting in truncated forms of IL-8 possessing either 77, 72, 71, 70, or 69 amino acids *(54)*. Each of these processed forms of IL-8 possesses biologic activity.

The cysteine amino acids are not only important in naming the chemokine family, but they are critically important to the stability of the molecule. The addition of 1% 2-mercaptoethanol to C-X-C chemokines leads to unfolding of the protein and inactivation of the biologic characteristics of the molecules. However, the addition of 0.5% sodium dodecyl sulfate, extremes of pH and temperature, 2 *M* lithium chloride, 6 *M* guanidinium, and mild enzymatic treatment do not dramatically impact the activity of these chemokines *(36)*. These physicochemical characteristics all support a role for C-X-C chemokines as persistent leukocyte-activating factors that can survive in the inflammatory milieu.

One of the intriguing aspects of many C-X-C chemokines is that these polypeptides are synthesized by a variety of cells. For example, IL-8 has been identified as a product of monocytes, alveolar macrophages, neutrophils, mast cells, eosinophils, lymphocytes, natural killer (NK) cells, fibroblasts, endothelial cells, epithelial cells, smooth muscle cells, keratinocytes, hepatocytes, mesothelial cells, and mesangial cells *(6,14,24,30,38,42,46,47,50,51)* (Table 3). In summation, most nucleated cells of the body, when appropriately stimulated, can express certain chemokines. Not only is the cellular source of the chemokines varied, but the activating agents are also quite different, as cytokines (IL-1, TNF, and interferons), bacterial products, viruses, and other chemotactic factors (C5a and leukotriene B_4) can serve as stimuli for chemokine expression.

**Table 3
C-X-C Chemokines a Product of Many
Cell Types, Including Mononuclear Phagocytes,
Fibroblasts, and Epithelial Cells**

Chemotactic cytokines	Cellular source
IL-8	Phagocytes/nonimmune cells
NAP-2	Platelets
GRO/MGSA	Various cells
ENA-78	Various cells
GCP-2	Various cells

Although the majority of the C-X-C chemokines have been studied in the context of neutrophil activation, a variety of investigations have shown that IL-8 and other members of this family possess activity for other leukocyte populations. Both IL-8 and the GRO family can dose dependently, induce a rise in cytosolic calcium, and induce chemotaxis in basophils. Furthermore, IL-8 and NAP-2 both can induce significant histamine release from IL-3-treated basophils. These studies suggest that certain C-X-C chemokines may play an important role in mediating basophil activation and migration at the site of inflammation. Eosinophils have also been reported to respond to IL-8 with a rise in cytosolic calcium, a change in cell shape, and exocytosis of eosinophil peroxidase. Pretreatment with pertussis toxin (PTx) attenuates this activation, demonstrating that G proteins are also involved in the signal-coupling events in the eosinophil. IL-8 has been reported to be chemotactic for T-lymphocytes; however, this activity is limited compared to C-C chemokines. IL-8 does have an effect on NK cells, but the biologic effect was identified as the induction of random migration rather than directed chemotaxis. Interestingly, IL-8 has been reported to have potent effects on B-lymphocytes, as it can selectively inhibit the ability of IL-4 to induce the expression of IgE or IgG4, but not other immunoglobulin isotypes.

3.2. The C-C Chemokine Family

The related C-C chemokine family also displays four highly conserved cysteine amino acid residues; however, in contrast to the C-X-C family, the C-C chemokines do not have a separating amino acid between the two cysteines in the amino terminal domain. Like the C-X-C chemokines, the C-C family members are also cationic, small mol wt polypeptides, 7–10 kDa, which bind heparin. While the C-X-C chemokines possess chemotactic activity for neutrophils, this chemokine family appears to have specificity for the directed movement of monocytes, lymphocytes, eosinophils, and basophils. The genes encoding these chemokines are clustered at 17 q11.2-112, and their proteins possess 28–45% amino acid homology *(3,28,35,41,48)*. Between the C-X-C and C-C subfamilies of chemokines, there is approx 20–45% homology at the amino acid level *(3,28,35)*. A growing list of C-C chemokines has been discovered and includes monocyte chemoattractant proteins 1,2,3,4,5 (MCP1–5), macrophage inflammatory protein-1α and -β (MIP-1α, -β), RANTES, eotaxin, C-10, and 1-309 *(3,28,35,48)* (Table 4). Many of these polypeptides were originally isolated from

Table 4
C-C Chemokines Belong to a Related Supergene Family of
Mediators Possessing a Conserved C-C Amino Acid Motif

C-C Chemokines
　　Monocyte chemoattractant protein-1,2,3,4,5 (MCP-1,2,3,4,5)
　　Macrophage inflammatory protein-1α (MIP-1α)
　　Macrophage inflammatory protein-1β (MIP-1β)
　　C-10
　　I-309
　　RANTES
　　TCA-3

tumors or tumor-derived cell lines, which has created an interesting enigma regarding the biologic activity of these chemokines.

Like the C-X-C chemokines, the C-C family genes also have three exons and two introns. The first, second, and third exons encode the 5′ untranslated region and the signal peptide, the amino terminal half of the polypeptide, and the carboxyl terminal half of the polypeptide plus the 3′ untranslated region, respectively *(31,34)*. The two chemokine families appear to have diverged from a common ancestral gene, because the splice junction between the second and third exons occurs at the same position in all the chemokines. The 5′ flanking region of C-C chemokine genes contain CCAAT and TATA box structures and possess a number of potential binding sites for nuclear transcription factors. Both NF-κB and NF-IL-6 sites have been identified in the promoter region of these genes *(31)*.

The prototype C-C chemokine is MCP-1. This polypeptide is synthesized as a 99 amino acid precursor, but is secreted as a 76 amino acid protein, as are many of the C-C chemokines. MCP-1 appears to be produced in two isoforms from the same gene with mol wt of 13 and 9 kDa *(19)*. The 13-kDa isoform contains the disaccharide galactose-beta 1-3D-*N*-acetyl galactosamine, whereas the 9-kDa isoform does not possess this glycosylation. However, the glycosylation of MCP-1 does not appear to affect the monocyte chemotactic activity of this protein. Although glycosylation of MCP-1 does not alter the activity of MCP-1, reduction and alkylation of the paired disulfide bridges greatly reduces the ability of MCP-1 to act as a chemotactic factor. Furthermore, both the amino and carboxyl termini of MCP-1 are particularly important for biologic activity as deletion of either amino acid residues 2–8 or truncation of the carboxyl terminus greatly abrogates the chemotactic activity of MCP-1 *(55)*.

The binding of C-C chemokines to their respective receptors results in a signal-coupled event that is similar to that induced by many known chemotactic factors. The C-C chemokines can activate monocytes and induce a rise in cytosolic calcium, respiratory burst, and chemotactic activity *(39,49)*. Furthermore, MCP-1, RANTES, and MIP-1α can modulate the expression of adhesion molecules on the surface of monocytes. These C-C chemokines can upregulate the β2 integrins CD11b/CD18 and CD11c/CD18, but not CD11a/CD18 in a similar concentration range and potency as f-met-leu-phe, and LTB$_4$. By contrast, these small mediators were not able to induce the expression of the β1 integrin, VLA-4, on the surface of monocytes. The mechanism for β2-integrin expression is related to microtubule formation and the mobilization of calcium. MCP-1, RANTES, and MIP-1α have also been shown to activate other functional activities of monocytes, such as induction of chemotaxis and release of arachidonic acid. Both of these events are related to G protein–coupled signals, as treatment with PTx can abrogate these responses.

While MCP-1 has been identified as a potent activator of monocytes for their participation in host defense against infectious agents, this factor also appears to play an important role in augmenting monocyte-dependent tumoricidal activity *(45)*. Specifically, MCP-1 has been observed to prime monocytes/macrophages and heighten the tumoricidal activity of monocytes when stimulated with lipopolysaccharide. Similar observations have been made in an in vivo situation; melanoma or Chinese hamster ovary cells transfected with MCP-1 cDNA resulted in a significant modification of the subsequent tumor growth. The expression of MCP-1 in vivo was associated with a rise in macrophage accumulation at the tumor site and a reduction in tumor burden.

Several investigations have shown that C-C chemokines, as compared with C-X-C chemokines, are potent agents for the activation and chemotaxis of basophils and eosinophils *(22,4,40)*. Recent studies have demonstrated that MCP-1, MCP-3, MIP-1α, and RANTES can activate and induce the chemotaxis of basophils, and that eotaxin, MCP-3, MCP-4, MIP-1α, and RANTES induce the directed migration of eosinophils. Interestingly, MIP-1β failed to activate either basophils or eosinophils. Unprimed basophils treated with either MCP-1 or MCP-3 were able to induce the release of histamine, whereas IL-3-primed basophils were responsive to MCP-1, MCP-3, and RANTES, but not MIP-1α. These investigations support the notion that the order of chemokine-induced, basophil activation proceeds as follows: RANTES = MCP-3 >> MCP-1 > MIP-1α for chemotaxis and MCP-1 = MCP-3 >> RANTES > MIP-1α for histamine release and the production of LTC_4. These studies support the idea that MCP-3 may be one of the most important C-C chemokines for basophil activation, leading to chemotaxis and histamine release.

The migration of mononuclear cells toward sites of antigen-induced inflammation is important in the evolution of the host's immune response. The ability of certain leukocyte chemotactic factors to elicit specific subsets of cells to a site of inflammation has provided the impetus to study the role of chemokines as specific leukocyte chemotactic factors. A number of C-C chemokines have been shown to be chemotactic not only for monocytes but also T-lymphocytes, B-lymphocytes, and NK cells. RANTES was one of the first chemokines to be characterized as a T-lymphocyte chemotactic chemokine. This polypeptide was found to induce specific migration of memory CD4[+] T-cells (CD45RO[+]), as compared with naive T-cells (CD45RA[+]), in a dose-dependent manner *(43)*. Although this study did not address the lymphocyte chemotactic activity of other members of the C-C chemokine family, it did suggest that RANTES may be notable for its ability to recruit specific subsets of CD4[+] T-cells to a site of immune reactivity. In further studies, MIP-1α and MIP-1β have been demonstrated to induce the predominant migration of CD8[+] and CD4[+] T-cells, respectively; but, neither chemokine was able to elicit the migration of quiescent T-cells. Both of these C-C chemokines were shown to augment the adhesion of either subset of T-cells to endothelial monolayers, suggesting that these factors were not only important in inducing directed T-cell movement, but could also localize the cells to the activated vasculature for subsequent transendothelial cell migration. The concept of chemokines being involved in binding leukocyte subpopulations to the endothelium is further supported by the observation that either soluble MIP-1α, RANTES, or MIP-1β anchored to subendothelial cell extracellular matrix (ECM) enhanced the binding of CD4+ T-cells to the ECM.

While the original focus of early MCP-1 studies demonstrated that it was a monocyte chemotactic factor, subsequent investigations have also shown this chemokine to be a potent lymphocyte chemotactic factor *(7)*. This finding has been supported by additional investigations showing that not only is MCP-1 chemotactic for T-cells but MCP-2 and MCP-3 are also potent lymphocyte chemotactic factors. A comparison study has demonstrated that MCP-1, MCP-2, MCP-3, MIP-1α, MIP-1β, and RANTES all can induce the directed migration of CD4+ and CD8+ T-cell clones. However, the chemotactic response of T-cells to MCP-1, MCP-2, and MCP-3 was more pronounced, as compared with MIP-1α, MIP-1β, and RANTES. The migration of lymphocytes was not only assessed in in vitro analyses; investigations using a model of in vivo human T-cell migration found that human CD3+ T-cells, which were intraperitoneally injected into severe combined immunodeficient mice, migrated to sites subcutaneously injected with MCP-1. Similar findings for the recruitment of T-cells in vivo were identified using RANTES as the challenging chemokine. One caveat is that several investigations have examined the participation of C-C chemokines in lymphocyte recruitment, and, in certain instances, these studies have contradicted each other. The major differences in these investigations may likely be related to differences in the isolation techniques of the lymphocytes, differences in donor populations of T-cells, the "age" of the T-cells used in the chemotactic assay, the use of cloned T-cells, or the use of different extracellular matrix molecules to coat the filters in the chemotaxis assay.

4. CHEMOKINES IN EXPERIMENTAL MODELS OF DISEASE

4.1. The Role of Chemokines in Infectious Processes

The treatment of infectious diseases has become more difficult for a variety of reasons, including the emergence of multidrug-resistant pathogens, the increased incidence of acquired immunodeficiency disorders, human immunodeficiency virus infection, and the increased use of immunosuppressive drugs. Therefore, an intense effort to understand and take advantage of an activated host response is becoming an increasingly important avenue for potential therapy. It is well known that effective antimicrobial defenses require the generation of an efficacious leukocyte response, which involves the elicitation of neutrophils and mononuclear cells. The early clearance of an infectious agent is critical and is dependent on activated granulocytes and monocytes/macrophages. The recruitment of these highly phagocytic cells is directed, in part, by established concentration gradients of chemotactic factors, including members of the chemokine family.

To assess the participation of a C-X-C chemokine, MIP-2 (a functional homolog of IL-8 in the mouse) in the host defense effort, a murine model of bacterial pneumonia was established via an intratracheal inoculation with *Klebsiella pneumoniae*. Two days postbacterial challenge, the animals were in respiratory distress, which correlated with a substantial recruitment and accumulation of neutrophils into the lungs. The cytologic evidence of leukocyte accumulation was associated with a time-dependent expression of MIP-2 mRNA and protein, as maximal production of MIP-2 occurred by 48 h. Immunohistochemical analysis of the infected lungs demonstrated that alveolar macrophages were the predominant source of MIP-2. In an effort to establish the biologic contribution of MIP-2 to neutrophil recruitment to the lungs during the evolving pathology of *K. pneumoniae,* mice with developing pneumonia were passively immunized with neutralizing antibodies to MIP-2. Experimental animals treated with anti–MIP-2 antibodies demonstrated a 36% reduction in neutrophil accumulation within the lungs at the 48-h time point, as compared with the control animals. The reduction in neutrophil accumulation in the animals treated with anti-MIP-2 antibody correlated with an impaired clearance of bacteria and a subsequent decrease in survival of the challenged animals. These studies underscore the importance of neutrophil activation and the chemotactic response as a dynamic host defense factor against infectious agents.

While C-X-C chemokines have been identified as important mediators of acute bacterial infections, C-C chemokines have been shown to play an important role in the host's response to opportunistic fungal infections. Using an experimental model of *Cryptococcus neoformans*–induced pneumonia, investigations have shown that MCP-1 is an important chemokine in the clearance of Cryptococcus organisms *(18)*. Mice challenged with *C. neoformans* demonstrated an increase in the number of fungal colony forming units during the first week of infection, followed by a significant increase in the recruitment of leukocytes into the lungs. During the first 5 wk of infection, the numbers of mononuclear cells increased in the lungs, which correlated with the production of MCP-1. To assess the contribution of MCP-1 to the development of the host response, animals with developing fungal infections were treated with neutralizing antibodies to MCP-1. The depletion of MCP-1 had profound effects on the recruitment of leukocytes, especially CD4[+] T-cells. Interestingly, MCP-1 depletion also reduced the numbers of neutrophils, B-cells, and CD8[+] T-cells normally recruited to the lungs in this model. These findings suggest that the early generation of MCP-1 can participate in both a direct and indirect manner leading to the elicitation of leukocytes. The reduction of leukocyte accumulation in the lungs resulted in a significant reduction in the clearance of Cryptococcus organisms, an increased dissemination of the infectious organisms to the brain, and a decrease in the survival of the animals.

4.2. The Role of Chemokines in Granulomatous Inflammation

Additional studies have indicated that the degree of MCP-1 participation in an immune/inflammatory response varies according to the immune status of the reaction and the extent of T-cell involvement. For example, in vivo studies assessing the development of interstitial lung granulomas induced by mycobacteria antigens have demonstrated that IFN-γ and TNF were necessary cytokines for lesion progression *(12)*. By contrast, pulmonary inflammation initiated by embolization of *Schistosoma mansoni* eggs was maintained by IL-4 *(11)*. These cytokine profiles suggest that interstitial delayed-type hypersensitivity granulomatous inflammation involves Th1 and/or Th2 cytokines *(12)*. In the context of interstitial lung inflammation, these observations served as the basis for the establishment of models that exhibit either a Th1 or Th2 inflammatory response within the lung. This was accomplished by presensitization of mice with Mycobacteria species (BCG) or *S. mansoni* eggs followed by pulmonary embolization of Sephadex (carbohydrate beads) coated with a known amount of soluble antigen, purified protein derivative (PPD), or schistosome egg antigen, derived from the respective organisms *(10)*. Granulomas formed in response to PPD were characterized by the appearance of IL-2 and IFN-γ in the lymph nodes and primarily IFN-γ at the site of the lung lesion. This pattern is consistent with previous reports that Th1 cells mediate the response to mycobacterial infections.

An assessment of the participation of chemokines in these models demonstrated that MCP-1 contributed more to the development of the Th2-type immune response than to the Th1 response. Although MCP-1 is likely not a pure Th2-related cytokine, it does appear to be heavily involved during Th2-type inflammatory responses. Investigations have shown that macrophages isolated from Th2-type granulomas have an enhanced ability to produce MCP-1, as compared with macrophages recovered from either foreign body or Th1-type lesions. The macrophages isolated from these cell-mediated immune responses are only one of the cellular sources for MCP-1; fibroblasts or myofibroblasts, endothelial cells, eosinophils, and vascular-associated stromal cells are also potential sources of MCP-1.

Further investigations have demonstrated that MCP-1 is more than just a chemotactic factor, because the in vivo studies have linked MCP-1 to the evolving Th2 response by showing that IL-4 can promote MCP-1 production by macrophages recovered from the Th2-type granuloma. The IL-4/MCP-1 connection has been previously identified in in vitro studies showing that IL-4 directly stimulates endothelial cells and macrophages to produce MCP-1. Interestingly, the crossregulatory activity between different Th1 and Th2 cytokines can influence the in vivo expression of MCP-1. To assess the contribution of these cytokines to local MCP-1 production, experimental animals, with developing Th1- or Th2-type granulomas, were treated with neutralizing antibodies to either IFN-γ, IL-12, or IL-4. Then, the macrophages were recovered and MCP-1 levels assayed. Although the anticytokine treatment protocols did not affect MCP-1 production from macrophages recovered from Th1-type granulomas, the treatment of animals with evolving Th2 responses with either anti–IFN-γ or anti–IL-4 antibodies did have interesting effects. Anti–IL-4 treatment reduced MCP-1 production in the Th2 response, whereas anti–IFN-γ treatment increased MCP-1 levels. Treatment with anti–IL-12 antibody failed to influence the production of MCP-1. The modulating effect of IL-4 and IFN-γ depletion was associated with corresponding changes in the size of the developing granulomatous lesions. In total, these studies indicate that MCP-1 expression is enhanced by Th2-type cytokines and that the production of this chemokine is subject to cross-regulatory inhibition by IFN-γ.

Recent reports have demonstrated that macrophages recovered from Th1 vs Th2 granulomas can be respectively characterized by augmented and impaired IL-12 production *(9)*. The IL-12 impairment appeared to be owing to the regulatory effects of IL-4 and IL-10; however, in view of the contribution of MCP-1 to the developing Th2-type granuloma, investigations were designed to determine whether IL-12 expression was also affected by MCP-1 depletion. Initial investigations demonstrated that macrophages isolated from Th2-type lesions were weak IL-12-producing cells, as compared to macrophages isolated from Th1-type lesions. Treatment of mice with anti–MCP-1 antibody reversed the impaired IL-12-producing capacity of Th2-type granuloma macrophages, whereas this same treatment protocol did not alter the IL-12

Table 5
Examples of Different Experimental Models of Immune/Inflammatory Diseases Possessing a Chemokine Component

Disease model	Chemokine involved
Liver ischemia/reperfusion (rat)	ENA-78
Lung ischemia/reperfusion (rabbit)	IL-8
Asthma	RANTES, MIP-1α, eotaxin
Bacterial pneumonia (mouse)	MIP-2
Cecal ligation and puncture (sepsis)	MIP-2
Allergic encephalomyelitis	MIP-1α
Arthritis, type II collagen induced (mouse)	MIP-2, MIP-1α
Mycobacteria-induced granuloma	MIP-1α
Schistosoma-induced granuloma	MCP-1

producing capacity of macrophages isolated from Th1-type lesions. These data suggest that MCP-1 plays a role in regulating IL-12 expression and, coupled with the modulating effects of IL-4 and IL-10, may further contribute to the immunoregulation of various types of cell-mediated immune responses. Investigations into the role of various chemokines, such as MCP-1, demonstrate that these factors contribute, in a selective way, to the potential differentiation and expression of cytokine profiles associated with particular responses (Table 5). The differential expression and contribution of the chemokines raises the possibility that these factors may be targeted for therapeutic intervention to alter various types of inflammation.

4.3. The Role of Chemokines in Noninfectious Disorders

The activation and elicitation of leukocytes in response to an infectious process are clearly natural sequelae of a normal physiologic host response. While this process is essential to the pathology of infectious disease, the recruitment of leukocytes in response to noninfectious disorders, such as asthma, ischemia/reperfusion, and autoimmune concerns, may have unwanted consequences. The activation and elicitation of specific leukocyte populations during allergic airway inflammation is dependent on the interactions between the inciting antigen and the subsequent cascade of activating inflammatory mediators. One of the most prominent events during the evolution of allergic inflammation is the activation and recruitment of eosinophils. These cells have been implicated as the major leukocyte population responsible for bronchial injury and airway obstruction. The specific mechanisms involved in eosinophil activation and chemotaxis are still enigmatic; however, recent information suggests that C-C chemokines are involved in these processes *(25)*. Eotaxin, MCP-3, RANTES, and MIP-1α are all potent eosinophil chemotactic factors in vitro, and elevated levels of MIP-1α have been identified in the bronchoalveolar lavage fluid of asthmatics.

To identify a causal relationship between C-C chemokine expression and allergic airway disorders, experimental models have been developed. Intratracheal challenge with the identical antigen used to sensitize mice resulted in a time-dependent rise in eosinophil accumulation to the airways. A chemokine profile demonstrated that both RANTES and MIP-1α were expressed coincident with the elicitation of eosinophils.

To assess the contribution of these chemokines to the development of asthma, mice were passively immunized with neutralizing antibodies to either MIP-1α or RANTES. In this experimental system, animals depleted with MIP-1α or RANTES demonstrated a specific reduction in eosinophil recruitment by 50% and 60%, respectively. These results begin to establish a causal role for specific C-C chemokines in eosinophil-dependent inflammatory disorders and open potentially novel avenues for the development of useful therapeutic modalities.

Autoimmune diseases, such as rheumatoid arthritis, are usually regarded as noninfectious processes that are extremely debilitating. Rheumatoid arthritis is characterized by inflammation and destruction of the joints related to the sequestration of leukocytes into both a developing pannus and the synovial space. A variety of investigations have determined that both C-C and C-X-C chemokines can be found associated with human rheumatoid arthritis. While the involvement of these chemokines in the pathology of rheumatoid arthritis is not entirely clear, studies have shown that IL-8, ENA-78, GRO, MCP-1, RANTES, and MIP-1α are expressed in this disease and account for a significant portion of neutrophil and mononuclear cell chemotactic activity. The role of specific chemokines in the pathology of rheumatoid arthritis has been partially elucidated using an experimental model of type II collagen–induced arthritis *(4,21)*. By 36 d after receiving a second immunization of type II collagen, most experimental animals developed clinical and histopathologic evidence of arthritis. The levels of both MIP-2 and MIP-1α in the joint paralleled the incidence and magnitude of arthritis, with peak levels of the two chemokines occurring at d 44. Immunohistochemical analyses of the joint tissue revealed that chondrocytes, macrophages, and fibroblasts of the developing pannus were the major sources of chemokine production. The contribution of MIP-2 and MIP-1α was assessed via passively immunizing rheumatoid arthritis animals with $F(ab')_2$ fragments every other day from d 24 to 32 post primary immunization with type II collagen. Depletion of either MIP-2 or MIP-1α, in this manner, resulted in a significant reduction in both the arthritic index and the overall incidence of arthritis. This reduction in joint inflammation suggests that chemokines may play a key role in the evolution of chronic joint inflammation.

Ischemia/reperfusion injury is another medical disorder that involves the activation and recruitment of leukocytes as part of the pathologic process. However, the mechanisms involved in neutrophil activation and elicitation in ischemia/reperfusion have not been fully studied. Investigations have shown that anoxia/hyperoxia can induce the expression of IL-8, which was dependent on the activation of the transcription factor NF-κB activation. Subsequent experiments using experimental models demonstrated that IL-8 may be a major neutrophil activation factor during ischemia/reperfusion. Using a rabbit lung model of ischemia/reperfusion, IL-8 was identified as a significant mediator of reperfusion injury. Passive immunization with neutralizing antibodies to rabbit IL-8 before reperfusion of the ischemic lung prevented neutrophil elicitation and tissue injury. Chemokines have also been shown to play a role in both liver and lung injury subsequent to liver ischemia/reperfusion injury. Tissue damage after hepatic ischemia/reperfusion was dependent on a TNF-α-directed network and resulted in the expression of C-X-C chemokines, such as ENA-78, in the liver and lungs. Levels of the chemokines directly correlated with the recruitment of neutrophils and injury, and passive immunization with neutralizing antichemokine antibody blocked a significant portion of the pathology *(13)*. In total, these studies demonstrate that various chemokines are expressed during ischemia/reperfusion processes and likely contribute to the underlying pathology.

5. CONCLUSION

Investigation into chemokine biology is a rapidly growing area of research, which has impacted a diversity of disciplines such as physiology, immunology, and virology. Recent studies have underscored the importance of chemokines in directing immune reactivity using a variety of models of inflammation. These investigations have illustrated the contribution of chemokines via either their ability to promote the inflammatory response and increase host survival during infectious processes or to augment the pathology of noninfectious disorders. There is little doubt that the future for chemokine biology holds exciting promise for the development of novel therapeutic strategies to treat many diseases whose current treatments are inadequate.

ACKNOWLEDGMENTS

These investigations were supported in part from National Institutes of Health grants 1P50HL46487, NL31963, HL35276, HL58200, and AA10571

REFERENCES

1. Ansiowicz, A., D. Zajchowski, G. Stenman, and R. Sager. 1988. Functional diversity of gro gene expression in human fibroblasts and mammary epithelial cells. *Proc. Natl. Acad. Sci. USA* **85:** 9645–9649.
2. Baggiolini, M., A. Walz, and S. L. Kunkel. 1989. NAP-1/IL-8, a novel cytokine that activates neutrophils. *J. Clin. Invest.* **57:** 2837–2841.
3. Baggiolini, M., B. Dewald, and B. Moser. 1994. Interleukin-8 and related chemotactic cytokines CXC and CC chemokines. *Adv. Immunol.* **55:** 97–179.
4. Bischoff, S. C., M. Krieger, T. Brunner, A. Rot, V. von Tscharner, M. Baggiolini, and C. A. Dahinden. 1993. RANTES and related chemokines activate human basophil granulocytes through different G protein-coupled receptors. *Eur. J. Immunol.* **23:** 761–767.
5. Boyden, S. 1962. The chemotactic effect of mixtures of antibody and antigens on polymorphonuclear leukocytes. *J. Exp. Med.* **115:** 453–460.
6. Brown, Z., M. E. Gerritsen, W. W. Carly, R. M. Strieter, S. L. Kunkel, and J. Westwick. 1989. Chemokine gene expression and secretion by cytokine-activated human microvascular endothelial cells: differential regulation by MCP-1 and IL-8 in regulation of MCP-1 IL-8 in response to interferon-gamma. *Am. J. Pathol.* **145:** 913–921.
7. Carr, M. W., S. J. Roth, E. Luther, S. S. Ross, and T. A. Springer. 1994. Monocyte chemoattractant protein-1 acts as a T lymphocytes chemoattractant. *Proc. Natl. Acad. Sci. USA* **91:** 3652–3656.
8. Chang, M. S., J. McNinch, R. Basu, and S. Simonet. 1994. Cloning and characterization of the human neutrophil-activating peptide 78 (ENA-78) gene. *J. Biol. Chem.* **269:** 25,277–25,282.
9. Chensue, S. W., J. H. Ruth, K. Warmington, P. Lincoln, and S. L. Kunkel. 1995. In vivo regulation of macrophage IL-12 production during type 1 and type 2 cytokine-mediate granuloma formation. *J. Immunol.* **155:** 3546–3551.
10. Chensue, S. W., K. Warmington, J. Ruth, P. Lincoln, M. C. Kuo, and S. L. Kunkel. 1994. Cytokine responses during mycobacterial and schistosomal antigen-induced pulmonary granuloma formation: production of Th1 and Th2 cytokines and relative contribution of tumor necrosis factor. *Am. J. Pathol.* **145:** 1105–1113.

11. Chensue, S. W., K. S. Warmington, J. Ruth, P. M. Lincoln, and S. L. Kunkel. 1994. Crossregulatory role of gamma interferon, IL-4, and IL-10 in schistosome egg granuloma formation: in vivo regulation of Th activity and inflammation. *Clin. Exp. Immunol.* **98:** 395–400.

12. Chensue, S. W., K. S. Warmington, J. H. Ruth, P. Lincoln, and S. L. Kunkel. 1995. Cytokine function during mycobacterial and schistosomal antigen-induced pulmonary granuloma formation. *J. Immunol.* **154:** 5969–5976.

13. Colletti, L. M., S. L. Kunkel, A. Walz, M. Burdick, R. G. Kunkel, C. A. Wilke, and R. M. Strieter. 1996. The role of cytokine networks in the local liver injury following hepatic ischemia/reperfusion in the rat. *Hepatology.* **23:** 506–514.

14. Elner, S. G., R. M. Strieter, V. M. Elner, B. J. Rollins, M. A. Del Monte, and S. L. Kunkel. 1991. Monocyte chemotactic protein gene expression by cytokine treated human retinal pigment epithelial cells. *Lab. Invest.* **64:** 819–825.

15. Farber, J. M. 1993. HuMIG: a new member of the chemokine family of cytokines. *Biochem. Biophys. Res. Commun.* **192:** 223–230.

16. Fernandez, H. N., P. M. Henson, A. Otani, and T. E. Hugli. 1978. Chemotactic response to human C3a and C5a anaphylatoxins. I. Evaluation of C3a and C5a leukotaxis in vitro and under stimulated in vivo conditions. *J. Immunol.* **120:** 109–115.

17. Ford-Hutchinson, A. W., M. A. Bray, M. V. Doig, and M. J. Smith. 1980. Leukotriene B$_4$ a potent chemokinetic and aggregating substance released from polymorphonuclear leukocytes. *Nature* **286:** 262–265.

18. Huffnagle, G. B., R. M. Strieter, T. J. Standiford, R. A. McDonald, M. D. Burdick, S. L. Kunkel, and G. B. Toews. 1995. The role of monocyte chemotactic protein-1 (MCP-1) in the recruitment of monocyte and CD4+ T cell during a pulmonary *Cryptococcus neoformans* infection. *J. Immunol.* **155:** 4790–4797.

19. Jiang, Y., L. A. Tabak, A. J. Valente, and D. T. Graves. 1991. Initial characterization of the carbohydrate structure of MCP-1. *Biochem. Biophys. Res. Commun.* **178:** 1400–1404.

20. Kaplan, G., A. D. Luster, G. Hancock, and Z. Cohen. 1987. The expression of a gamma interferon-induced protein (IP-10) in delayed immune responses in human skin. *J. Exp. Med.* **166:** 1098–1108.

21. Kasama, T., R. M. Strieter, N. W. Lukacs, P. M. Lincoln, M. D. Burdick, and S. L. Kunkel. 1995. Interleukin-10 expression and chemokine regulation during the evolution of murine type II collagen-induced arthritis. *J. Clin. Invest.* **95:** 2868–2876.

22. Leonard, E. J., A. Skeel, and T. Yoshimura. 1991. Biological aspects of monocyte chemoattractant protein-1 (MCP-1). *Adv. Exp. Med. Biol.* **305:** 57–64.

23. Leonard, E. J., and T. Yoshimura. 1990. Human monocyte chemoattractant protein-1 (MCP-1). *Immunol. Today* **11:** 97–100.

24. Lukacs, N. W., S. W. Chensue, R. E. Smith, R. M. Strieter, K. Warmington, C. Wilke, and S. L. Kunkel. 1994. Production of monocyte chemoattractant protein-1 and macrophage inflammatory protein-1 alpha by inflammatory granuloma fibroblasts. *Am. J. Pathol.* **144:** 711–718.

25. Lukacs, N. W., R. M. Strieter, S. W. Chensue, and S. L. Kunkel. 1996. Activation and regulation of chemokines in allergic airway inflammation. *J. Leuk. Biol.* **59:** 13–17.

26. Majundar, S., D. Gonder, B. Koutsis, and M. Poncz. 1991. Characterization of the beta-thromboglobulin gene: comparison with the gene for platelet factor 4. *J. Biol. Chem.* **266:** 5785–5789.

27. Matsushima, K., K. Morishita, T. Yoshimura, E. J. Leonard, and J. J. Oppenheim. 1988. Molecular cloning of a human monocyte-derived neutrophil chemotactic factor (MDNCF) and the induction of MDNCF mRNA by interleukin-1 and tumor necrosis factor. *J. Exp. Med.* **167:** 1883–1893.

28. Matsushima, K., and J. J. Oppenheim. 1990. Interleukin-8 and MCAF: novel inflammatory cytokines inducible by IL-1 and TNF. *Cytokine* **1:** 2–13.

29. Miller, M. D., and M. S. Krangel. 1992. Biology and biochemistry of the chemokines: a family of chemotactic and inflammatory cytokines. *Crit. Rev. Immunol.* **12:** 17–46.
30. Miller, M. D., S. Hata, R. deWaal Malefyt, and M. S. Krangel. 1989. A novel polypeptide secreted by activated human T lymphocytes. *J. Immunol.* **143:** 2907–2916.
31. Miller, M. D., S. D. Wilson, M. E. Dorf, H. N. Seuanez, S. J. O'Brien, and M. S. Krangel. 1990. Sequence and chromosomal location of the I-309 gene: relationship to genes encoding a family of inflammatory cytokines. *J. Immunol.* **145:** 2737–2744.
32. Modi, W. S., M. Dean, H. N. Seuanez, N. Mukaida, K. Matsushima, and S. J. O'Brien. 1990. Monocyte-derived neutrophil chemotactic factor (MDNCF/IL-8) resides in a gene cluster along with several other members of the platelet factor 4 gene superfamily. *Human Genet.* **84:** 185–187.
33. Mukaida, N., M. Shiroo, and K. Matsushima. 1994. Molecular mechanism of interleukin-8 gene expression. *J. Leuk. Biol.* **56:** 554–558.
34. Opdenakker, G., P. Fiten, G. Nys, G. Froyen, N. Van Roy, F. Speleman, G. Laureys, and J. Van Damme. 1994. The human MCP-3 gene (SCTA7): cloning, sequence analysis, and assignment to the C-C chemokine gene cluster on chromosome 17q11.2-q12. *Genomics* **21:** 403–408.
35. Oppenheim, J. J., O. C. Zachariae, N. Mukaida, and K. Matsushima. 1991. Properties of the novel proinflammatory supergene "intercrine" cytokine family. *Annu. Rev. Immunol.* **9:** 617–648.
36. Peveri, P., A. Walz, B. DeWald, and M. Baggiolini. 1988. A novel neutrophil-activating factor produced by human mononuclear phagocytes. *J. Exp. Med.* **167:** 1547–1559.
37. Proost, P., C. De Wolf-Peeters, R. Conings, G. Opdenakker, A. Billiau, and J. Van Damme. 1993. Identification of a novel granulocyte chemotactic protein (GCP-2) from human tumor cells: in vitro and in vivo comparison with natural forms of GRO-gamma, IP-10, and IL-8. *J. Immunol.* **150:** 1000–1010.
38. Rolfe, M. W., S. L. Kunkel, T. J. Standiford, M. B. Orringer, S. H. Phan, H. L. Evanoff, M. D. Burdick, and R. M. Strieter. 1992. Expression and regulation of human pulmonary fibroblast-derived monocyte chemotactic peptide (MCP-1). *Am. J. Physiol.* **263:** L536–L545.
39. Rollins, B. J., A. Walz, and M. Baggiolini. 1991. Recombinant human MCP-1/JE induces chemotaxis, calcium flux, and the respiratory burst in human monocytes. *Blood* **8:** 1112–1116.
40. Rot, A., M. Krieger, T. Brunner, S. C. Bischoff, T. J. Schall, and C. A. Dahinden. 1992. RANTES and macrophages inflammatory protein-1 alpha induce the migration and activation of normal human eosinophil granulocytes. *J. Exp. Med.* **176:** 1489–1495.
41. Schall, T. J. 1991. Biology of the RANTES/sis family. *Cytokine* **3:** 165–183.
42. Schall, T. J., J. Jongstra, B. J. Dyer, J. Jorgensen, C. Clayberger, M. M. Davis, and A. M. Krensky. 1988. A human T cell-specific molecule is a member of a new gene family. *J. Immunol.* **141:** 1018–1025.
43. Schall, T. J., K. Bacon, K. J. Koy, and D. V. Goeddel. 1990. Selective attraction of monocytes and T lymphocytes of the memory phenotype by cytokine RANTES. *Nature* **347:** 669–671.
44. Shiffman, E., B. A. Corcoran, and S. M. Wahl. 1975. N-formylmethionyl peptides as chemoattractants for leukocytes. *Proc. Natl. Acad. Sci. USA* **72:** 1059–1062.
45. Singh, R., K. Berry, K. Matsushima, K. Yasumoto, and I. J. Fidler. 1993. Synergism between human monocyte chemotactic and activating factor and bacterial products for activation of tumoricidal properties in murine macrophages. *J. Immunol.* **151:** 2786–2793.
46. Standiford, T. J., S. L. Kunkel, S. H. Phan, B. J. Rollins, and R. M. Strieter. 1991. Alveolar macrophage-derived cytokines induce monocyte chemoattractant protein-1 expression from human pulmonary type II like epithelial cells. *J. Biol. Chem.* **266:** 9912–9918.
47. Strieter, R. M., R. Wiggins, S. H. Phan, B. L. Wharram, H. J. Showell, D. G. Remick, S. W.

Chensue, and S. L. Kunkel. 1989. Monocyte chemotactic protein gene expression by cytokine-treated human fibroblasts and endothelial cells. *Biochem. Biophys. Res. Commun.* **162:** 694–700.

48. Taub, D. D., and J. J. Oppenheim. 1994. Chemokines, inflammation, and the immune system. *Ther. Immunol.* **1:** 229–246.
49. Vaddi, K, and R. C. Newton. 1994. Regulation of monocyte integrin expression by beta-family chemokines. *J. Immunol.* **153:** 4721–4732.
50. Van Damme, J., P. Proost, W. Put, S. Arens, J. P. Lenaerts, R. Coning, G. Opdenakker, H. Heremans, and A. Billiau. 1994. Induction of monocyte chemotactic protein MCP-1 and MCP-2 in human fibroblasts and leukocytes by cytokines and cytokine inducers: chemical synthesis of MCP-2 and development of specific RIA. *J. Immunol.* **152:** 5495–5502.
51. Van Otteren, G. M., T. J. Standiford, S. L. Kunkel, J. M. Danforth, M. D. Burdick, L. V. Abruzzo, and R. M. Strieter. 1994. The expression and regulation of macrophage inflammatory protein-1 alpha by murine alveolar and peritoneal macrophages. *Am. J. Respir. Cell Mol. Biol.* **10:** 8–15.
52. Walz, A., and M. Baggiolin. 1990. Generation of the neutrophil-activating peptide NAP-2 from platelet basic protein or connective tissue-activating peptide III through monocyte proteases. *J. Exp. Med.* **171:** 449–454.
53. Ward, P. A., and L. J. Newman. 1969. A neutrophil chemotactic factor from human C′5. *J. Immunol.* **102:** 93–99.
54. Yoshimura, T., E. A. Robinson, E. Apella, K. Matsushima, S. D. Showalter, A. Skeel, and E. J. Leonard. 1989. Three forms of monocyte-derived neutrophil chemotactic factor (MDNCF) distinguished by different lengths of the amino-terminal sequence. *Mol. Immunol.* **26:** 87–93.
55. Zhang, Y. J., B. J. Rutledge, and B. J. Rollins. 1994. Structure/activity analysis of human monocyte chemoattractant protein-1 (MCP-1) by mutagenesis: identification of a mutated protein that inhibits MCP-1 mediated monocyte chemotaxis. *J. Biol. Chem.* **269:** 15,918–15,924.
56. Zigmond, S. H., and J. G. Hirsch. 1973. Leukocyte locomotion and chemotaxis: new methods for evaluation and demonstration of cell-derived chemotactic factor. *J. Exp. Med.* **137:** 387–393.

2

Chemokine Receptors and Ligand Specificity

Understanding the Enigma

Craig Gerard

Chemokine receptors are now well established as a large gene family within the superfamily of G-protein-coupled receptors. Despite the fact that chemokines themselves are relatively large ligands, many fundamental features of the receptors are similar to those for all members of the superfamily. These features include multiple affinity states for ligand, isomerization to forms that preferentially interact with the signal transduction apparatus, phosphorylation and desensitization, and internalization.

The peptide receptors, however, have some specialized features. Characterizing the biochemistry of chemokines and receptors has led to the realization that "sharing" of ligands and receptors occurs. Yet, genetic-disruption experiments targeting chemokines and receptors have indicated that the biology of these molecules is nonredundant in vivo. In this chapter, the enigma of chemokine/receptor promiscuity is examined as a form of biological control, with parallels in the neuropeptide receptor system.

1. INTRODUCTION

Since the first chemokines were described as growth-factor-inducible genes and chemotactic factors over a decade ago (*1*), there has been an astonishing growth in the understanding of these molecules as fundamental migration signals for a variety of cells. Originally thought to be limited to effects on bone-marrow-derived cells, we now recognize that many epithelial, endothelial, parenchymal, mesothelial, and neuronal cells express chemokines and their receptors. The picture emerging in late 1998 is that the chemokine/receptor system probably began as a system to control cell migration during embryogenesis and has been adapted by the immune system and perhaps other cells as well (epithelial, endothelial) to regulate both basal and activated cell trafficking.

As chemokines and their receptors were characterized, a mystifying overlap began to be appreciated whereby multiple chemokines were capable of activating a single receptor, and multiple receptors were capable of recognizing a single ligand. This is diagrammed in Fig. 1.

Occasionally, a single ligand has been demonstrated to be specific for a single receptor (e.g., SDF-1α and CXCR4) but these instances are likely to be either exceptions that prove the rule or a result of incomplete sampling of the genome. Recently, for

From: *Chemokines and Cancer*
Edited by: B. J. Rollins © Humana Press Inc., Totowa, NJ

RECEPTOR	LIGAND
CCR1	MIP-1α, Rantes, MCP-3
CCR2	MCP-1-5
CCR3	Eotaxin, MCP2-5, RANTES
CCR4	TARC, MDC
CCR5	MIP 1α, MIP1β, Rantes
CCR6	LARC, MIP3α, Exodus
CCR7	ELC, MIP3β, SLC
CCR8	1309
CCR9	"Promiscuous"
CCR10	TECK
CXCR1	IL-8
CXCR2	IL-8, ENA78, Groα,β,γ, NAP-1
CRCR3	IP-10, MIG, ITAC, (Eotaxin, MCP-4, SLC)
CSCR4	SDF-1α
CXCR5	BLC-1
CX3CR$_1$	Fractalkine
C-1	Lymphotactin

Fig. 1

example, it has been reported that GRP-2 is a full agonist at CXCR-1, which ends IL-8's reign as unique ligand for this receptor.

Thus, the concept of receptor/ligand promiscuity has been a redundant enigma to most chemokinologists. However, chemokine aficionados are not alone in their confusion; a model for this phenomenon has already been described for the tachykinin receptors. In this chapter we interpret chemokine ligand/receptor redundancy as a mechanism for combinatorial control, whereby expression of ligands, receptors, and their admixture may differentially affect a biological outcome.

2. THE CHEMOKINE RECEPTORS: G PROTEIN COUPLED

As might have been predicted based on the structure of the major chemotactic receptors for bacterial N-formylated peptides and C5a anaphylatoxin that were cloned earlier *(2)*, the first cloned chemokine receptors were found to be members of the seven transmembrane segment (7TMS) spanning (or serpentine) receptors. The 7TMS cell surface receptors are likely to be the largest superfamily in the genome. In broadest terms, the G-protein-coupled receptors represent a fundamental solution to the problem of how a cell can "sense" its environment. Their basic structure, from opsins through chemokine receptors, is believed to be primarily the same; the specificity of a given 7TMS receptor for a ligand from a small molecule such as a catecholamine or volatile odorant through large polypeptides, is governed by primary amino acid sequence changes primarily in the extracellular regions. Similarly, changes in the primary amino acid sequences of the intracellular regions dictate specificity of coupling

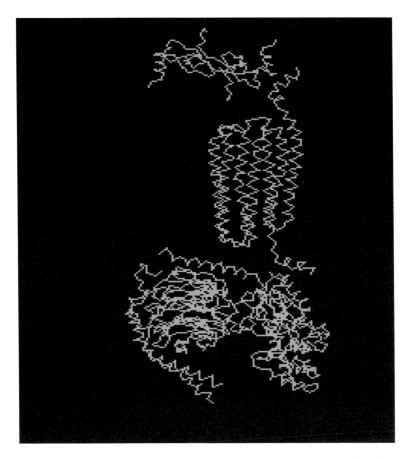

Fig. 2. A model for chemokine/receptor/G protein complexes. Known dimeric structure for RANTES is positioned at a theoretical model, based on rhodopsin, for CCR5. The known structure of $G_1\alpha\beta\gamma$ is oriented to position the lipid modified residues as facing the cell membrane (not shown) and receptor.

to different G proteins. The basic components of the system are portrayed in Fig. 2. Interestingly, it has been hypothesized that the tertiary structure and mechanism of activation of all 7TMS receptors is inherently similar. Precise contacts between residues in the transmembrane helices (particularly transmembrane helix 3 and transmembrane helix 6) change upon ligand binding; this pivoting of the helices in relation to the other imparts to the intracellular loops and coupled G protein a conformational signal for GTP–GDP exchange by the alpha subunit and dissociation of complex of G protein and receptor.

Pharmacologically, the chemokine receptors are coupled to G proteins, which generally inhibit adenylate cyclase, and are referred to as Giα. The alpha subunit has the ability to bind either GDP or GTP. When ligand binds the receptor, the G protein exchanges GDP for GTP and dissociates from the complex with the receptor and βγ subunits. While binding GTP, the alpha subunit is locked in a conformation that can interact with a wide variety of intracellular effectors, including adenylate cyclase, phospholipase C and A2, certain ion channels, and a number of serine/threonine and tyrosine

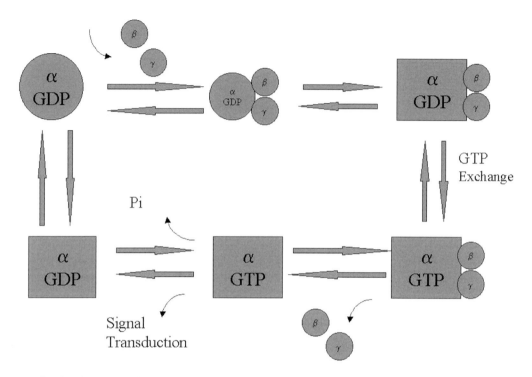

Fig. 3. The G protein activation cycle. The α subunit binds GTP with high affinity. This form serves as a docking site for βγ subunit dimers. Upon ligand binding to the receptor, a guanine nucleotide exchange of GDP by GTP occurs; importantly, it is the equilibrium for this reaction that is ligand-driven. The GTP-bound α subunit dissociates from the receptor and βγ dimer. Both the GTP-bound form of the α subunit and the βγ subunits function in signal transduction. The " lifetime" of the α subunit is limited by intrinsic GTPase activity. Upon hydrolysis to GDP, the α subunit reassociates with the receptor and βγ subunits to complete the cycle.

kinases. Giα has intrinsic GTPase activity, and after hydrolysis of GTP to GDP and release of inorganic phosphate, the GDP-bound form associates again with βγ subunit and an unoccupied 7-TMS receptor (see Fig. 3).

As demonstrated in extremely detailed studies on visual rhodopsin and later on the beta adrenergic receptor *(3,4)*, the conformational state of the receptor associated with G protein activation is an excellent substrate for serine/threonine kinases that rapidly phosphorylate intracellular segments, predominantly at the C-terminus. As a consequence of receptor phosphorylation, the receptor is "desensitized." For example, desensitization of the adrenergic receptor involves specific phosphorylation by GRKs (G-protein-related kinases), which then facilitates the association of the receptor with a second molecule, known as an Arrestin. This latter protein interferes with the association of the receptor with G proteins, thus blocking ligand-induced agonist activity. A second consequence of phosphorylation is receptor internalization and sequestration within intracellular vesicular compartments that may allow proteolysis and/or recycling of the reception to the plasma membrane.

This mechanism describes ligand-specific (homologous) desensitization such as MCP-1 desensitizing CCR2 to a second challenge with MCP-1. In the case of many members of the serpentine receptor family, agonist-induced "cross-desensitization" (better referred to as heterologous desensitization) may be observed among receptors of a particular structural group. For example, a subset of chemoattractant receptors has been demonstrated to undergo heterologous desensitization with a hierarchical order (formyl peptide~=C5a>IL-8) *(5)*. The biological significance of desensitization is quite obvious; in addition to providing a way to terminate a sensory response, it frequently serves as a mechanism for clearing ligand through internalization. In the special case of chemoattractant receptors, the ability to discriminate among multiple ligands in an inflammatory locus may also depend upon relative affinities and desensitization responsiveness. This will become clearer when the receptor/ligand promiscuity issue is discussed below.

3. THE TACHYKININS AND THEIR RECEPTORS; A PARADIGM APPLICABLE TO THE CHEMOKINE FAMILY

Before the promiscuity of chemokines and their receptors was fully appreciated, a well-characterized neuropeptide system puzzled neuropharmacologists for similar reasons. As a paradigm directly applicable to the chemokines, the insights gained from this system will be detailed below.

The tachykinins are a family of small peptides, 11 residues in length, produced in neural cells and some myeloid cells such as macrophages and eosinophils. Three classic tachykinins are known in mammals: substance p, neurokinin A (substance k), and neurokinin B (neuromedin K). Tachykinins bind to G-protein-coupled receptors known as NK1, NK2, and NK3 *(6)*, which are the only known tachykinin receptors and account pharmacologically for all tachykinin effects. The range of sequence homology runs between ~35% and 50% overall between NK1, 2, and 3 receptors with the greatest divergence in the extracellular segments and the highest homologies in the transmembrane segments. The NK1 receptor has a rank agonist potency of substance p > substance K > neurokinin b. The NK2 receptor recognizes the order substance K > neurokinin B > substance p. Finally, NK3 sees neurokinin b > neurokinin A > substance p *(7)*.

The relative agonist potency qualitatively parallels the apparent binding affinity when assessed in heterologous binding assays. By heterologous binding assay we refer to the technique of using one agonist as the tracer, in competition with multiple unrelated agonists. For example, on the NK1 receptor, the apparent affinity for substance p is ~0.35 n*M,* while the apparent affinities determined by heterologous competition for substance k and neurokinin B are 100-fold and 500-fold lower, respectively *(8)*. Quantitatively, however, the range of potencies is less than 10–100-fold different when assessed by inositol phosphate formation in transfected CHO cells *(9)*. Thus, while the qualitative rank order binding affinities for each tachykinin receptor correlates with the selectivity of the receptors pharmacologically, it is clear that there is a quantitative discrepancy between heterologous binding and signal transduction. Signal transduction is more sensitive than the binding assay. Perhaps this results from occupancy of a relatively low number of receptors, poorly detected in the binding assay, amplified by the G proteins into a detectable signal. Finally, a valuable NK1 receptor probe was described as an NK1 antagonist. This compound, CP-96,345, was demonstrated to be a competitive inhibitor for substance p, but noncompetitive for substance K and Neurokinin A at the NK1 receptor *(10)*. This latter finding is in conflict with "classical" assumptions for receptor function, which would posit a single binding site for all three tachykinin ligands with varying affinities depending on the ligand structure, which were competitively blocked at a single site by the antagonist compound.

In trying to understand this model, a rich literature evolved around receptor-mutation studies using chimeric and point-mutated tachykinin receptors. NK1/NK2 and NK1/NK3 chimeras were made by serial substitution of one receptor by progressively longer segments of a related receptor defined by common restriction sites. Such studies suggested that the regions comprising the N-terminus through TM4 dictate ligand binding selectivity, while TM5 through TM7 dictate the functional outcome *(11)*, conforming to the "message/address" hypothesis of Schwyzer for peptidergic receptors. This hypothesis posits that a region of receptor is common for related ligand structures (address site) while some unique sequences in the ligand activate the receptor (message site).

An important caveat in the interpretation of the chimeric receptor approach was provided by an elegant series of studies from the laboratories of Fong and Strader at Merck *(12)*. The binding of nonpeptide antagonists such as CP-96,345 was unaffected by the same loop swaps that dramatically affected peptide binding. This latter finding was independently confirmed by other investigators, and agreed with the observation that NK1 antagonists interacted critically with a histidine residue at the extracellular/TM5 junction *(13,14)*. Some point-mutant studies confirmed the chimera experiments implicating the second and third extracellular loops. However, dramatic differences in affinities caused by other segment swaps within the second extracellular loop (between TM4-5) were not confirmed by single or double point-mutants, which either eliminated electrostatic properties of individual residues or introduced NK3 residues into the NK1 receptor. Since the binding of nonpeptide antagonists was unchanged and receptor signal transduction was maintained, albeit at lower potency, the authors suggested that conformational differences between the chimeric receptors could account for the discrepancies.

Overall, the conclusion from extensive studies with promiscuous tachykinin receptors may be summarized as follows:

1. The three tachykinins—substance p, substance K, and neurokinin B—bind to three tachykinin receptors—NK1, NK2, and NK3—and elicit signal transduction. Each receptor favors one of the ligands by the criteria of both binding affinity and potency.
2. The peptide ligands interact with all four extracellular domains in some fashion, as well as residues near the cytoplasmic surface of the TM segments.
3. The peptide ligands do not interact with the same receptor residues in each case, but rather with domains that overlap to a degree.
4. Small-molecule nonpeptide NK1 antagonists interact with a different set of residues than the ligand, predominantly in the TM5–7 region proximal to the cytoplasmic surface.
5. The behavior of small-molecule NK1 antagonists is competitive with respect to substance p binding, but noncompetitive with respect to the other tachykinins, neurokinin A and neurokinin B.
6. The interpretation of chimeric receptor studies must be cautioned by effects that are apparently conformational in nature that perturb some, but not all, aspects of ligand binding.

4. THE PROBLEM OF HETEROLOGOUS BINDING ASSAYS

An important observation alluded to in the opening discussion was that the rank order of potency for tachykinins on each of their cellular receptors matched qualitatively but not quantitatively their apparent affinities using [^{125}I]-labeled substance p as a probe. Hastrup and Schwartz *(15)* confirmed an earlier report that a series of point mutants on the inner-facing (hydrophilic) face of the TM2 segment had apparently micromolar avidity for substance p when radiolabeled antagonist was used as the tracer. Yet when radiolabeled substance p was used as the tracer, or substance p itself was assayed in signal transduction, nanomolar affinity was observed *(16)*. This apparent contradiction can be resolved when one understands what is being probed in homologous versus heterologous binding assays. When substance p is used as a tracer, NK1 binds substance p with high affinity (50 p*M* Kd) and "marks" a selective binding conformation of the receptor for which the other tachykinins have low affinity (> 100 n*M*). On the other hand, although radiolabeled substance k also reveals a high affinity binding state (Kd 500 p*M*) substance p is still a very capable competitor, because it selectively sees the high (50 p*M*) site as well as the second high affinity state (500 p*M* apparent Kd). The antagonist compound has high affinity for the form of the receptor that recognizes all tachykinins with low affinity. Thus, point mutants in TM2 described above apparently interfered with the ability of the receptors to interconvert between the high affinity forms recognizing either the antagonist or the agonist. Figure 4 depicts a model that incorporates these concepts.

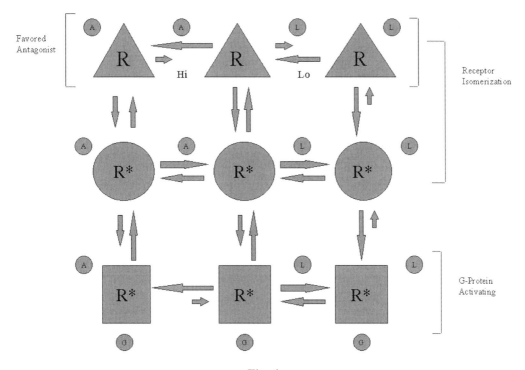

Fig. 4.

This model extends the previously described paradigm for the adrenergic receptors *(17)*. The receptor may exist in a number of conformational states, either by itself or in multimeric form. The antagonist molecule (A) binds with high affinity to a form of the receptor that binds native ligand (L) with low affinity. (The binding sites for ligand and antagonist are not identical.) When labeled antagonist is used, it selectively binds and drives the equilibrium toward the form of the receptor that binds agonist with low affinity and is uncoupled from G proteins. Receptor may also interconvert (isomerize) to a form (depicted R^*) that recognizes agonist ligand with high affinity. This form also couples and activates the G protein, a process that is driven in an equilibrium sense by ligand. Nonetheless, a small portion of R^* may interact with G protein *even in the absence of ligand.* This is a small population of receptors in steady state, although so-called "constitutively active" point mutants have been made, which likely favor this conformer.

5. THE TACHYKININ RECEPTOR MODEL EXTENDS TO THE CHEMOKINE RECEPTORS

The recent literature on the biochemistry of the chemokine receptors is replete with experiments that confirm the paradigm described above for the "promiscuous" tachykinin receptors.

Work with chimeric receptors derived from CXCR1 and CXCR2 had been reported as "surprising" because the chimeric receptors did not recapitulate the binding of either parent receptor *(18)*. Given the caveats described above for the tachykinin receptors, these results are not unanticipated and underscore the need to perform confirmatory point-mutant experiments. Since the receptors can exist in multiple affinity states that may interconvert, and each agonist "sees" each conformer with different apparent avidity, the construction of mutants may effect changes that are related not to agonist binding but rather to receptor isomerization, as described above for the NK1 receptor TM2 mutants. Nonetheless, this report strongly suggests that the binding of various alpha chemokines to CXCR2 occurs at nonidentical sites.

A second report from Ahuja and Murphy catalogued exactly the sort of data described above for heterologous versus homologous binding of IL-8, Gro, ENA78, and NAP2 to CXCR1 and CXCR2 *(19)*. These authors demonstrated that CXCR1 bound IL-8 with high affinity in homologous binding assays, which were weakly competed by NAP-2, Gro proteins, and ENA78. Additionally, calcium flux and desensitization assays indicated 50–100 nM EC50 values for ELR chemokines other than IL-8. Thus, CXCR1 is a relatively selective receptor for IL-8. The highest affinity binding isoform recognizes IL-8 selectively, although lower affinity isoforms can transduce signals to ENA-78 and Gro peptides. In homologous binding assays, these ligands were of too low affinity to register detectable binding at the concentration of tracer offered (0.1 nM). Had these authors used a higher concentration of tracer (on the order of 5 nM), the lower affinity binding sites on CXCR1 that transduce signals most likely would have been detected.

CXCR2 presented a striking analogy to the NK1 paradigm presented above. When CXCR2 was probed with $[^{125}I]$IL-8 as probe, a population of receptor was detected that had high (5 nM) affinity for IL-8, but 500 nM for NAP-2, 100 nM for Groβ, and 125 nM

for ENA-78. Groα and Groγ competed with similar high affinities at 8 and 14 nM, respectively. When ENA-78, however, was used as the radiolabeled probe, a population of receptors was detected that competed with extremely high (<1 nM) affinity for all ELR chemokines. Thus, for the tachykinins, the concept was put forth that the NK1 receptor is "optimized" for substance p, but has additional conformers that recognize substance k and neurokinin b with high affinity. Here, with CXCR2, the data argue that ENA-78 may be the ligand for which CXCR2 is "optimized," with a relatively selective lower affinity conformer which recognizes IL-8 more selectively.

6. BIOLOGICAL MEANING FOR RECEPTOR PROMISCUITY

It is probably apparent to most investigators that the redundancy among chemokines and their receptors provides an elegant mechanism for biological control. First, consider the results of heterologous versus homologous binding assays. In real terms, the high affinity of ENA-78 at CXCR2 in homologous binding assays (using labeled ENA-78) means that, in the absence of IL-8, this is a perfectly respectable ligand and agonist, as are NAP2, and the Gro proteins. Consider the heterologous assay conditions with radiolabeled IL-8 as probe. Here, CXCR2 requires greater than 100 nM ENA-78 to compete for IL-8 binding, making the receptor essentially "blind" to ENA-78. Thus, the level of ENA-78 and IL-8 protein expression in a given locale will dictate which agonist is utilized. Each chemokine may have different kinetics or stimuli for induction of its expression, different levels of its expression, and different biological half-lives. This scenario just as easily extends to CXCR3, CCR1-7 at present.

A second implication of receptor promiscuity is that each chemokine receptor has evolved to favor a particular chemokine agonist. The multiple states or conformations in which a receptor exists in the membrane each may have particular bound water molecules, ions, posttranslational modifications, and oligomeric states that favor a particular equilibrium condition among these populations of receptors. The preferred ligand at a given receptor is likely to have evolved along with the receptor to accomplish a specific biological task. For example, there are at least five known ligands for CCR2 in the mouse. Yet MCP-1 and its mouse orthologue JE are the dominant partners of CCR2. This is evidenced by the fact that the knockout for CCR2 recapitulates the major aspects of the phenotype for the knockout of MCP-1/JE *(20,21)*. This is in spite of the fact that a higher degree of sequence homology between MCP-1 (human) and MCP-5 (murine) exists. However, under conditions of *expression* (for example, after PDGF stimulation) the dominant chemokine produced in a human is MCP-1 and JE in the mouse. Thus, the receptor–ligand pairs have evolved in a given species to capitalize on combinations that most benefit the host in a given situation. Thus, in some models, we might expect to see a divergence in the phenotype of CCR2 knockouts when compared with the MCP-1/JE knockout. In such a situation, an alternative chemokine (MCP-2,3,4,5?) might be expressed in favor of JE/MCP-1.

Another implication of the ligand redundancy for a given chemokine receptor may be understood in terms of the model recently put forth by Butcher and colleagues *(22)*, who found that in gradients produced by heterologous chemoattractants a hierarchy was observed which presumably relates to the fact that in a given milieu, a cell must discriminate among a number of signals to finally execute its appointed task.

7. CONCLUSION

Interactions between chemokines and their receptors are quite consistent with other models of peptidergic receptors, such as those for tachykinins and C5a. Peptidergic ligands have a "message" sequence which may be common among groups of related agonists (for example, the ELR sequence in CXC chemokines), which is important for *both* binding and signal transduction. The "address" sequence is that part of the peptide structure which participates in high affinity receptor *selectivity* but does not in itself elicit signal transduction *(23)*. As antagonists are developed against chemokine receptors, we will undoubtedly see more parallels with the tachykinin paradigm. We will also have tools more powerful than gene knockout to investigate the roles of chemokines in biology. The concepts advanced in this chapter, however, have implications for drug discovery. Choosing the right assay system to select for small molecules may involve more than screening for competitive binding antagonists. Perhaps a more fruitful approach, given the nature of the binding equilibria involved, might be to design assays that select for the receptor's low affinity binding state which recognizes the greatest number of ligands.

REFERENCES

1. Rollins B. J. 1997. Chemokines. *Blood* **90:** 909–928.
2. Gerard C., and Gerard N. P. 1994. C5a anaphylatoxin and its seven transmembrane-segment receptor. *Annu. Rev. Immunol.* **12:** 775–808.
3. Khorana H. G. 1992. Rhodopsin, photoreceptor of the rod cell. An emerging pattern for structure and function. *J. Biol. Chem.* **267:** 1–4.
4. Freedman N. J., and Lefkowitz R. J. 1996. Desensitization of G protein-coupled receptors. *Rec. Prog. Hormone Res.* **51:** 319–325.
5. Didsbury J. R., Uhing R. J., Tomhave E., Gerard C., Gerard N. P., and Snyderman, R. 1991. Receptor class-specific desensitization identified using cloned leukocyte chemoattractant receptors. *Proc. Natl. Acad. Sci. USA* **88:** 11564–11568.
6. Maggi C. A. 1995. The mammalian tachykinin receptors. *Gen. Pharmacology* **26:** 911–944.
7. Nakanishi S., Nakajima Y., and Yokota Y. 1993. Signal transduction and ligand-binding domains of tachykinin receptors. *Reg. Peptides* **46:** 37–42.
8. Fong T. M., Yu H., Huang R. R., and Strader C. D. 1992. The extracellular domain of the NK-1 receptor is required for high-affinity bindings of peptides. *Biochemistry* **31:** 11806–11811.
9. Nakajim Y., Tsuchida K., Negishi M., Ito S., and Nakanishi S. 1992. Direct linkage of three tachykinin receptors to stimulation of both phosphatidyl inositol hydrolysis and cycle AMP cascades in trasfected Chinese hamster ovary cells. *J. Biol. Chem.* **267:** 2437–2442.
10. Gether U., Lowe J. A. 3rd, and Schwartz T. W. 1995. Tachykinin non-peptide antagonists: binding domain and molecular mode of action. *Biochemistry Society Transactions* **23:** 96–102.
11. Gether U., Johansen T. E., and Schwartz T. W. 1993. Chimeric NK1 (substance P)/NK3 (neurokinin B) receptors. Identification of domains determining the binding specificity of tachykinin agonists. *J. Biol. Chem.* **268:** 7893–7898.
12. Huang R. R., Yu H., Strader C. D., and Fong T. M. 1994. Localization of the ligand binding site of the neurokinin-1 receptor: interpretation of chimeric mutations and single-residue substitutions. *Mol. Pharmacol.* **45:** 690–695.
13. Gether U., Johansen T. E., Snider R. M., Lowe J. A. 3rd, Nakanishi S., and Schwartz T. W. 1993. Different binding epitopes on the NK1 receptor for substance P and non-peptide antagonist. *Nature* **362:** 345–348.

14. Fong T. M., Cascieri M. A., Yu H., Bansal A., Swain C., and Strader C. D. 1993. Amino-aromatic interaction between histidine 197 of the neurokinin-1 receptor and CP 96345. *Nature* **362:** 350–353.

15. Hastrup H., and Schwartz T. W. 1996. Septide and neurokinin A are high-affinity ligands on the NK-1 receptor: evidence from homologous versus heterologous binding analysis. *FEBS Letters* **399:** 264–266.

16. Rosenkilde M. M., Cahir M., Gether U., Hjorth S. A., and Schwartz T. W. 1994. Mutations along transmembrane segment II of the NK-1 receptor affect substance P competition with non-peptide antagonists but not substance P binding. *J. Biol. Chem.* **269:** 28160–28164.

17. Samama P., Cotecchia S., Costa T., and Lefkowitz R. J. 1993. A mutation-induced activated state of the beta 2-adrenergic receptor. Extending the ternary complex model. *J. Biol. Chem.* **268:** 4625–4636.

18. Ahuja S. K., Lee J. C., and Murphy P. M. 1996. CXC chemokines bind to unique sets of selectivity determinants that can function independently and are broadly distributed on multiple domains of human interleukin-8 receptor B. Determinants of high affinity binding and receptor activation are distinct. *J. Biol. Chem.* **271:** 225–232.

19. Ahuja S. K., and Murphy P. M. 1996. The CXC chemokines growth-regulated oncogene (GRO) alpha, GRObeta, GROgamma, neurophil-activating peptide-2, and epithelial cell-derived neutrophil-activating peptide-78 are potent agonists of the type B, but not the type A, human interleukin-8 receptor. *J. Biol. Chem.* **271:** 20545–20550.

20. Gu L., Okada Y., Clinton S. K., Gerard C., Sukhova G. K., Libby P., and Rollins B. J. 1998. Absence of monocyte chemoattractant protein-1 reduces atherosclerosis in low density lipoprotein receptor-deficient mice. *Mol. Cell* **2:** 275–281.

21. Boring L., Gosling J., and Charol F. 1998. Decreased lesion formation in CCR2(-1-) mice reveals a role for chemokines in the initiation of atherosclerosis. *Nature* **394:** 894–897.

22. Foxman E. F., Campbell J. J., and Butcher E. C. 1997. Multistep navigation and the combinatorial control of leukocyte chemotaxis. *J. Cell Biol.* **139:** 1349–1360.

23. Schwyzer R. 1987. Membrane-assisted molecular mechanism of neurokinin receptor subtype selection. *EMBO Journal* **6:** 2255–2259.

II

Tumor Infiltration by Leukocytes

3

Tumors as a Paradigm for the In Vivo Role of Chemokines in Leukocyte Recruitment

Alberto Mantovani, Annunciata Vecchi, Silvano Sozzani, Antonio Sica, and Paola Allavena

1. INTRODUCTION

Ever since the first description by Virchow in 1863, histopathologists have recognized the occurrence of host leukocytes in tumor tissues and/or at their periphery. Interestingly, Virchow felt that the frequent presence of a lymphoreticular infiltrate in human neoplasms reflected the origin of cancer at sites of previous chronic inflammation. In 1907 Hardley reported that normal cell infiltration in malignant melanoma indicated a "regressive process." This observation marked a complete change in the general opinion as to the significance of the "lymphoreticular infiltrate," a change reflected by a number of reports on pathology and prognosis. These opposite ways of looking at the relationship between leukocyte infiltration and malignancy have polarized views in the field but, indeed, reflect the pleiotropic, ambivalent functions of infiltrating cells.

Mononuclear phagocytes are an important component of the stroma of neoplastic tissues often underestimated in conventional histologic sections *(26,44,92)*. Solid tumors consist of malignant cells and stroma. These two compartments are discrete and interdependent, in that malignant cells elicit stroma formation and that this is essential for neoplastic growth and progression. Components of the tumor stroma include new blood vessels, matrix components as well as cells responsible for their production, a fibrin-gel matrix, and inflammatory leukocytes *(25)*. Tumor-associated macrophages (TAMs) can interact with both the neoplastic and the stromal components of tumor tissues.

Interest in cells of the mononuclear phagocyte lineage in relation to neoplasia stemmed largely from the observation that these effector cells, when appropriately activated, are able to kill neoplastically transformed target cells in vitro and that normal cells are usually relatively resistant to killing by activated macrophages. The cytotoxic function of activated macrophages on transformed target cells led to the hypothesis (to date, not adequately tested) that they represent a mechanism of nonspecific surveillance against neoplasia *(1,35)*. It has been more recently shown that the spectrum of the cytotoxic action of activated mononuclear phagocytes encompasses tumor cells with various forms of resistance to chemotherapeutic agents, an observation with obvious implications for combined therapies *(2)*.

From: *Chemokines and Cancer*
Edited by: B. J. Rollins © Humana Press Inc., Totowa, NJ

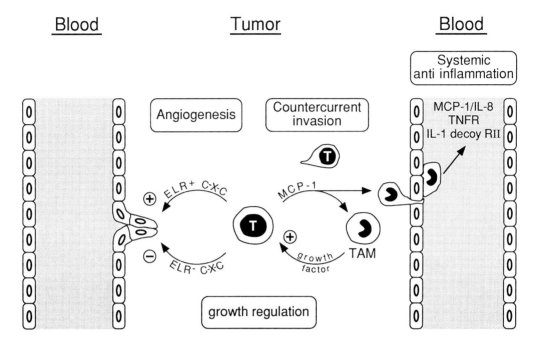

Fig. 1. A schematic overview of the role of chemokines in the regulation of tumor growth and metastasis. T, tumor cell; TAM, tumor-associated macrophages; ELR⁺ and ELR⁻ C-X-C, C-X-C chemokines with or without the ELR motif; TNFR and IL-1 RII, TNF and IL-1 receptor. MCP-1 is indicated as a prototypic C-C chemokine. Countercurrent invasion as well as direct attraction for tumor cells may explain a positive role for MCP-1 in metastasis under certain conditions *(45,59,95).*

The in vivo relevance of the in vitro cytotoxic interaction of activated macrophages with tumor cells has not been unequivocally demonstrated, even under conditions in which macrophages are likely to have antitumor activity. Tissue-destructive reactions centered on vascular elements, induced by mononuclear phagocytes via their secretory products (e.g., tumor necrosis factor [TNF], interleukin-12 [IL-12], or interferon-γ-inducible protein-10 [IP-10]), are likely to represent an important mechanism of antitumor activity in vivo *(46).*

Macrophages express diverse functions essential for tissue remodeling, inflammation, and immunity. Analysis of TAMs, using the tools of cellular and molecular biology, suggests that these pleiotropic cells have the capacity to affect diverse aspects of the immunobiology of neoplastic tissues, including vascularization, growth rate and metastasis, stroma formation, and dissolution (Fig. 1). As discussed subsequently, there is evidence that in some neoplasms, including common human cancers, the protumor functions of TAMs prevail. In certain tumors, neutrophils can exert the same tumor promoting function as TAMs *(63).* The "macrophage balance" hypothesis *(44)* emphasizes the dual potential of TAMs to influence neoplastic growth and progression in opposite directions, with a prevailing protumor activity in the absence of therapeutic intervention in many neoplasms.

The search for tumor-derived chemotactic factors (TDCFs), which could account for recruitment of mononuclear phagocytes in neoplastic tissues, represented one pathway that led to the identification of the prototypic CC chemokine monocyte chemoattractant protein-1 (MCP-1) *(13)*.

This chapter reviews evidence that chemokines, MCP-1 in particular, play an important role in regulating macrophage recruitment in tumors and explains how chemokines active on activated natural killer (NK) cells and on dendritic cells may provide tools to activate specific immunity against neoplasms *(90,97–99)*.

2. CHEMOKINES IN THE REGULATION OF TAM LEVELS

2.1. *Murine Tumors*

The percentage of TAMs for each tumor is usually maintained as a relatively stable "individual" property during tumor growth and on transplantation in syngeneic hosts. Transplant of xenogeneic human (but not allogeneic murine) tumors is associated with a different pattern of distribution of TAMs within the lesion, i.e., peripheral rather than diffuse *(16)*. Macrophages also infiltrate metastatic lesions, although TAMs have been less extensively studied in secondary foci *(43,44)*. Even at macrophage-rich anatomic sites such as the liver, macrophage infiltration in metastasis depends, to a large extent, on the recruitment of monocytic precursors *(34)*. Experiments in which tumors were transplanted in hosts with defective T-cell or NK cell immunity suggest that, for many neoplasms, specific immunity is not a major determinant of macrophage infiltration, and that factors derived from the tumor itself play a pivotal role in the regulation of macrophage levels in poorly immunogenic metastatic tumors *(44)*.

Analysis of the mechanisms of macrophage recruitment in tumors was one pathway that led to the identification of MCP-1 *(13,30,44,90,97,98,98,99)*. Several lines of evidence suggest that MCP-1 can represent an important determinant of the levels of TAMs *(44,59)*. In early studies with murine tumors or human tumors in nude mice, a correlation was found between MCP-1 bioactivity and the percentage of TAMs, a finding confirmed in subsequent experiments measuring MCP-1 mRNA levels *(94)*. Subcutaneous inoculation of tumor-derived human MCP-1, MCP-2, and MCP-3 led to macrophage infiltration *(36,90,99)*. Finally, and conclusively, transfer of the mouse or human *MCP-1* gene was associated with augmented levels of macrophage infiltration *(15,71)*. High expression of MCP-1 was associated with abrogation of tumorigenicity of Chinese hamster ovary cells *(71)* but not of malignant mouse tumors *(15)*. At low tumor inocula, MCP-1 gene transfer was associated with higher tumorigenicity and lung-colonizing ability, despite a lower growth rate of resulting lesions *(15,45)*. These findings were interpreted as reflecting the dual influence that TAMs can exert on tumor growth *(44,59)*. Expression of MCP-1/JE was also detected in various rat tumors *(97)*. Using markers selective for monocyte-derived vs tissue macrophages, MCP-1/JE gene transfer caused recruitment of mononuclear phagocytes from the blood compartment *(97)*. Evidence for a role of MCP-1 in recruitment was also obtained in human tumor xenografts *(49)*.

Leukocyte infiltration in murine tumors is associated with the administration of cytokines such as interferons, IL-2, or IL-4, by conventional routes or following gene transfer. Interferons, IL-12, and IL-2 induce endogenous chemokines in renal and colon cancer models *(83,89)*. Thus, secondary induction of chemokines may play a pivotal role in leukocyte recruitment in tumors treated with cytokines other than chemokines.

2.2. Human Tumors

Various human tumor lines express MCP-1 in vitro spontaneously or after exposure to inflammatory signals, and some do so in vivo. The latter include gliomas, histiocytomas, sarcomas, and melanomas *(29,88,98,99)*. The expression of MCP-1 was recently found in Kaposi's sarcoma (KS) in vivo and in KS-derived spindle cell cultures *(78)*. Since KS is characterized by a conspicuous macrophage infiltrate and is believed to represent a cytokine-propelled disease, production of MCP-1 may be particularly significant in this disease. Interestingly, human herpesvirus 8, likely involved in the pathogenesis of KS, encodes a constitutively active chemokine receptor that stimulates cell proliferation *(6)*.

Human tumor lines of epithelial origin (breast, colon, ovary) *(12,13)* release small mol wt chemoattractant(s). A TDCF in ovarian carcinoma was recently identified as MCP-1 *([54]*, see Subheading 2.1.).

The expression of MCP-1 in relation to cervical cancer has been investigated by in vitro and in vivo approaches *(36,69)*. Somatic cell hybrids were generated between human papillomavirus type 18 (HPV-18) cells and normal cells. Only nontumorigenic hybrids expressed MCP-1, whereas it was undetectable in tumorigenic segregants and in HPV-positive cervical carcinoma lines. By *in situ* hybridization, MCP-1 was detected in certain human cervical cancers. In high-grade squamous intraepithelial lesions, MCP-1 expression was detected in normal, dysplastic, and neoplastic epithelia, as well as in macrophages and endothelial cells. MCP-1 expression was most prominent at epithelial-mesenchymal junctions and was associated with macrophage infiltration. In intraepithelial lesions, expression of MCP-1 and of the HPV oncogenes E6/E7 tended to be mutually exclusive, whereas in squamous cell carcinoma, MCP-1 was expressed in the presence of transcriptionally active E6/E7.

Various human tumors express chemokines of the C-X-C family. Some neoplasms of the melanocyte lineage express growth-related oncogene-α (GRO-α), and the related molecule, IL-8, which induce proliferation and migration of melanoma cells *(8,76,96)*. Transfer of the *GRO-α* gene in an untransformed melanocytic line rendered it competent to form tumors in immunodeficient mice *(8):* this effect could be related to direct growth stimulation or to promotion of an inflammatory reaction, which would, in turn, favor tumor formation (see Subheading 3.). Inflammation and wound healing have, in fact, been implicated in the initial steps of melanocyte oncogenesis *(48,50)*. IL-8 is produced by various human tumor lines in vitro, in particular, carcinomas and brain tumors, either spontaneously or after exposure to IL-1 and TNF *(74,91)*. It has been speculated that IL-8 may contribute to lymphocytic infiltration in brain tumors *(91)*. In addition, IL-8 has angiogenic activity *(38),* and could thus enhance tumor angiogenesis. A novel member of the C-X-C chemokine family, GCP-2, was recently identified in the supernatants of stimulated sarcoma cells *(68)*. Direct evidence that C-X-C chemokines containing the ELR motif *(see* Chapter 1) play a positive role in tumor angiogenesis has been obtained in non-small cell lung cancer *(5,80)*. In this human tumor, angiogenesis appears to be regulated by a balance between pro- and antiangiogenic chemokines including, among the latter, IP-10 *(5)*.

Table 1
Chemokines as Mediators of a Systemic Antiinflammatory State

Reverse gradient
Receptor desensitization
Rapid shedding of the IL-1 decoy RII *(16)*
Rapid shedding of the TNFR *(44)*

3. DEFECTIVE SYSTEMIC IMMUNITY AND INFLAMMATION IN CANCER PATIENTS: A ROLE FOR CHEMOKINES?

In terms of mounting immunoinflammatory reactions, neoplastic disorders constitute, in a way, a paradox. As discussed previously, many, if not all, tumors produce chemoattractants and are infiltrated by leukocytes; yet, it has long been known that neoplastic disorders are associated with immunosuppression and a defective capacity to mount inflammatory reactions at sites other than the tumor *(81)*. It has often been demonstrated that circulating monocytes from cancer patients have defects in their ability to respond to chemoattractants *(10,20,55–57,82,86)*. We have speculated that tumor-derived chemokines may play a role in the two seemingly contradictory aspects of monocyte function in neoplasia (Table 1) *(43)*. Chemokines released continuously from a growing tumor may, beyond a certain tumor size, leak into the systemic circulation. Chemoattractants are classically known to cause desensitization that, depending on the time of exposure, can be restricted to agents that use the same receptor (homologous desensitization) or can involve other seven-transmembrane domain receptors (heterologous desensitization). Therefore, continuous exposure to tumor-derived chemoattractants may paralyze leukocytes. A more subtle antiinflammatory action of chemoattractants depends on their effect on the receptors of the primary cytokines IL-1 and TNF *(23,66)*. Chemotactic agents cause rapid shedding of the TNF receptors, most efficiently RII/p75, and of the type II IL-1 "decoy" receptor.

IL-8 was also able to induce rapid decoy RII release, though less efficiently than FMLP or C5a *(23)*. However, IL-8 had additive effects with other elements in the cascade of recruitment such as platelet activating factor (Orlando, S., unpublished data). Most likely, rapid shedding of the TNFR and of the IL-1 decoy R serves to buffer primary proinflammatory cytokines leaking from sites of inflammation. Consistent with the concept of the antiinflammatory potential of chemokines, systemic IL-8 inhibits local inflammatory reactions *(33)*, and transgenic mice overexpressing MCP-1 have impaired resistance to intracellular pathogens *(73)*. Thus, chemoattractant-induced continuous release of these molecules able to block IL-1 and TNF may contribute to a defective capacity to mount an inflammatory response systemically, coexisting with continuous leukocyte recruitment at the tumor site.

4. MONOCYTE FUNCTIONS OTHER THAN CHEMOTAXIS

C-C chemokines, MCP-1 in particular, affect several functions of mononuclear phagocytes related to recruitment or to effector activity. Interaction with, and localized digestion of, extracellular matrix components is essential for phagocyte extravasation and migration in tissues. MCP-1 induces production of gelatinase and of urokinase-type plasminogen activator (uPA) *(47,60)*. Concomitantly, MCP-1 augments expression of the cell surface receptor for uPA. Induction of gelatinase was also observed in response to MCP-2 and MCP-3 *(90)*. Thus, C-C chemokines arm monocytes with the molecular tools that allow local and polarized digestion of extracellular matrix components during recruitment. In tumor tissues, the release of lytic enzymes by MCP-1-stimulated TAMs may provide a ready-made pathway for invasion of tumor cells (countercurrent invasion) and thus contribute to augmented metastasis associated with inflammation *(47,58–60,90)*. Accordingly, in one mouse model, MCP-1 gene transfer augmented lung-colony formation *(45)*. Moreover, tissue-derived MCP-1 was implicated in the homing of lymphoma cells at specific anatomic sites *(95)*.

MCP-1 induces a respiratory burst in human monocytes, though it is a weak stimulus compared to other agonists *(37,99)*. Natural MCP-1 was reported to induce IL-1 and IL-6 but not TNF production *(37)*. In another study, recombinant MCP-1 had little effect on IL-6 release (Sironi, M., et al., unpublished data). Human MCP-1 induced monocyte cytostasis for a tumor line *(99)* or synergized with bacterial products (but not with interferon-γ [IFN-γ]) in the stimulation of mouse macrophage cytotoxicity *(7,79)*. In an intriguing recent study, human MCP-1 inhibited induction of the nitric oxide (NO) synthase in the macrophage cell line J774 *(70)*. Since TAMs have reduced NO synthase activity *(24)*, this finding, if confirmed, would suggest that MCP-1 could account for both recruitment and concomitant partial functional deactivation of TAMs.

5. OVARIAN CANCER AS A PARADIGM FOR CHEMOKINES IN NEOPLASIA

Ovarian carcinoma is the one human tumor that has been most extensively studied for cytokine circuits between tumor cells and infiltrating leukocytes *(17)*. These studies have also led to the design of therapeutic strategies targeted to TAMs, which gave encouraging results *(3,22)*. The role of chemokines in the reciprocal interactions between ovarian carcinoma cells and macrophages has been discussed elsewhere *(26)*. Freshly isolated ovarian carcinoma cells, primary cultures, and some established cell lines were shown in early studies to release TDCF activity *(12–14)*. These observations were recently revisited *(54)*. Immunohistochemistry and *in situ* hybridization demonstrated that ovarian carcinoma cells, as well as stromal elements in some tumors, express MCP-1. High levels of MCP-1 were measured in the ascites (but not in blood) of patients with ovarian cancer, and was absent in the peritoneal fluid of patients with nonmalignant conditions. Production of MCP-1 and recruitment of TAMs are likely to play important roles in the progression of this disease because macrophage-derived cytokines promote the growth of ovarian carcinoma and its secondary implantation on peritoneal surfaces *(43)*.

6. THERAPEUTIC POTENTIAL OF CHEMOKINES: ANTIANGIOGENESIS

In general, the spectrum of action of chemokines tends to be restricted to leukocytes, but recent evidence suggests that some members of this superfamily of inflammatory mediators may affect endothelial cell function. IL-8, GRO-α, and other C-X-C chemokines have been reported to induce endothelial cell migration and proliferation in vitro and to be angiogenic in vivo *(38)*. However, the expression of high-affinity receptors on endothelial cells and their responsiveness to IL-8 have been the subjects of conflicting results *(64,77)*.

In common with platelet factor 4, IP-10 was shown to have angiostatic properties in vivo and to represent the ultimate mediator of the antiangiogenic activity of IL-12 *(93)*, although conflicting results have been obtained as to its capacity to inhibit basic fibroblast growth factor–induced proliferation of human umbilical vein endothelial cells in vitro *(4,40)*. A three-amino-acid motif (ELR), is conserved in members of the C-X-C family that activate neutrophils. Recent results, including the action of molecules with or without the ELR motif and the activity of IL-8 muteins, suggest that the presence or absence of an ELR motif dictates whether C-X-C chemokines induce or inhibit angiogenesis *(87)*. However, the observation that GRO-β inhibits angiogenesis is not consistent with this model of function *(18)*.

Three types of chemokine binding sites have been identified. The presence and type of high-affinity chemokine receptors on endothelial cells that transduce signals is controversial *(38,64,77)*. The promiscuous chemokine receptor identical to the Duffy blood group antigen, which does not appear to transduce intracellular signals, is expressed by endothelial cells at postcapillary venules in vivo, but not by endothelial cells in vitro *(62)*. Finally, heparin and heparin-like proteoglycans on endothelial cells present some chemokines to leukocytes in the multistep process of recruitment *(72)*.

Thus, certain chemokines such as IP-10 have antiangiogenic activity, and represent the ultimate mediator in the antitumor action of a cytokine cascade involving IL-12 and IFN-γ. After gene transfer in certain tumors, other cellular targets (e.g., T-cells with a type I cytokine profile; *[11]*) may play a role in the antitumor activity of IP-10.

7. THERAPEUTIC POTENTIAL OF CHEMOKINES: ATTRACTION OF DENDRITIC CELLS

Cytokine gene transfer into tumor cells has resulted in tumor rejection in experimental systems and is undergoing evaluation in human tumors. The antitumor activity of cytokine gene transfer is associated with distinct patterns of leukocyte infiltration (for review see ref. *52*). Although it is likely that chemokines play a pivotal role in determining the timing, type, and amount of infiltrate under these conditions, detailed analysis is at present lacking.

Chemokines have been used in gene transfer studies. Depending on the tumor type, MCP-1 gene transfer has been associated with abrogation of tumorigenicity, reduced growth rate, augmented tumor take or metastasis, or no effect *(15,21,36,45,61)*. Antitumor activity and activation of specific immunity have been observed after gene transfer of MCP-1, IP-10, TCA3, RANTES, lymphotactin, and MCP-3 *(27,39,41,42,51,52)*.

A major goal of immunotherapeutic approaches to neoplasia is activation of specific antitumor immunity. In this perspective, dendritic cells may be a crucial determinant of success or failure. Recent results suggest that dendritic cells express receptors for and respond to chemokines *(28,85)*.

Dendritic cell precursors originate in the bone marrow and subsequently migrate into peripheral tissues and primary lymphoid organs, where they efficiently take up and process soluble antigens. After capture of antigen in tissues, dendritic cells migrate via the afferent lymphatics to draining lymph nodes or via blood to spleen, where they stimulate T-cells *(9,19)*. As the molecules controlling these events are unknown, we

Table 2
Chemoattractants Active on Dendritic Cells[a]

Family	Active	Inactive
C-X-C	SDF-1	IL-8, GRO-β, IP-10
C-C	MCP-3, MCP-4, MIP-1α, MIP-1β, MIP-5, RANTES, MDC, LARC[b]	MCP-1, MCP-2, eotaxin
C	—	Lymphotactin
Classical, peptides	C5a, fMLP	—
Classical, lipids	PAF	Oxolipids

[a]Data from refs. *32,67,84,85.*

[b]LARC/MIP-3α/exodus is active on CD34 cell-derived dendritic cells but not on monocyte-derived dendritic cells. This pattern of differential responsiveness correlates with CCR6 expression *(31,67).* SDF-1, stromal-derived factor; LARC, liver and activation-regulated chemokine; MDC, macrophage-derived chemokine.

investigated which chemotactic factors could attract this cell population and regulate their trafficking in tissues *(85).*

For these experiments, dendritic cells were obtained from peripheral blood precursor cells cultured in the presence of granulocyte-macrophage colony-stimulating factor (GM-CSF) and IL-4 or IL-13 *(65,75).* These cells were CD1a[+], major histocompatibility complex (MHC) class II[++], CD14[−], CD3[−], and CD20[−] and behaved as classical immature dendritic cells being active in eliciting the proliferation of naive T-lymphocytes and showing a strong ability to take up fluorescein isothiocyanate–dextran *(65).* In a microwell chemotaxis assay, these cells migrated in response to a selected pattern of C-C chemokines, such as MCP-3, RANTES, and macrophage inflammatory protein-1α (MIP-1α) and to two prototypic chemotactic factors, formyl-methione-leucine-proline (fMLP) and C5a *(85)* (Table 2). MCP-1 and MCP-2, two other C-C chemokines, and all the C-X-C chemokines tested (IL-8, IP-10, and GRO-β) were inactive. Peak active concentrations and the percentage of input dendritic cells migrating in response to C-C chemokines were comparable to those observed with monocytes.

MCP-3, MIP-1α, and RANTES showed a complex pattern of cross-desensitization suggesting the presence of multiple promiscuous receptors on these cells. In Northern blot studies, it was found that dendritic cells express the CCR1, CCR2, and CCR5, as well as CXCR2 and CXCR4. Dendritic cells respond to SDF-1 but not to IL-8 and MCP-1 in vitro, in spite of expressing CCR2 and CXCR2 mRNA.

Transgenic mice, in which MCP-1 is constitutively expressed in the epidermis under the control of human keratin 14 promoter, respond to a contact hypersensitivity challenge with an increased lichenoid infiltration of monocytes, T-lymphocytes, and CD45[+], Ia[+] cells that assumed a dendritic morphology *in situ (53).* We speculate that MCP-1 may attract monocytes to the skin, where these cells find an environment (e.g., GM-CSF) conducive to dendritic cell differentiation.

Macrophage-derived chemokine (MDC) is a recently identified C-C chemokine, which, unlike related molecules, is located on chromosome 16 and has a rather distant relationship with other family members *(28).* We recently found that MDC has an ED_{50} 100-fold lower for activated NK cells and dendritic cells than for monocytes *(28).*

Moreover, it is expressed by dendritic cells in addition to macrophages. We speculate that molecules such as SDF-1 and MDC may contribute to directing the "normal" trafficking of dendritic cells in the absence of antigen or inflammation, whereas inducible chemokines may underlie the dramatic changes in route and trafficking after exposure to antigenic or inflammatory stimulation.

In the context of our interest in chemokines and dendritic cells, we recently transfected tumor cells with MCP-3 *(27)*. After MCP-3 gene transfer, P815 mastocytoma cells grew, but underwent rejection. MCP-3-elicited rejection was associated with resistance to subsequent challenge with parental cells. MCP-3-elicited rejection was associated with profound alterations of leukocyte infiltration. TAMs were already present in copious number, but T-cells, eosinophils, and neutrophils increased in tumor tissues after MCP-3 gene transfer. Dendritic cells (e.g., Dec205+, high MHC class II+ cells) did not increase substantially in the tumor mass. However, in peritumoral tissues, dendritic cells accumulated in perivascular areas. In contrast to their behavior in immunocompetent mice, MCP-3-transfected tumor cells grew normally in nude mice. Increased accumulation of macrophages and polymorphonuclear leukocytes (PMNs) was evident also in nude mice. Antibodies against CD4, CD8, and IFN-γ, but not against IL-4, inhibited rejection of MCP-3-transfected P815 cells. An anti-PMN monoclonal antibody caused only a retardation of MCP-3-elicited tumor rejection. Thus, MCP-3 gene transfer elicits tumor rejection by activating type 1 T-cell-dependent immunity. It is tempting to speculate that altered trafficking of antigen-presenting cells, which express receptors and respond to MCP-3, together with recruitment of activated T-cells, underlies the activation of specific immunity by MCP-3-transfected cells.

8. CONCLUSION

Chemokines play a dual role in the regulation of tumor growth and metastasis. Certain chemokines are produced by tumor cells and, by attracting macrophages and endothelial cells, provide optimal conditions for tumor growth and progression. We speculate that chemokines leaking from sites of tumor growth may contribute to systemic impairment of the capacity to mount immune and inflammatory reactions, a situation frequently observed in advanced neoplasia. Conversely, the antiangiogenic activity of chemokines and their capacity to recruit and activate immunocompetent cells can be exploited therapeutically in gene transfer studies.

A better understanding of the physiologic role of chemokines in directing the traffic of dendritic cells and NK cells, crucial for the activation and orientation of specific immunity, may provide a basis for a less empirical design of chemokine-based therapeutic strategies.

ACKNOWLEDGMENTS

This work was supported by the Italian Association for Cancer Research, Milan, Italy. The authors thank Mrs. Antonella Palmiero for invaluable help in the preparation of this manuscript.

REFERENCES

1. Adams, D. O., and R. Snyderman. 1979. Do macrophages destroy nascent tumors? *J. Natl. Cancer Inst.* **62:** 1341–1745.

2. Allavena, P., M. Grandi, M. D'Incalci, O. Geri, F. C. Giuliani, and A. Mantovani. 1987. Human tumor cell lines with pleiotropic drug resistance are efficiently killed by interleukin-2 activated killer cells and by activated monocytes. *Int. J. Cancer* **40:** 104–107.
3. Allavena, P., F. Peccatori, D. Maggioni, A. Erroi, M. Sironi, N. Colombo, A. Lissoni, A. Galazka, W. Meiers, C. Mangioni, and A. Mantovani. 1990. Intraperitoneal recombinant gamma-interferon in patients with recurrent ascitic ovarian carcinoma: modulation of cytotoxicity and cytokine production in tumor-associated effectors and of major histocompatibility antigen expression on tumor cells. *Cancer Res.* **50:** 7318–7323.
4. Angiolillo, A. L., C. Sgadari, D. D. Taub, F. Liao, J. M. Farber, S. Maheshwari, H. K. Kleinman, G. H. Reaman, and G. Tosato. 1995. Human interferon-inducible protein 10 is a potent inhibitor of angiogenesis in vivo. *J. Exp. Med.* **182:** 155–162.
5. Arenberg, D. A., S. L. Kunkel, P. J. Polverini, S. B. Morris, M. D. Burdick, M. C. Glass, D. T. Taub, M. D. Iannettoni, T. I. Whyte, and R. M. Strieter. 1996. Interferon-gamma-inducible protein 10 (IP-10) is an angiostatic factor that inhibits human non-small cell lung cancer (NSCLC) tumorigenesis and spontaneous metastases. *J. Exp. Med.* **184:** 981–992.
6. Arvanitakis, L., E. GerasRaaka, A. Varma, M. C. Gershengorn, and E. Cesarman. 1997. Human herpesvirus KSHV encodes a constitutively active G-protein-coupled receptor linked to cell proliferation. *Nature* **385:** 347–350.
7. Asano, T., T. An, S. F. Jia, and E. S. Kleinerman. 1996. Altered monocyte chemotactic and activating factor gene expression in human glioblastoma cell lines increased their susceptibility to cytotoxicity. *J. Leukocyte Biol.* **59:** 916–924.
8. Balentien, E., B. E. Mufson, R. L. Shattuck, R. Derynck, and A. Richmond. 1991. Effects of MGSA/GRO alpha on melanocyte transformation. *Oncogene* **6:** 1115–1124.
9. Bancherau, J., and R. M. Steinman. 1998. Dendritic cells and the control of immunity. *Nature* **392:** 245–252.
10. Boechter, D., and E. J. Leonard. 1974. Abnormal monocyte chemotactic response in mice. *J. Natl. Cancer Inst.* **52:** 1091–1099.
11. Bonecchi, R., G. Bianchi, P. Panina Bordignon, D. D'Ambrosio, R. Lang, A. Borsatti, S. Sozzani, P. Allavena, P. A. Gray, A. Mantovani, and F. Sinigaglia. 1998. Differential expression of chemokine receptors and chemotactic responsiveness of Th1 and Th2 cells. *J. Exp. Med.* **187:** 129–134.
12. Bottazzi, B., P. Ghezzi, G. Taraboletti, M. Salmona, N. Colombo, C. Bonazzi, C. Mangioni, and A. Mantovani. 1985. Tumor-derived chemotactic factor(s) from human ovarian carcinoma: evidence for a role in the regulation of macrophage content of neoplastic tissues. *Int. J. Cancer* **36:** 167–173.
13. Bottazzi, B., N. Polentarutti, R. Acero, A. Balsari, D. Boraschi, P. Ghezzi, M. Salmona, and A. Mantovani. 1983. Regulation of the macrophage content of neoplasms by chemoattractants. *Science* **220:** 210–212.
14. Bottazzi, B., N. Polentarutti, A. Balsari, D. Boraschi, P. Ghezzi, M. Salmona, and A. Mantovani. 1983. Chemotactic activity for mononuclear phagocytes of culture supernatants from murine and human tumor cells: evidence for a role in the regulation of the macrophage content of neoplastic tissues. *Int. J. Cancer* **31:** 55–63.
15. Bottazzi, B., S. Walter, D. Govoni, F. Colotta, and A. Mantovani. 1992. Monocyte chemotactic cytokine gene transfer modulates macrophage infiltration, growth, and susceptibility to IL-2 therapy of a murine melanoma. *J. Immunol.* **148:** 1280–1285.
16. Bucana, C. D., A. Fabra, R. Sanchez, and I. G. Fidler. 1992. Different patterns of macrophage infiltration into allogeneic-murine and xenogeneic-human neoplasms growing in nude mice. *Am. J. Pathol.* **141:** 1225–1236.
17. Burke, F., M. Relf, R. Negus, and F. Balkwill. 1996. A cytokine profile of normal and malignant ovary. *Cytokine* **8:** 578–585.
18. Cao, Y. H., C. Chen, J. A. Weatherbee, M. Tsang, J. Folkman. 1995. gro-beta, a -C-X-C-

chemokine, is an angiogenesis inhibitor that suppresses the growth of Lewis lung carcinoma in mice. *J. Exp. Med.* **182:** 2069–2077.

19. Caux, C., Y. J. Liu, and J. Banchereau. 1995. Recent advances in the study of dendritic cells and follicular dendritic cells. *Immunol. Today* **16:** 2–4.

20. Cianciolo, G. J., J. Hunter, J. Silva, J. S. Haskill, and R. Snyderman. 1981. Inhibitors of monocyte responses to chemotaxins are present in human cancerous effusions and react with monoclonal antibodies to the P15(E) structural protein of retroviruses. *J. Clin. Invest.* **68:** 831–844.

21. Clauss, M., M. Gerlach, H. Gerlach, J. Brett, F. Wang, P. C. Familletti, Y. C. Pan, J. V. Olander, D. T. Connolly, and D. Stern. 1990. Vascular permeability factor: a tumor-derived polypeptide that induces endothelial cell and monocyte procoagulant activity, and promotes monocyte migration. *J. Exp. Med.* **172:** 1535–1545.

22. Colombo, N., F. Peccatori, C. Paganin, S. Bini, M. Brandely, C. Mangioni, A. Mantovani, and P. Allavena. 1992. Anti-tumor and immunomodulatory activity of intraperitoneal IFN-gamma in ovarian carcinoma patients with minimal residual tumor after chemotherapy. *Int. J. Cancer* **51:** 42–46.

23. Colotta, F., S. Orlando, E. J. Fadlon, S. Sozzani, C. Matteucci, and A. Mantovani. 1995. Chemoattractants induce rapid release of the interleukin 1 type II decoy receptor in human polymorphonuclear cells. *J. Exp. Med.* **181:** 2181–2188.

24. DiNapoli, M. R., C. L. Calderon, and D. M. Lopez. 1996. The altered tumoricidal capacity of macrophages isolated from tumor-bearing mice is related to reduced expression of the inducible nitric oxide synthase gene. *J. Exp. Med.* **183:** 1323–1329.

25. Dvorak, H. F. 1986. Tumors: wounds that do not heal. Similarities between tumor stroma generation and wound healing. *N. Engl. J. Med.* **315:** 1650–1659.

26. Evans, R. 1972. Macrophages in syngeneic animal tumours. *Transplantation* **14:** 468–470.

27. Fioretti, F., D. Fradelizi, A. Stoppacciaro, L. Ruco, A. Minty, S. Sozzani, A. Vecchi, and A. Mantovani. 1998. Reduced tumorigenicity and augmented leukocyte infiltration after MCP-3 gene transfer: perivascular accumulation of dendritic cells in peritumoral tissue and neutrophil recruitment within the tumor. *J. Immunol.* **161:** 342–346.

28. Godiska, R., D. Chantry, C. J. Raport, S. Sozzani, P. Allavena, D. Leviten, A. Mantovani, and P. W. Gray. 1997. Human macrophage derived chemokine (MDC)—a novel chemoattractant for monocytes, monocyte derived dendritic cells, and natural killer cells. *J. Exp. Med.* **185:** 1595–1604.

29. Graves, D. T., R. Barnhill, T. Galanopoulos, and H. N. Antoniades. 1992. Expression of monocyte chemotactic protein-1 in human melanoma in vivo. *Am. J. Pathol.* **140:** 9–14.

30. Graves, D. T., Y. L. Jiang, M. J. Williamson, and A. J. Valente. 1989. Identification of monocyte chemotactic activity produced by malignant cells. *Science* **245:** 1490–1493.

31. Greaves, D. R., W. Wang, D. J. Dairaghi, M. C. Dieu, B. de Saint-Vis, K. Franz-Bacon, D. Rossi, C. Caux, T. McClanahan, S. Gordon, A. Zlotnik, and T. J. Schall. 1997. CCR6, a CC chemokine receptor that interacts with macrophage inflammatory protein 3 alpha and is highly expressed in human dendritic cells. *J. Exp. Med.* **186:** 837–844.

32. Hallmann, R., D. N. Mayer, E. L. Berg, R. Broermann, and E. C. Butcher. 1995. Novel mouse endothelial cell surface marker is suppressed during differentiation of the blood brain barrier. *Dev. Dynamics* **202:** 325–332.

33. Hechtman, D. H., M. I. Cybulsky, H. J. Fuchs, J. B. Baker, and M. A. J. Gimbrone. 1991. Intravascular IL-8: inhibitor of polymorphonuclear leukocyte accumulation at sites of acute inflammation. *J. Immunol.* **147:** 883–892.

34. Heuff, G., M. B. van der Ende, H. Boutkan, W. Prevoo, L. G. Bayon, G. J. Fleuren, R. H. Beelen, S. Meijer, and C. D. Dijkstra. 1993. Macrophage populations in different stages of induced hepatic metastases in rats: an immunohistochemical analysis. *Scand. J. Immunol.* **38:** 10–16.

35. Hibbs, J. B. 1976. The macrophage as a tumoricidal effector cell: a review of in vivo and in vitro studies on the mechanism of the activated macrophage nonspecific cytotoxicity reaction. In: *The macrophage and neoplasia* (M. A. Fink, ed.), Academic Press, New York, pp. 83–98.

36. Hirose, K., M. Hakozaki, Y. Nyunoya, Y. Kobayashi, K. Matsushita, T. Takenouchi, A. Mikata, N. Mukaida, and K. Matsushima. 1995. Chemokine gene transfection into tumour cells reduced tumorigenicity in nude mice in association with neutrophilic infiltration. *Br. J. Cancer* **72:** 708–714.

37. Jiang, Y., D. I. Beller, G. Frendl, and D. T. Graves. 1992. Monocyte chemoattractant protein-1 regulates adhesion molecule expression and cytokine production in human monocytes. *J. Immunol.* **148:** 2423–2428.

38. Koch, A. E., P. J. Polverini, S. L. Kunkel, L. A. Harlow, L. A. DiPietro, V. M. Elner, S. G. Elner, and R. M. Strieter. 1992. Interleukin-8 as a macrophage-derived mediator of angiogenesis. *Science* **258:** 1798–1801.

39. Laning, J., H. Kawasaki, E. Tanaka, Y. Luo, and M. E. Dorf. 1994. Inhibition of in vivo tumor growth by the beta chemokine, TCA3. *J. Immunol.* **153:** 4625–4635.

40. Luster, A. D., S. M. Greenberg, and P. Leder. 1995. The IP-10 chemokine binds to a specific cell surface heparan sulfate site shared with platelet factor 4 and inhibits endothelial cell proliferation. *J. Exp. Med.* **182:** 219–231.

41. Luster, A. D., and P. Leder. 1993. IP-10, a -C-X-C- chemokine, elicits a potent thymus-dependent antitumor response in vivo. *J. Exp. Med.* **178:** 1057–1065.

42. Manome, Y., P. Y. Wen, A. Hershowitz, T. Tanaka, B. J. Rollins, D. W. Kufe, and H. A. Fine. 1995. Monocyte chemoattractant protein-1 (MCP-1) gene transduction: an effective tumor vaccine strategy for non-intracranial tumors. *Cancer Immunol. Immunother.* **41:** 227–235.

43. Mantovani, A. 1994. Tumor-associated macrophages in neoplastic progression: a paradigm for the in vivo function of chemokines. *Lab Invest.* **71:** 5–16.

44. Mantovani, A., B. Bottazzi, F. Colotta, S. Sozzani, and L. Ruco. 1992. The origin and function of tumor-associated macrophages. *Immunol. Today* **13:** 265–270.

45. Mantovani, A., B. Bottazzi, S. Sozzani, G. Peri, P. Allavena, Q. G. Dong, A. Vecchi, and F. Collotta. 1993. Cytokine regulation of tumour-associated macrophages. *Res. Immunol.* **144:** 280–283.

46. Mantovani, A., F. Bussolino, and E. Dejana. 1992. Cytokine regulation of endothelial cell function. *FASEB J.* **6:** 2591–2599.

47. Mantovani, A., S. Sozzani, B. Bottazzi, G. Peri, F. L. Sciacca, M. Locati, and F. Colotta. 1993. Monocyte chemotactic protein-1 (MCP-1): signal transduction and involvement in the regulation of macrophage traffic in normal and neoplastic tissues. *Adv. Exp. Med. Biol.* **351:** 47–54.

48. Medrano, E. E., J. Z. Farooqui, R. E. Boissy, Y. L. Boissy, B. Akadiri, and J. J. Nordlund. 1993. Chronic growth stimulation of human adult melanocytes by inflammatory mediators in vitro: implications for nevus formation and initial steps in melanocyte oncogenesis. *Proc. Natl. Acad. Sci. USA* **90:** 1790–1794.

49. Melani, C., S. M. Pupa, A. Stoppacciaro, S. Menard, M. I. Colnaghi, G. Parmiani, and M. P. Colombo. 1995. An in vivo model to compare human leukocyte infiltration in carcinoma xenografts producing different chemokines. *Int. J. Cancer* **62:** 572–578.

50. Mintz, B., and W. K. Silvers. 1993. Transgenic mouse model of malignant skin melanoma. *Proc. Natl. Acad. Sci. USA* **90:** 8817–8821.

51. Mulé, J. J., M. Custer, B. Averbook, J. C. Yang, J. S. Weber, D. V. Goeddel, S. A. Rosenberg, and T. J. Schall. 1996. RANTES secretion by gene-modified tumor cells results in loss of tumorigenicity *in vivo:* role of immune cell subpopulations. *Hum. Gene Ther.* **7:** 1545–1553.

52. Musiani, P., A. Modesti, M. Giovarelli, F. Cavallo, M. P. Colombo, P. L. Lollini, and

G. Forni. 1997. Cytokines, tumor-cell death and immunogenicity: a question of choice. *Immunol. Today* **18**: 32–36.

53. Nakamura, K., I. R. Williams, and T. S. Kupper. 1995. Keratinocyte-derived monocyte chemoattractant protein 1 (MCP-1): analysis in a transgenic model demonstrates MCP-1 can recruit dendritic and langerhans cells to skin. *J. Invest. Dermatol.* **105**: 635–643.

54. Negus, R. P., G. W. Stamp, M. G. Relf, F. Burke, S. T. Malik, S. Bernasconi, P. Allavena, S. Sozzani, A. Mantovani, and F. R. Balkwill. 1995. The detection and localization of monocyte chemoattractant protein-1 (MCP-1) in human ovarian cancer. *J. Clin Invest.* **95**: 2391–2396.

55. Normann, S. J., M. Schardt, and E. Sorkin. 1981. Biphasic depression of macrophage function after tumor transplantation. *Int. J. Cancer* **28**: 185–190.

56. Normann, S. J., and E. Sorkin. 1976. Cell-specific defect in monocyte function during tumor growth. *J. Natl. Cancer Inst.* **57**: 135–140.

57. Normann, S. J., and E. Sorkin. 1977. Inhibition of macrophage chemotaxis by neoplastic and other rapidly proliferating cells in vitro. *Cancer Res.* **37**: 705–711.

58. Opdenakker, G., G. Froyen, P. Fiten, P. Proost, and J. Van Damme. 1993. Human monocyte chemotactic protein-3 (MCP-3): molecular cloning of the cDNA and comparison with other chemokines. *Biochem. Biophys. Res. Commun.* **191**: 535–542.

59. Opdenakker, G., and J. Van Damme. 1992. Chemotactic factors, passive invasion and metastasis of cancer cells. *Immunol. Today* **13**: 463–464.

60. Opdenakker, G., and J. Van Damme. 1992. Cytokines and proteases in invasive processes: molecular similarities between inflammation and cancer. *Cytokine* **4**: 251–258.

61. Pardoll, D. M. 1995. Paracrine cytokine adjuvants in cancer immunotherapy. *Annu. Rev. Immunol.* **13**: 399–415.

62. Peiper, S. C., Z. X. Wang, K. Neote, A. W. Martin, H. J. Showell, M. J. Conklyn, K. Ogborne, T. J. Hadley, Z. H. Lu, J. Hesselgesser, and R. Horuk. 1995. The Duffy antigen receptor for chemokines (DARC) is expressed in endothelial cells of Duffy negative individuals who lack the erythrocyte receptor. *J. Exp. Med.* **181**: 1311–1317.

63. Pekarek, L. A., B. A. Starr, A. Y. Toledano, and H. Schreiber. 1995. Inhibition of tumor growth by elimination of granulocytes. *J. Exp. Med.* **181**: 435–440.

64. Petzelbauer, P., C. A. Watson, S. E. Pfau, and J. S. Pober. 1995. IL-8 and angiogenesis: evidence that human endothelial cells lack receptors and do not respond to IL-8 in vitro. *Cytokine* **7**: 267–272.

65. Piemonti, L., S. Bernasconi, W. Luini, Z. Trobonjaca, A. Minty, P. Allavena, and A. Mantovani. 1995. IL-13 supports differentiation of dendritic cells from circulating precursors in concert with GM-CSF. *Eur. Cytokine Network* **6**: 245–252.

66. Porteu, F., and C. Nathan. 1990. Shedding of tumor necrosis factor receptor by activated human neutrophils. *J. Exp. Med.* **172**: 599–607.

67. Power, C. A., D. J. Church, A. Meyer, S. Alouani, A. E. I. Proudfoot, I. Clark-Lewis, S. Sozzani, A. Mantovani, and T. N. C. Wells. 1997. Cloning and characterization of a specific receptor for the novel CC chemokine MIP-3 alpha from lung dendritic cells. *J. Exp. Med.* **186**: 825–835.

68. Proost, P., C. De Wolf Peeters, R. Conings, G. Opdenakker, A. Billiau, and J. Van Damme. 1993. Identification of a novel granulocyte chemotactic protein (GCP-2) from human tumor cells: in vitro and in vivo comparison with natural forms of GRO, IP-10, and IL-8. *J. Immunol.* **150**: 1000–1010.

69. Riethdorf, L., S. Riethdorf, K. Gutzlaff, F. Prall, and T. Loning. 1996. Differential expression of the monocyte chemoattractant protein-1 gene in human papillomavirus-16-infected squamous intraepithelial lesions and squamous cell carcinomas of the cervix uteri. *Am. J. Pathol.* **149**: 1469–1476.

70. Rojas, A., R. Delgado, L. Glaria, and M. Palacios. 1993. Monocyte chemotactic protein-1

inhibits the induction of nitric oxide synthase in J774 cells. *Biochem. Biophys. Res. Commun.* **196:** 274–279.

71. Rollins, B. J., and M. E. Sunday. 1991. Suppression of tumor formation in vivo by expression of the JE gene in malignant cells. *Mol. Cell. Biol.* **11:** 3125–3131.

72. Rot, A. 1992. Endothelial cell binding of NAP-1/IL-8: role in neutrophil emigration. *Immunol. Today* **13:** 291–294.

73. Rutledge, B. J., H. Rayburn, R. Rosenberg, R. J. North, R. P. Gladue, C. L. Corless, and B. J. Rollins. 1995. High level monocyte chemoattractant protein-1 expression in transgenic mice increases their susceptibility to intracellular pathogens. *J. Immunol.* **155:** 4838–4843.

74. Sakamoto, K., T. Masuda, S. Mita, T. Ishiko, Y. Nakashima, H. Arakawa, H. Egami, S. Harada, K. Matsushima, and M. Ogawa. 1992. Interleukin-8 is constitutively and commonly produced by various human carcinoma cell lines. *Int. J. Clin. Lab. Res.* **22:** 216–219.

75. Sallusto, F., and A. Lanzavecchia. 1994. Efficient presentation of soluble antigen by cultured human dendritic cells is maintained by granulocyte/macrophage colony-stimulating factor plus interleukin-4 and downregulated by tumor necrosis factor-alpa. *J. Exp. Med.* **179:** 1109–1118.

76. Schadendorf, D., A. Moller, B. Algermissen, M. Worm, M. Sticherling, and B. M. Czarnetzki. 1993. IL-8 produced by human malignant melanoma cells in vitro is an essential autocrine growth factor. *J. Immunol.* **151:** 2667–2675.

77. Schonbeck, U., E. Brandt, F. Petersen, H. D. Flad, and H. Loppnow. 1995. IL-8 specifically binds to endothelial but not to smooth muscle cells. *J. Immunol.* **154:** 2375–2383.

78. Sciacca, F. L., M. Stürzl, F. Bussolino, M. Sironi, H. Brandstetter, C. Zietz, D. Zhou, C. Matteucci, G. Peri, S. Sozzani, R. Benelli, M. Arese, A. Albini, F. Colotta, and A. Mantovani. 1994. Expression of adhesion molecules, platelet-activating factor, and chemokines by Kaposi's sarcoma cells. *J. Immunol.* **153:** 4816–4825.

79. Singh, R. K., K. Berry, K. Matsushima, K. Yasumoto, and I. J. Fidler. 1993. Synergism between human monocyte chemotactic and activating factor and bacterial products for activation of tumoricidal properties in murine macrophages. *J. Immunol.* **151:** 2786–2793.

80. Smith, D. R., P. J. Polverini, S. L. Kunkel, M. B. Orringer, R. I. Whyte, M. D. Burdick, C. A. Wilke, and R. M. Strieter. 1994. Inhibition of IL-8 attenuates angiogenesis in bronchogenic carcinoma. *J. Exp. Med.* **179:** 1409–1415.

81. Snyderman, R., and G. J. Cianciolo. 1984. Immunosuppressive activity of the retroviral envelope protein P15E and its possible relationship to neoplasia. *Immunol. Today* **5:** 240–244.

82. Snyderman, R., and M. C. Pike. 1976. An inhibitor of macrophage chemotaxis produced by neoplasms. *Science* **192:** 370–372.

83. Sonouchi, K., T. A. Hamilton, C. S. Tannenbaum, R. R. Tubbs, R. Bukowski, and J. H. Finke. 1994. Chemokine gene expression in the murine renal cell carcinoma, renca, following treatment in vivo with interferon-alpha and interleukin-2. *Am. J. Pathol.* **144:** 747–755.

84. Sozzani, S., W. Luini, A. Borsatti, N. Polentarutti, D. Zhou, L. Piemonti, G. D'Amico, C. A. Power, T. N. Wells, M. Gobbi, P. Allavena, and A. Mantovani. 1997. Receptor expression and responsiveness of human dendritic cells to a defined set of CC and CXC chemokines. *J. Immunol.* **159:** 1993–2000.

85. Sozzani, S., F. Sallusto, W. Luini, D. Zhou, L. Piemonti, P. Allavena, J. Van Damme, S. Valitutti, A. Lanzavecchia, and A. Mantovani. 1995. Migration of dendritic cells in response to formyl peptides, C5a and a distinct set of chemokines. *J. Immunol.* **155:** 3292–3295.

86. Stevenson, M. M., and M. S. Meltzer. 1976. Depressed chemotactic responses in vitro of peritoneal macrophages from tumor-bearing mice. *J. Natl. Cancer Inst.* **57:** 847–852.

87. Strieter, R. M., P. J. Polverini, S. L. Kunkel, D. A. Arenberg, M. D. Burdick, J. Kasper, J. Dzuiba, J. Van Damme, A. Walz, D. Marriott, S. Y. Chan, S. Roczniak, and A. B. Shanafelt. 1995. The functional role of the ELR motif in CXC chemokine-mediated angiogenesis. *J. Biol. Chem.* **270:** 27,348–27,357.
88. Takeya, M., T. Yoshimura, E. J. Leonard, T. Kato, H. Okabe, and K. Takahashi. 1991. Production of monocyte chemoattractant protein-1 by malignant fibrous histiocytoma: relation to the origin of histiocyte-like cells. *Exp. Mol. Pathol.* **54:** 61–71.
89. Tannenbaum, C. S., N. Wicker, D. Armstrong, R. Tubbs, J. Finke, R. M. Bukowski, and T. A. Hamilton. 1996. Cytokine and chemokine expression in tumors of mice receiving systemic therapy with IL-12. *J. Immunol.* **156:** 693–699.
90. Van Damme, J., P. Proost, J. P. Lenaerts, and G. Opdenakker. 1992. Structural and functional identification of two human, tumor-derived monocyte chemotactic proteins (MCP-2 and MCP-3) belonging to the chemokine family. *J. Exp. Med.* **176:** 59–65.
91. Van Meir, E., M. Ceska, F. Effenberger, A. Walz, E. Grouzmann, I. Desbaillets, K. Frei, A. Fontana, and N. de Tribolet. 1992. Interleukin-8 is produced in neoplastic and infectious diseases of the human central nervous system. *Cancer Res.* **52:** 4297–4305.
92. van Ravenswaay Claasen, H. H., P. M. Kluin, and G. J. Fleuren. 1992. Tumor infiltrating cells in human cancer: on the possible role of CD16+ macrophages in antitumor cytotoxicity. *Lab. Invest.* **67:** 166–174.
93. Voest, E. E., B. M. Kenyon, M. S. O'Reilly, G. Truitt, R. J. D'Amato, and J. Folkman. 1995. Inhibition of angiogenesis in vivo by interleukin-12. *J. Natl. Cancer Inst.* **87:** 581–586.
94. Walter, S., B. Bottazzi, D. Govoni, F. Colotta, and A. Mantovani. 1991. Macrophage infiltration and growth of sarcoma clones expressing different amounts of monocyte chemotactic protein/JE. *Int. J. Cancer* **49:** 431–435.
95. Wang, J. M., O. Chertov, P. Proost, L. Jian-Jian, P. Menten, L. Xu, S. Sozzani, A. Mantovani, W. Gong, V. Schirrmacher, J. Van Damme, and J. J. Oppenheim. 1998. Purification and identification of chemokines potentially involved in kidney-specific metastasis by a murine lymphoma variant: induction of migration and NFκB activation. *Int. J. Cancer* **75:** 900–907.
96. Wang, J. M., G. Taraboletti, K. Matsushima, J. Van Damme, and A. Mantovani. 1990. Induction of haptotactic migration of melanoma cells by neutrophil activating protein/interleukin-8. *Biochem. Biophys. Res. Commun.* **169:** 165–170.
97. Yamashiro, S., M. Takeya, T. Nishi, J. Kuratsu, T. Yoshimura, Y. Ushio, and K. Takahashi. 1994. Tumor-derived monocyte chemoattractant protein-1 induces intratumoral infiltration of monocyte-derived macrophage subpopulation in transplanted rat tumors. *Am. J. Pathol.* **145:** 856–867.
98. Yoshimura, T., E. A. Robinson, S. Tanaka, E. Appella, J. Kuratsu, and E. J. Leonard. 1989. Purification and amino acid analysis of two human glioma-derived monocyte chemoattractants. *J. Exp. Med.* **169:** 1449–1459.
99. Zachariae, C. O., A. O. Anderson, H. L. Thompson, E. Appella, A. Mantovani, J. J. Oppenheim, and K. Matsushima. 1990. Properties of monocyte chemotactic and activating factor (MCAF) purified from a human fibrosarcoma cell line. *J. Exp. Med.* **171:** 2177–2182.

4

Novel Monocyte Chemoattractants in Cancer

Ghislain Opdenakker and Jo Van Damme

1. INTRODUCTION: C-C CHEMOKINES DERIVED FROM CANCER CELLS

1.1. Cancer Cells Produce Chemokines: Early Observations

The in vivo infiltration of tumors with leukocytes is an old histopathologic observation, but only recently have insights been obtained in the molecular mechanisms that govern this type of leukocyte recruitment *(39)*. Along the same line, the similarities between a chronic inflammatory process and the phenomena occurring at the invasive front of a malignant tumor have been recognized for a long time. Only recently has the molecular dissection begun to demonstrate the fine-detailed differences between these two types of pathologic processes *(55)*. Originally it was thought that tumor-associated leukocytes (TALs) recognize tumor-specific antigens *(16)*. Most often these TALs were mononuclear cells. An active mechanism of monocyte recruitment by chemoattractants was postulated later and Botazzi et al. *(7)* identified a specific chemoattractant for monocytes. Then, it was documented that a monocyte chemotactic factor from smooth muscle cells was serologically related to that of various tumor cells *(22)*. For example, in the latter study, it was observed that MG-63 osteosarcoma cells abundantly produce monocyte chemotactic proteins (vide infra).

The recruitment of TAMs by mononuclear cell C-C chemokines has emerged as a central theme in tumor biology. It is, however, equally important to indicate that tumor-associated neutrophils (TANs) and tumor-associated lymphocytes (TALys) are also recognizable on histopathologic examination. It is clear that for each individual leukocyte type, specific chemokines exist (*see* Chapters 1 and 2) and that the total TAL load at any moment results from the concerted action of the differential temporospatial expression of chemokine mixtures. With the advent of new technology to test the biologic activities of specific chemokines, many tumor cells, both primary cultures and cell lines, have been used to produce chemokines in vitro. Since the late 1980s, many chemokines have been purified to homogeneity from these sources, and the availability of natural, recombinant, and synthetic chemokines, and cDNA probes and specific antisera, made it possible to study the regulation of these factors in normal and tumor cells *(15,21,23,24,47,70,84,87,88)*.

From: *Chemokines and Cancer*
Edited by: B. J. Rollins © Humana Press Inc., Totowa, NJ

1.2. Simultaneous Production of Several Chemokines

Although it was—and often still is—not clear what the meaning of chemokine production by tumor cells is, a variety of secreted products, including glycoprotein hormones, cytokines, and colony-stimulating factors, may be produced as ectopic factors and lead to paraneoplastic effects. Chemokines are not an exception. Thus, in the 1970s, in our laboratory, primary cultures of human tumors were screened for the ectopic production of fibroblast interferon, and the 63rd specimen of such a tumor (in Dutch, Menselijk Gezwel-63 [MG-63], which means human tumor-63), an osteosarcoma, was not only prolific but also produced considerable amounts of interferon-β (IFN-β) (6). This same MG-63 tumor cell line (deposited as ATCC.CRL 1427) was later used to identify and isolate a hybridoma growth factor as interleukin-6 (IL-6) (79). Furthermore, MG-63 cells were the source for the purification of a number of C-X-C chemokines, including the neutrophil chemoattractants IL-8 (78,82) and granulocyte chemotactic protein-2 (GCP-2); growth-related oncogene-α (GRO-α), GRO-γ, interferon-γ-inducible protein-10 (58); the C-C chemokines monocyte chemoattractant protein-1, -2, and -3 (MCP-1, MCP-2, MCP-3) (60,80); and RANTES (66).

The example of the MG-63 tumor cell line as a cytokine source might be extreme, but it nonetheless clearly illustrates that one particular tumor may produce many chemokines and cytokines simultaneously, presumably through the action of common second-messenger pathways and shared transcription factors. This example also shows that the expression of C-X-C and C-C chemokines in tumor biology are not mutually exclusive, which implies that TAMs, TANs, and TALys may coincide in individual tumors. Although this section emphasizes the structures and biologic functions of the C-C chemokines in cancer, the interrelations with the C-X-C and other chemoattractants such as lymphotactins, complement factors, and virus-encoded peptides (2,5,65) must be kept in mind. The simultaneous production of various chemokines by cancer cells and the interrelation in vivo is also observed in mouse tumor cells (35,85).

2. THE COUNTERCURRENT MODEL OF INVASION

2.1. The Paradox: Cancer Cells Produce Immunostimulators

The immunochemists who purified and identified chemokines from tumor cells might have provided indirect evidence for the molecular mechanisms that lead in vivo to TALs, but they remain faced with many unresolved questions: Why do the tumor cells produce chemokines and what are the regulatory mechanisms involved? What is the advantage for the tumor? Which forces influence the in vivo selection of chemokine-secreting tumor cells? Is the observation of TALs a coincidence? Although many more studies will be needed to answer these questions and to confirm or contradict current models, one of the older hypotheses—that TALs are eliminating the cancer—seems unlikely. If this hypothesis were correct, there would exist a negative correlation between chemokine production and malignancy, a statement that remains unproven.

We have interpreted the production of chemokines by tumor cells in the opposite way (54,55). Several studies indicated a positive correlation between (C-X-C) chemokine expression and invasiveness (56,68), whereas some others indicated the opposite (69). Our interpretation was born from the observation that the most malignant tumors seem to produce the highest amounts and the broadest range of chemokines.

Many relevant recent studies complement our original picture of a countercurrent model of invasion by chemokine-secreting tumors *(54)*. This picture may be adapted depending on the type of chemokines that are produced. Tumors that attract neutrophils by secreting chemokines (IL-8, GCP-2, GRO-α, -β, -γ, etc.) enhance the local protease load. Indeed, the chemoattracted neutrophils are activated to degranulate quite rapidly *(42,58)*, and the secreted enzymes locally dissolve the extracellular matrix. This leads to solubilization of the intercellular matrix and a trypsinizing effect on cell–cell contacts (the so-called sheddase activity) that facilitate the routing of tumor cells toward the vessels (from where the neutrophils come). The countercurrent mechanism *(54)* also explains the *direction of invasion* of chemokine-producing tumors (*see* Fig. 1). In addition, neutrophils produce platelet-activating factors, which result in transforming growth factor-β and platelet-derived growth factor (PDGF) release from platelets. These trophic factors might directly influence the tumor and also might indirectly regulate the production of MCPs *(18,20,30,56)*. Tumors that produce only monocyte chemoattractants locally recruit TAMs, which deliver trophic factors and produce cellular interactions with the tumor. When compared to the abundant release of neutrophilic enzymes by C-X-C chemokines *(52)*, MCPs are relatively weak in inducing *de novo* synthesis of proteases in monocytes *(51,80)*, but the recruited TAMs and the tumor cells might be well activated to produce GCPs. The cohabitation among TAMs, TANs, and the tumor increases the local protease load and the remodeling of the extracellular matrix *(55,61)*. This may also influence the invasion and metastasis of tumor cells *(40)*.

Virus–host interactions often stand as models for host–tumor interactions. The study of retroviruses and the discovery of host oncogenes have enormously contributed to understanding the basic mechanisms of tumorigenesis. Similarly, in the chemokine field there is an important cross-fertilization between virology and immunology. A number of examples have illustrated this cross-fertilization. First, the recent discovery of chemokine receptors as cofactors for human immunodeficiency virus infection (*[14,57]; see also* Chapter 2) shows that adaptable viruses use the chemokine machinery for their own profit. In line with such a theory, in a malignant tumor, particular tumor cell clones might be selected that use the chemokine machinery for their advantage. Second, several viruses mimic chemokine receptors or chemokine activities *(2)*. As such, these viruses do not stimulate immunity, but instead misuse our immune cells for the virus spread and replication. For instance, viruses that produce chemokine-like molecules might attract permissive host cells. Alternatively, chemokine receptor-producing viruses might absorb chemokines and thus prevent phagocyte recruitment. Similarly, chemokine-producing tumors might use this mechanism for their growth and invasion. Although not yet documented, it might well be that there also exist tumors that, by chemokine receptor production, have a positive advantage in preventing tumor immune rejection. In line with such a theorem is the recent observation that CXCR2 expressing melanoma cells become independent of serum for their growth *(43,48)*.

2.2. Interactions Between Tumor-Produced Chemokines and the Host

There are at least three effector functions of chemokines that have a major impact on tumorigenesis and tumor cell spread: cell recruitment, angiogenesis, and regulation of matrix degradation.

Tumor cell-derived C-C chemokines *recruit monocytes* and other mononuclear cells (e.g., dendritic cells, lymphocytes, natural killer [NK] cells) *(36,37,71,72,80,86)* that are the sources of many trophic factors. Indeed, monocytes, when appropriately stimulated, produce growth factors, angiogenesis factors, and enzymes that might influence tumor growth and invasion. Of particular interest is the observation that monocytes also produce neutrophil chemokines such as IL-8 *(78,82)*. The latter and similar C-X-C chemokines affect angiogenesis and enzyme release. A second aspect is that cell recruitment leads to better chances for direct cell–cell contacts, a phenomenon that has been shown to be essential for the efficient release of growth factors and enzymes by mononuclear and other cell types *(31)*. By the recruitment of leukocytes, cancers might take advantage of all the molecular devices that are provided by these recruited cells. This implies also a number of similarities between chronic inflammation and an invasive cancer *(55,61)*. In an infection or disease-limiting inflammation, in response to local C-C chemokines, the attracted monocytes regulate the activities of the neutrophils by secreting C-X-C chemokines, and all these phagocytic cell types try to eliminate the parasite or foreign body. Similarly, if the tumor is recognized as a foreign body (e.g., by the expression of potent tumor antigens), it may be eliminated by immune surveillance mechanisms. In such a case, chemokines most probably are produced by nontumor host cells. In comparison, many malignant tumors, which by themselves produce chemokines, are not rejected (possibly owing to the absence of tumor antigens or immune-deviation mechanisms). These tumors act as dictators on chemoattracted monocytes to enhance tumor growth and invasion, eventually by stimulating TAMs to produce IL-8, which then recruits the neutrophils filled with enzymes. As outlined previously, C-X-C chemokines might also be produced directly or indirectly by the tumor.

An important function of C-X-C chemokines is the *control of angiogenesis (4,69)*, which enhances the supply of oxygen and nutrients to the growing tumor (*see* Chapters 11 and 12). However, neovascularization also has an effect on metastasis. Indeed, by microvessel outgrowth toward the tumor, the escape of invasive clones into the circulation is facilitated.

A third mechanism, which is essential both for neovascularization and for invasion and metastasis of tumor cells, is the *release of matrix remodeling enzymes*. Here, again, the induced C-X-C chemokines are at the forefront. IL-8 and related molecules act on neutrophils as secretagogues and induce the immediate release of matrix metalloproteinases such as gelatinase B *(42,58,85)*. In addition, some C-X-C chemokines have been reported to possess direct enzymatic activity on matrix components and, e.g., degrade heparan sulfates *(26)*. All these elements can be summarized in the "countercurrent model" of chemokine-producing tumors (*[54]*; Fig. 1).

3. THE STRUCTURES OF THE CHEMOKINE GENE CLUSTERS

3.1. The Growing Family of Human Monocyte Chemokines from Cancer Cells

The discovery of the first monocyte chemotactic factors from tumor cells was based on in vitro assays of chemotaxis. Several variations of these assays exist *(76)*, e.g., migration of monocytes under agarose, through micropore membranes, and through endothelia. Finally, the intradermo assay of pure chemokines in rabbit skin optimally

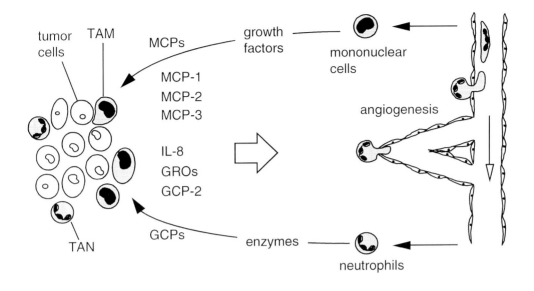

TUMOR   CHEMOKINES   TROPHISM   VESSELS

Fig. 1. The countercurrent principle of invasion and metastasis. Tumor cells produce chemoattractants for mononuclear cells (MCPs) and granulocytes (GCPs). These chemokines recruit TAMs or TANs. The attracted cells also may include lymphocytes or other leukocyte types and are the source of trophic factors and enzymes. Chemokines (GCPs) induce angiogenesis in the direction of the tumor. Invasion and metastasis of cancer cells is in the direction that is countercurrent to that of the chemoattracted leukocytes. (Adapted from ref. *54.*)

mimics the tumor-associated recruitment of monocytes in vivo *(58,80)*. With chemotaxis as a readout system, MCP-1 and later MCP-2 and MCP-3 were identified by amino acid sequence analysis and shown to act in vitro and in vivo *(80)*.

Molecular cloning technology has helped to complement the classical biochemical studies in various ways. The mouse MCP-1 cDNA was cloned first by subtraction hybridization as the JE competence gene, induced by PDGF, quite some time before its function was known *(12,62,89)*. Nevertheless, the natural mouse JE/MCP-1 protein was also purified from tumor cells *(77)*. Other mouse C-C chemokines *(73)* were later identified by cloning with the use of probes from other species. Another example of the early contributions of recombinant DNA technology to chemokine research is the LD78 cDNA cloning done in the late 1980s *(45,49)*.

A number of human C-C chemokine cDNAs and genes were cloned *(50,51)* on the basis of protein sequences. The genes were mapped in the human genome and were found to cluster in one area at 17q11.2 *([46,50]; Table 1)*. More recently, novel C-C chemokines have been discovered by bioinformatics. These may be localized at other chromosomal sites. For instance, the lymphocyte-specific C-C chemokine LARC is on human chromosome 2 *([25]; see Table 1)*. Similarly, the chemokine receptor gene families are clustered in the human genome. Therefore, C-C chemokines and the receptors are also becoming an interesting topic for evolutionary biologists and geneticists.

Table 1
Human C-C Chemokines

Gene symbol[a]	Literature symbols[b]	Gene accession number[b] (DNA segment)	Sequence length[c] (bp)
SCYA1	I-309	M57506 (gene)	3709
SCYA2	MCP-1/MCAF/hJE/HC11	D26087 (promoter)	2776
		M37719 (gene)	
SCYA3/SCYA3L1	LD78a/AT464-1/GOS19-1	D90144 (gene)	3176
	LD78b/AT464-2/GOS19-2	D90145 (gene)	3112
SCYA3L2	LD78g/GOS19-3	D12592 (gene)	2038
		M96851 (promoter)	4106
SCYA4/SCYA4L1	Act-2/LAG-1/HC21/G26	X53682 (gene)	
	AT744/hMIP-a/H400/SIS-γ	S56704 (promoter)	1199
SCYA5	RANTES	S64885 (promoter)	1016
SCYA6	ND	ND	
SCYA7	MCP-3/NC28/HC14	X72309 (gene)	2885
		X93215 (promoter)	4301
SCYA8	MCP-2	X99886 (gene)	2991
SCYA9/SCYA10	ND	ND	
SCYA11	Eotaxin	U46573 (cDNA)	839
SCYA12	ND	ND	
SCYA13	MCP-4/NCC-1	U46767 (cDNA)	825
SCYA14	HCC-1/HCC-3/NCC-2	Z49269 (gene)	4037
SCYA15	HCC-2/MIP-5/NCC-3	Z70293 (cDNA)	973
SCYA16	NCC-4	ND	
SCYA17 (16q13)	TARC	D43767 (cDNA)	538
SCYA18	PARC/MIP-4/DC-CK1	AB00021 (cDNA)	
SCYA19 (9p13)	MIP-3β/ELC	U77180 (cDNA)	545
SCYA20 (2q33)	LARC/MIP-3α/exodus	D86955 (cDNA)	789

[a] The listed genes are all on human chromosome 17q11.2, except *SCYA17, SCYA19,* and *SCYA20,* of which the chromosome location is indicated in parentheses.

[b] ND, not determined.

[c] Details refer to the longest gene or cDNA sequence available. For a number of gene (or cDNA) segments, shorter sequences have been deposited under other accession numbers in the databases.

In the mouse genome, the C-C chemokines are clustered on chromosome 11 (Table 2). The mapping of chemokine genes to a particular genomic region is currently used as a strong criterion of classification. Other criteria include the conservation of cysteines and other residues and functional characteristics. Therefore, we favor the notion that the C-C chemokine nomenclature is based on such practical criteria and that the best way to nominate the chemokines would be by using the human genome-based nomenclature; this avoids the difficulties encountered with the many acronyms. For clarity, Tables 1 and 2 give an overview of the identified molecules, the abbreviations used, and the accession numbers of the longest sequence that were deposited in the databases.

More recently, combinatorial technology has been used to identify randomly or specifically novel chemotactic proteins. The *random approach* uses motif recognition in data libraries of expressed sequence tags. In particular, the conservation of the four

Table 2
Mouse C-C Chemokines

Gene symbol	Literature symbols	Accession numbers[a]	Sequence length (bp)
Scya1	TCA3/P500	X52401 (gene)	4282
Scya2	JE	M19681 (gene)	244
Scya3	SCI/MIP-1α	X53372 (gene)	1988
		M73061 (gene)	3574
Scya4	MIP-1β/H400	X62502 (gene)	2961
Scya5	RANTES	U02298 (gene)	5859
Scya6	C10/MRP-1	L11237 (gene)	5129
Scya7	MARC/FIC/MCP-3	S71251 (cDNA)	808
		X70058 (gene)	2559
Scya8	MCP-2	ND	
Scya9/Scya10	MRP-2/CCF18/MIP-γ	U15209 (cDNA)	1255
Scya11	Eotaxin	U40672 (cDNA)	982
Scya12	MCP-1-related	U50712 (cDNA)	540

[a]The longest gene or mRNA species is described; shorter sequences with other accession numbers exist; ND, not determined.

cysteine spacings in peptides is used to recognize homologs deposited in the data libraries *(5,25)*. By this approach, several new C-C chemokines (NCCs) have been identified *(46)* and further characterized (NCC-1, TARC, LARC, PARC, MCP-4, MCP-5) *(17,25,46,64)*. The *specific approach* consists of generating and using degenerate polymerase chain reaction primers, based on the MCP-consensus sequences and amplifying novel sequences from the gene contig of human chromosome 17q11.2. With this approach, the human eotaxin and MCP-2 genes were recently identified *(74,75)*. This development in technology implies that at present several novel C-C chemokines have been cloned (sequenced and expressed), but that less information exists about their cell specificity and physiologic relevance and that the functions in tumor–host interactions remain elusive and a challenge for future cancer research. Bioinformatics technology thus rapidly advanced the identification of new C-C chemokines, and novel gene(s) (clusters) have been identified on chromosomes different from chromosome 17 (*[25];* Table 1).

3.2. Chromosomal Breaks Near or in the C-C Chemokine Gene Cluster

Regions of chromosomal instability (breakpoint cluster regions [BCRs]) are associated with tumorigenesis. In a simplified way, at the BCR a tumor suppressor gene is possibly inactivated by, e.g., a chromosomal translocation. Alternatively, the DNA-recombinatorial rearrangement events might enhance tumor growth by generating fusion proteins that directly (e.g., growth factors, growth factor receptors) or indirectly (e.g., transcription factors) yield a positive selection benefit in favor of the cells with the rearranged DNAs. Figure 2 shows the MCP chemokine gene cluster and the breakpoints associated with oncogenesis. In particular, two major regions, associated with oncogenesis, have been found near this region: centromerically from the C-C chemokine gene cluster resides the neurofibromatosis type I suppressor gene (NF-1),

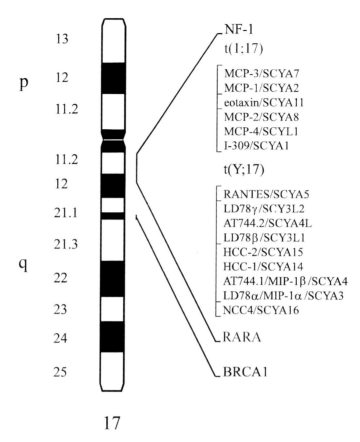

Fig. 2. The C-C chemokine gene cluster on human chromosome 17. The chemokine genes are ordered in relation to the centromere and are divided in two groups that are separated by a t(Y;17) breakpoint locus *(46)*. A constitutional t(1;17) breakpoint, associated with neuroblastoma oncogenesis, is located between the MCP-3 locus and the neurofibromatosis gene-1 *(NF-1)*. At the telemoric side, the area is flanked by the retinoic acid receptor-α gene *(RARA) (34)*.

and at the telomeric side a tumor suppressor gene associated with breast cancer *(BRCA1)* is located. As indicated, the C-C chemokine gene cluster can be divided into two subregions spanning in total about 2 cM (~2 Mbp). A breakpoint t(Y;17) has been localized between these two subregions *(46)*.

Are there particular tumors associated with altered chemokine gene structures and protein functions? Neuroblastoma is the most frequent solid childhood cancer. Although similar mechanisms of tumor suppression as in retinoblastoma and nephroblastoma (Wilms' tumor) have been postulated, a single neuroblastoma tumor suppressor has not yet been found. Most often constitutional translocations (preferentially reciprocal ones with minimal loss of genetic material) have indicated the gene locations of tumor suppressors. A neuroblastoma tumor suppressor gene was postulated at 1p36, a region that now harbors several putative suppressor genes. With the description of the first constitutional reciprocal translocation t(1;17) in a neuroblastoma patient, the focus has also been on chromosome 17q11.2 *(33)*. In addition to the constitutional reciprocal t(1;17), many neuroblastoma tumor karyotypes possess alterations at 1p36 and at 17q11.2 *(83)*. The flanking markers for the 1p36 break in the t(1;17) are an adenovirus integration site, which is also found in the NGP neuroblastoma cell line *(10)* and the pronatriodilatin gene *(34)*. The flanking markers for the 17q11.2 breakpoint are the NF-1 gene and *SCYA7*, the gene for MCP-3 *(34,50)*. Note that both regions at 1p36 and 17q11.2 are rather complex in nature. Because the 1p36 contains repetitive sequences (e.g., encoding tRNAs), hybridization experiments by Southern blot or fluorescent *in situ* hybridization should be interpreted with caution. A recently identified candidate gene for the 1p36 break is the *RIZ* gene, a rather large gene sequence encoding a zinc-finger protein *(9)*. Another candidate is p73, which shares homology with p53 *(29)*. Comparably, a member of the large C-C chemokine gene cluster might be involved in the 17q11.2 break. Similar to findings for other tumor suppressor genes, such a large gene segment might explain the possible heterogeneity of breaks (also found in other tumors). It is not yet known whether chemokine gene expression is altered as a result of any of the aforementioned translocations.

Recently, a YAC contig of the 17q11.2 region has been generated that includes all the known, and a number of novel, C-C chemokines. Within this 2-Mbp YAC contig, another chromosomal breakpoint, t(Y;17), has been localized *(46)*. This illustrates that DNA recombinations occur within this chemokine gene cluster. The further dissection of this YAC contig will indicate whether the t(1;17) neuroblastoma-associated breakpoint involves chemokine genes.

4. THE FUNCTIONS OF THE CHEMOKINE GENE CLUSTER

4.1. Are Chemokines Tumor Suppressors?

A tumor suppressor functionally inhibits tumor formation or progression (including enhancement of the invasive phenotype). At the structural level, a tumor suppressor is usually encoded by genes associated with recessive traits. Because of the redundancy of the C-C chemokine genes, compensatory mechanisms are expected to act when both alleles of one chemokine gene are inactivated. Therefore, and because there complementary mechanisms might exist, single chemokine gene knockout experiments might not yield clear insights into the functional roles of chemokines as tumor suppressors; one might have to inactivate a whole part of the chemokine gene cluster to obtain phenotypes with altered tumor suppression. How can we then interpret the current data on chemokine overexpression and altered tumor phenotypes? The examples of MCP-1 gene transfer indicate tumor suppression *(8,13,27,28,32,38,63,67)* (Table 3). However, in all the available examples secondary signals were involved. For instance, in addition to the MCP-1 overexpression in syngeneic colon carcinoma cells, the tumoricidal macrophages were activated by lipopolysaccharides (LPSs) *(27)*, or fibroblasts or immunogenic tumors were used. In the first study Chinese hamster ovary (CHO) cells expressing MCP-1 were compared with the parental CHO cell line for tumorigenic effects in nude mice *(63)*. Even in the latter animal model, a second signal is delivered to the host in terms of altered tumor cell surface molecules. Indeed, almost any cell type that overexpresses recombinant proteins alters the glycosylation machinery and thus the antigenicity of the overexpressing cell. Carbohydrate–lectin interactions are well established as an immune-recognition mechanism and might well contribute to the activation of macrophages/monocytes, NK cells, neutrophils, and lymphocytes.

Table 3
Overexpression of C-C Chemokines in Tumor Cells and In Vivo Effects

Name	Gene	Species	Recruited cells	Tumor type	Expression[a] In vitro	In vivo	Effect on host[a]	Reference
JE	*Scya2*	Mouse	Monocytes, eosinophils	CHO	ND	Impaired growth	Necessary for tumor suppression in vivo	63
MCP-1	SCYA2	Mouse	Macrophages	Melanoma B78/H1	Similar	Slower tumor growth	ND	8
MCAF/MCP-1	SCYA2	Mouse	Macrophages	Melanoma K-1735 clones	ND	ND	Tumor-specific lysis by LPS-stimulated Mφ, synergism with MCP-1 in vitro	67
JE/MCP-1	*Scya2*	Mouse	Macrophages	Colon carcinoma CT-26	Similar	Fewer lung metastasis	Macrophage-mediated cytotoxicity induced by LPS in vivo	27
JE/MCP-1	*Scya2*	Mouse	Macrophages	Renal adenocarcinoma (RENCA) expression in fibroblasts	Similar	Fewer lung metastasis	Synergistic effect of LPS and MCP-1 in vivo	28
MCP-1	SCYA2	Rat	Macrophages	Gliosarcoma 9L	Similar	Regression of intradermal tumors	Enhancing effect on tumor vaccination	38
TCA3	*Scya1*	Mouse	Monocytes, neutrophils	Myeloma P3X and J558	Similar	Impaired growth	Tumor necrosis tumor-specific immunity in vivo	32

[a]ND, not determined

On the basis of the cytogenetic and molecular data on the association between alterations in or near the chemokine gene cluster and neuroblastoma development, chemokines might be considered to yield a permissive oncogenic effect on this childhood tumor: alterations at both sites of the t(1;17), in particular at chromosomal subbands 1p36 and 17q11.2, are associated with tumorigenesis. Chemokines might be involved in the recruitment of Schwann cells, which deliver trophic factors for neuroblastoma development *(3)*. As such, the countercurrent model *(54)* might explain some mechanisms at the origin of neuroblastoma. This type of association does not seem to be restricted to neuroblastoma as similar speculations may be made for other tumor types.

In conclusion, the dual role of TAMs *(39)*, currently translated into the dual roles of chemokines in tumorigenesis and tumor development, is not yet fully understood. It is worthwhile to indicate that IL-1, a potent physiologic inducer of chemokines and immunostimulators as well as a predicted cancer immunotherapeutic, when intravenously administered at high doses potentiated efficiently the invasive behavior of cancer cells *(11)*.

The molecular dissection of the chemokine gene cluster, the identification of the full range of C-C chemokines, and the establishment of all the biologic functions is a preamble to obtaining a clear insight on the suppressive and enhancing activities of chemokines in tumorigenesis.

Even with the complete knowledge of the whole chemokine gene ensemble and of all the chemokine functions at hand, it will remain impossible, without extensive in vivo testing, to answer the question of whether chemokines are tumor suppressors.

4.2. Differences in Chemokine Production Between Normal and Tumor Cells

If a chronic inflammation resembles an invasive tumor, what are the mechanisms that make the outcomes so different in both types of diseases? We assume here that the effector cells, i.e., the chemoattracted phagocytes, have the same characteristics in both instances. First and most obviously, the chemokine-producing cell is different. A normal tissue fibroblast will synthesize chemokines if appropriately stimulated by inflammatory cytokines such as IL-1, tumor necrosis factor-α, and IFN-γ, whereas a tumor cell might autonomously (without external stimulation, perhaps by autonomous activation of transcription) synthesize chemotactic factors. Second, the stimuli for production (here used as a general term to include activation of gene transcription, translation, processing, and secretion) of chemokines might differ considerably between normal and tumor cells. For instance, Table 4 illustrates that blood monocytes produce MCP-1 and MCP-2 when stimulated with virus or double-stranded RNA (dsRNA), whereas myelomonocytic leukemia THP-1 cells (a cell line often used as the prototype for well-differentiated monocytes that is also chemotactically responsive to MCPs) produce these chemokines after stimulation with completely different inducers (IFN-γ and endotoxin). This responsiveness is linked to the presence of membrane receptors, signal transduction pathways, and transcription factors that are developmentally regulated. It is an adage that the fading from normal to dysplastic to neoplastic cells is a transition to an earlier stage of development. It can be deduced that the regulation signals (cytokines) in the tissues may be incorrectly interpreted by the tumor cells. What about the signals that are sent out by the tumor, in particular the chemokines?

Table 4
Induction of Human MCP-1 and MCP-2 by Monocytic Cells (Values Are in ng/mL)[a]

Induction		THP-1		Monocytes	
Stimulus	Dose	MCP-1	MCP-2	MCP-1	MCP-2
Measles virus	10^5 TCID$_{50}$/mL	5.3	1.1	83	1.4
dsRNA	100 µg/mL	2.5	0.5	7.9	0.7
LPS	5 µg/mL	187	7.1	6.3	0.2
IFN-γ	100 ng/mL	98	8.1	2.8	0.2
Control	—	0.6	0.4	2.5	0.1

[a]Cell cultures were stimulated with the indicated inducers for 48 h. MCP-1 and MCP-2 were measured by specific enzyme-linked immunosorbent assay (81); values represent the mean of four independent experiments.

So far there is a lack of information about the genetic signals that govern chemokine biosynthesis and about the differences between chemokines produced by normal vs malignant cells. There is an urgent need for detailed studies of chemokine gene promoters in tumor cells (44). Obviously, the documented examples indicate that the protein sequences of purified chemokines from normal and cancer cells are identical. Still, the possibility exists that posttranslational processing, e.g., aminoterminal or carboxyterminal clipping or glycosylation, might be different and might have profound effects on function (19,41).

More investigation about this processing is fraught with difficulties because it is laborious and expensive to produce sufficient amounts of pure, natural chemokines from large-scale mammalian cell cultures, and the analytic tools at the appropriate scale are currently only in development (19,41,59). From the analysis of oligosaccharides of many molecules and the differences in the glycosylation pathways between normal and tumor cells (53), it is an educated guess that MCP-1 (with O-linked sugars) from tumor cells might possess other sugars and different specific activities, or even other responsive cell types. In line with these suggestions, is the observation that purified glycosylation variants of MCP-1 from murine fibroblastic cells and epithelial cells showed up to fivefold differences in chemotactic activity (35).

In conclusion, the molecular differences between a host-controlled chronic inflammation and an autonomous cancer process reside in the genetic alterations of the tumor cells, which might result in (1) altered expression levels and spectra of chemokines and (2) the generation of posttranslationally modified chemokine variants.

4.3. Tumor Cells Responsive to C-C Chemokines

Very much like normal leukocytes, many leukemic cells are responsive to chemokines. For instance, THP-1 cells have been used to replace primary monocytes in chemotaxis and calcium release assays (60). The relation of C-C chemokines and cancer might, however, go much further. Recently, a novel C-C chemokine, stromal cell–derived factor-1 has been implied in the homing of bone marrow–derived progenitor cells (CD34+ cells) (1), and the C-C chemokine PARC, which attracts lymphocytes, is highly expressed in lymph node dendritic cells and may help in the homing of normal lymphocytes to specific areas in the lymph nodes. It is a current dogma that the metastasis of primary cancers to particular organs (e.g., liver, lung, brain) is governed by the expression of specific surface molecules and by the ensuing sugar–lectin or adhesion molecule–ligand interactions. The recently discovered CX_3C membrane-bound chemokine-like molecule might operate within the context of this dogma *(5)*. Such molecules have a hybrid function in chemotaxis and cell–cell interactions. This dogma might, however, be complemented by an additional chemokine-based homing mechanism for cancer. Indeed, there exist C-C chemokines that are constitutively expressed in particular organs. LARC, the gene product of *SCYA16*, is expressed in the liver *(25)*, whereas PARC is primarily expressed in the lung *(see* Table 2). It may well be that the ectopic expression of the PARC and LARC receptors in some undifferentiated cancer cells causes organ-specific metastasis by their specific recruitment to the lung and liver, respectively.

5. CONCLUSION

We have herein formulated some theoretical models on how previously studied and novel C-C-type chemoattractants might function in cancer. The perspectives for chemokine research, related to cancer, are hopeful not only because so many questions remain to be answered, but also because more molecular tools become available to answer specific questions, to test new hypotheses, and to challenge some current dogmas. There is an urgent need for progress at three levels: the analytic, the experimental, and the clinical.

In the early 1990s, chemokines were characterized by functional assay systems. Currently, novel cDNAs and genes are cloned with increasing pace. In addition, by bioinformatics and by the combinatorial cloning technology, many "orphan" chemokines and chemokine receptors are identified and are currently waiting for their function(s) to be discovered. *Better analytic techniques* to test the orphan molecules need to be developed. Similarly, more *animal experiments* are necessary to obtain a clear view in which tumors C-C chemokines are beneficial or detrimental for the host. Similarly, a better *clinical understanding* of the importance of a "chemokine grading" (i.e., which chemokines are expressed in which kind of tumors) in human tumor biology is necessary. Well-defined clinical diagnostics and novel therapeutics, based on chemokine research, will, in the future, undoubtedly complement the currently available means to fight proliferative and invasive cancers. Chemokines may become useful as adjuvant tumor therapies especially in the case of tumors that express strong tumor antigens. In this respect, C-C chemokines may be more useful than C-X-C chemokines because the latter seem to enhance angiogenesis toward the tumor and invasion and metastasis of the cancer cells.

Note added in proof. At the Keystone Symposium "Chemokines and Chemokine Receptors," Keystone, Colorado, 18–23 January 1999, it was suggested to adapt the chemokine nomenclature and abbreviations on the basis of the gene symbols (see Tables 1 and 2). The DNA sequences, referred to in these tables, are those at the time of submission. These have meanwhile been complemented by novel expressed sequence tag (EST) and gene data.

ACKNOWLEDGMENTS

We thank the Fund for Scientific Research of Flanders, the Belgian Cancer Association, the Cancer Foundation of the General Savings and Retirement Fund (A.S.L.K.), and the InterUniversitaire Attractiepolen for support. We also thank René Conings for help with the drawings. Dominique Brabants for the typescript, and Jean-Pierre Lenaerts, Ilse Van Aelst, Pierre Fiten, and Dr. Els Van Coillie for experimental help. Dr. Hisayuki Nomiyama (Kumamoto University, Kumamoto, Japan) and Dr. Patricia Baldacci (Pasteur Institute, Paris, France) are thanked for advice about the human and mouse chemokine gene clusters.

REFERENCES

1. Aiuti, A., I. J. Webb, C. Bleul, T. Springer, and J. C. Gutierrez-Ramos. 1997. The chemokine SDF-1 is a chemoattractant for human CD34+ hematopoietic progenitor cells and provides a new mechanism to explain the mobilization of CD34+ progenitors to peripheral blood. *J. Exp. Med.* **185:** 111–120.
2. Alcami, A., and G. L. Smith. 1995. Cytokine receptors encoded by poxviruses: a lesson in cytokine biology. *Immunol. Today* **16:** 474–478.
3. Ambros, I. M., A. Zellner, B. Roald, G. Amann, R. Ladenstein, D. Printz, H. Gadner, and P. F. Ambros. 1996. Role of ploidy, chromosome 1p, and Schwann cells in the maturation of neuroblastoma. *N. Engl. J. Med.* **334:** 1505–1511.
4. Arenberg, D. A., S. L. Kunkel, P. J. Polverini, S. B. Morris, M. D. Burdick, M. C. Glass, D. T. Taub, M. D. Iannettoni, R. I. Whyte, and R. M. Strieter. 1996. Interferon-γ-inducible protein 10 (IP-10) is an angiostatic factor that inhibits human non-small cell lung cancer (NSCLC) tumorigenesis and spontaneous metastases. *J. Exp. Med.* **184:** 981–992.
5. Bazan, J. F., K. B. Bacon, G. Hardiman, W. Wang, K. Soo, D. Rossi, D. R. Greaves, A. Zlotnik, and T. J. Schall. 1997. A new class of membrane-bound chemokine with a CX$_3$C motif. *Nature* **385:** 640–644.
6. Billiau, A., V. G. Edy, H. Heremans, J. Van Damme, J. Desmyter, J. A. Georgiades, and P. De Somer. 1977. Human interferon: mass production in a newly established cell line, MG-63. *Antimicrob. Agents Chemother.* **12:** 11–15.
7. Bottazzi, B., N. Polentarutti, R. Acero, A. Balsari, D. Boraschi, P. Ghezzi, M. Salmona, and A. Mantovani. 1983. Regulation of the macrophage content of neoplasms by chemoattractants. *Science* **220:** 210–212.
8. Bottazzi, B., S. Walter, D. Govoni, F. Colotta, and A. Mantovani. 1992. Monocyte chemo-tactic cytokine gene transfer modulates macrophage infiltration, growth, and susceptibility to IL-2 therapy of a murine melanoma. *J. Immunol.* **148:** 1280–1285.
9. Buyse, I. M., G. Shao, and S. Huang. 1995. The retinoblastoma protein binds to RIZ, a zinc-finger protein that shares an epitope with the adenovirus E1A protein. *Proc. Natl. Acad. Sci. USA* **92:** 4467–4471.
10. Casciano, I., J. V. M. Marchi, R. Muresu, E. V. Volpi, C. Rozzo, G. Opdenakker, and M. Romani. 1996. Molecular and genetic studies on the region of translocation and dupli-cation in the neuroblastoma cell line NGP at the 1p36.13-p36.32 chromosomal site. *Oncogene* **12:** 2101–2108.
11. Chirivi, R. G. S., A. Garofalo, I. M. Padura, A. Mantovani, and R. Giavazzi. 1993. Interleukin 1 receptor antagonist inhibits the augmentation of metastasis induced by interleukin 1 or lipopolysaccharide in a human melanoma/nude mouse system. *Cancer Res.* **53:** 5051–5054.
12. Cochran, B. H., A. C. Reffel, and C. D. Stiles. 1983. Molecular cloning of gene sequences regulated by platelet-derived growth factor. *Cell* **33:** 939–947.
13. Colombo, M. P., and G. Forni. 1994. Cytokine gene transfer in tumor inhibition and tumor therapy: where are we now? *Immunol. Today* **15:** 48–51.
14. D'Souza, P., and V. A. Harden. 1996. Chemokines and HIV-1 second receptors: confluence of two fields generates optimism in AIDS research. *Nat. Med.* **2:** 1293–1300.
15. Desbaillets, I., M. Tada, N. De Tribolet, A.-C. Diserens, M.-F. Hamou, and E. G. Van Meir. 1994. Human astrocytomas and glioblastomas express monocyte chemoattractant protein-1 (MCP-1) *in vivo* and *in vitro*. *Int. J. Cancer* **58:** 240–247.

16. Eccles, S. A., and P. Alexander. 1974. Macrophage content of tumours in relation to metastatic spread and host immune reaction. *Nature* **250:** 667–669.
17. Garcia-Zepeda, E. A., Combadiere, M. E. Rothenberg, M. N. Sarafi, F. Lavigne, Q. Hamid, P. M. Murphy, and A. D. Luster. 1996. Human monocyte chemoattractant protein (MCP)-4 is a novel CC chemokine with activities on monocytes, eosinophils, and basophils induced in allergic and nonallergic inflammation that signals through the CC chemokine receptors (CCR)-2 and -3. *J. Immunol.* **157:** 5613–5626.
18. Gautam, S. C., C. J. Noth, N. Janakiraman, K. R. Pindolia, and R. A. Chapman. 1995. Induction of chemokine mRNA in bone marrow stromal cells: modulation by TGF-beta 1 and IL-4. *Exp. Hematol.* **23:** 482–491.
19. Gong, J.-H., and I. Clark-Lewis. 1995. Antagonists of monocyte chemoattractant protein-1 identified by modification of functionally critical NH_2-terminal residues. *J. Exp. Med.* **181:** 631–640.
20. Goppelt-Struebe, M., and M. Stroebel. 1995. Synergistic induction of monocyte chemoattractant protein-1 (MCP-1) by platelet-derived growth factor and interleukin-1. *FEBS Lett.* **374:** 375–378.
21. Graves, D. T., R. Barnhill, T. Galanopoulos, and H. N. Antoniades. 1992. Expression of monocyte chemotactic protein-1 in human melanoma *in vivo. Am. J. Pathol.* **140:** 9–14.
22. Graves, D. T., Y. L. Jiang, M. J. Williamson, and A. J. Valente. 1989. Identification of monocyte chemotactic activity produced by malignant cells. *Science* **245:** 1490–1493.
23. Graves, D. T., and A. J. Valente. 1991. Monocyte chemotactic proteins from human tumor cells. *Biochem. Pharmacol.* **41:** 333–337.
24. Gruss, H.-J., M. A. Brach, H.-G. Drexler, R. Bonifer, R. H. Mertelsmann, and F. Herrmann. 1992. Expression of cytokine genes, cytokine receptor genes, and transcription factors in cultured Hodgkin and Reed-Sternberg cells. *Cancer Res.* **52:** 3353–3360.
25. Hieshima, K., T. Imai, G. Opdenakker, J. Van Damme, J. Kusuda, H. Tei, Y. Sakaki, K. Takatsuki, R. Miura, O. Yoshie, and H., Nomiyama. 1997. Molecular cloning of a novel human CC chemokine LARC expressed in liver: chemotactic activity for lymphocytes and gene localization on chromosome 2. *J. Biol. Chem.* **272:** 5846–5853.
26. Hoogewerf, A. J., J. W. Leone, I. M. Reardon, W. J. Howe, D. Asa, R. L. Heinrikson, and S. R. Ledbetter. 1995. CXC chemokines connective tissue activating peptide-III and neutrophil activating peptide-2 are heparin/heparan sulfate-degrading enzymes. *J. Biol. Chem.* **270:** 3268–3277.
27. Huang, S., R. K. Singh, K. Xie, M. Gutman, K. K. Berry, C. D. Bucana, I. J. Fidler, and M. Bar-Eli. 1994. Expression of the JE/MCP-1 gene suppresses metastatic potential in murine colon carcinoma cells. 1994. *Cancer Immunol. Immunother.* **39:** 231–238.
28. Huang, S., K. Xie, R. K. Singh, M. Gutman, and M. Bar-Eli. 1995. Expression of tumor growth and metastasis of murine renal adenocarcinoma by syngeneic fibroblasts genetically engineered to secrete the JE/MCP-1 cytokine. *J. Interferon Cytokine Res.* **15:** 655–665.
29. Kaghad, M., H. Bonnet, A. Yang, L. Creancier, J.-C. Biscan, A. Valent, A. Minty, P. Chalon, J.-M. Lelias, X. Dumont, P. Ferrara, F. McKeon, and D. Caput. 1997. Monoallelically expressed gene related to p53 at 1p36, a region frequently deleted in neuroblastoma and other human cancers. *Cell* **90:** 809–819.
30. Kovacs, E. J., and L. A. DiPietro. 1994. Fibrogenic cytokines and connective tissue production. *FASEB J.* **8:** 854–861.
31. Lacraz, S., P. Isler, E. Vey, H. G. Welgus, and J. M. Dayer. 1994. Direct contact between T lymphocytes and monocytes is a major pathway for induction of metalloproteinase expression. *J. Biol. Chem.* **269:** 22,027–22,033.
32. Lanning, J., H. Kawasaki, E. Tanaka, Y. Luo, and M. E. Dorf. 1994. Inhibition of *in vivo* tumor growth by the β chemokine. TCA3. 1994. *J. Immunol.* **153:** 4625–4635.
33. Laureys, G., F. Speleman, G. Opdenakker, Y. Benoit, and J. Leroy. 1990. Constitutional translocation t(1;17)(p36;q12-21) in a patient with neuroblastoma. *Genes, Chromosomes Cancer* **2:** 252–254.

34. Laureys, G., F. Speleman, R. Versteeg, P. van der Drift, A. Chan, J. Leroy, U. Francke, G. Opdenakker, and N. Van Roy. 1995. Constitutional translocation t(1;17)(p36.31-p36.13;q11.2-q12.1) in a neuroblastoma patient: establishment of somatic cell hybrids and identification of PND/A12M2 on chromosome 1 and NF1/SCYA7 on chromosome 17 as breakpoint flanking single copy markers. *Oncogene* **10**: 1087–1093.

35. Liu, Z.-G., A. Haelens, A. Wuyts, S. Struyf, X.-W. Pang, P. Proost, W.-F. Chen, and J. Van Damme. 1996. Isolation of a lymphocyte chemotactic factor produced by the murine thymic epithelial cell line MTEC1: identification as a 30kDa glycosylated form of MCP-1. *Eur. Cytokine Netw.* **7**: 381–388.

36. Maghazachi, A. A., A. Al-Aoukaty, and T. J. Schall. 1994. C-C chemokines induce the chemotaxis of NK and IL-2-activated NK cells. *J. Immunol.* **153**: 4969–4977.

37. Maghazachi, A. A., A. Al-Aoukaty, and T. J. Schall. 1996. CC chemokines induce the generation of killer cells from CD56+ cells. *Eur. J. Immunol.* **26**: 315–319.

38. Manome, Y., P. Y. Wen, A. Hershowitz, T. Tanaka, B. J. Rollins, D. W. Kufe, and H. A. Fine. 1995. Monocyte chemoattractant protein-1 (MCP-1) gene transduction: an effective tumor vaccine strategy for non-intracranial tumors. *Cancer Immunol. Immunother.* **41**: 227–235.

39. Mantovani, A. 1994. Tumor-associated macrophages in neoplastic progression: a paradigm for the *in vivo* function of chemokines. *Lab. Invest.* **71**: 5–16.

40. Mareel, M. M., F. M. Van Roy, and M. E. Bracke. 1993. How and when do tumor cells metastasize? *Crit. Rev. Oncog.* **4**: 559–594.

41. Masure, S., L. Paemen, P. Proost, J. Van Damme, and G. Opdenakker. 1995. Expression of a human mutant monocyte chemotactic protein 3 in *Pichia pastoris* and characterization as an MCP-3 receptor antagonist. *J. Interferon Cytokine Res.* **15**: 955–963.

42. Masure, S., P. Proost, J. Van Damme, and G. Opdenakker. 1991. Purification and identification of 91-kDa neutrophil gelatinase: release by the activating peptide interleukin-8. *Eur. J. Biochem.* **198**: 391–398.

43. Mueller, S. G., W. P. Schraw, and A. Richmond. 1994. Melanoma growth stimulatory activity enhances the phosphorylation of the class II interleukin-8 receptor in non-hematopoietic cells. *J. Biol. Chem.* **269**: 1973–1980.

44. Murakami, K., H. Nomiyama, R. Miura, A. Follens, P. Fiten, E. Van Coillie, J. Van Damme, and G. Opdenakker. 1997. Structural and functional analysis of the promoter region of the human MCP-3 gene: transactivation of expression by novel recognition sequences adjacent to the transcription initiation site. *DNA Cell. Biol.* **16**: 173–183.

45. Nakao, M., H. Nomiyama, and K. Shimada. 1990. Structures of human genes coding for cytokine LD78 and their expression. *Mol. Cell. Biol.* **10**: 3646–3658.

46. Naruse, K., M. Ueno, T. Satoh, H. Nomiyama, H. Tei, M. Takeda, D. H. Ledbetter, E. Van Coillie, G. Opdenakker, N. Gunge, Y. Sakaki, M. Iio, and R. Miura. 1996. A YAC contig of the human CC chemokine genes clustered on chromosome 17q11.2. *Genomics* **34**: 236–240.

47. Negus, R. P. M., G. W. H. Stamp, M. G. Relf, F. Burke, S. T. A. Malik, S. Bernasconi, P. Allavena, S. Sozzani, A. Mantovani, and F. R. Balkwill. 1995. The detection and localization of monocyte chemoattractant protein-1 (MCP-1) in human ovarian cancer. *J. Clin. Invest.* **95**: 2391–2396.

48. Norgauer, J., B. Metzner, and I. Schraufstätter. 1996. Expression and growth-promoting function of the IL-8 receptor β in human melanoma cells. *J. Immunol.* **156**: 1132–1137.

49. Obaru, K., M. Fukuda, S. Maeda, and K. Shumada. 1986. A cDNA clone used to study mRNA inducible in human tonsillar lymphocytes by a tumor promoter. *J. Biochem.* **99**: 885–894.

50. Opdenakker, G., P. Fiten, G. Nys, G. Froyen, N. Van Roy, F. Speleman, G. Laureys, and J. Van Damme. 1994. The human MCP-3 gene (SCYA7): cloning, sequence analysis, and assignment to the C-C chemokine gene cluster on chromosome 17q11.2-q12. *Genomics* **21**: 403–408.

51. Opdenakker, G., G. Froyen, P. Fiten, P. Proost, and J. Van Damme. 1993. Human monocyte chemotactic protein-3 (MCP-3): molecular cloning of the cDNA and comparison with other chemokines. *Biochem. Biophys. Res. Commun.* **191:** 535–542.

52. Opdenakker, G., S. Masure, B. Grillet, and J. Van Damme. 1991. Cytokine-mediated regulation of human leukocyte gelatinases and role in arthritis. *Lymphokine Cytokine Res.* **10:** 317–324.

53. Opdenakker, G., P. M. Rudd, M. Wormald, R. A. Dwek, and J. Van Damme. 1995. Cells regulate the activities of cytokines by glycosylation. *FASEB J.* **9:** 453–457.

54. Opdenakker, G., and J. Van Damme. 1992. Chemotactic factors, passive invasion and metastasis of cancer cells. *Immunol. Today* **13:** 463, 464.

55. Opdenakker, G., and J. Van Damme. 1992. Cytokines and proteases in invasive processes: molecular similarities between inflammation and cancer. *Cytokine* **4:** 251–258.

56. Pekarek, L. A., B. A. Starr, A. Y. Toledano, and H. Schreiber. 1995. Inhibition of tumor growth by elimination of granulocytes. *J. Exp. Med.* **181:** 435–440.

57. Premack, B. A., and T. J. Schall. 1996. Chemokine receptors: gateways to inflammation and infection. *Nat. Med.* **2:** 1174–1178.

58. Proost, P., C. De Wolf-Peeters, R. Conings, G. Opdenakker, A. Billiau, and J. Van Damme. 1993. Identification of a novel granulocyte chemotactic protein (GCP-2) from human tumor cells: *in vitro* and *in vivo* comparison with natural forms of GRO, IP-10 and IL-8. *J. Immunol.* **150:** 1000–1010.

59. Proost, P., P. Van Leuven, A. Wuyts, R. Ebberink, G. Opdenakker, and J. Van Damme. 1995. Chemical synthesis, purification and folding of the human monocyte chemotactic proteins MCP-2 and MCP-3 into biologically active chemokines. *Cytokine* **7:** 97–104.

60. Proost, P., A. Wuyts, and J. Van Damme. 1996. Human monocyte chemotactic proteins-2 and -3: structural and functional comparison with MCP-1. *J. Leukoc. Biol.* **59:** 67–74.

61. Raghow, R. 1994. The role of extracellular matrix in postinflammatory wound healing and fibrosis. *FASEB J.* **8:** 823–831.

62. Rollins, B. J., E. D. Morrison, and C. D. Stiles. 1988. Cloning and expression of *JE*, a gene inducible by platelet-derived growth factor and whose product has cytokine-like properties. *Proc. Natl. Acad. Sci. USA* **85:** 3738–3742.

63. Rollins, B. J., and M. E. Sunday. 1991. Suppression of tumor formation *in vivo* by expression of the JE gene in malignant cells. *Mol. Cell. Biol.* **11:** 3125–3131.

64. Sarafi, M. N., E. A. Garcia-Zepeda, J. A. MacLean, I. F. Charo, and A. D. Luster. 1997. Murine monocyte chemoattractant protein (MCP)-5: a novel CC chemokine that is a structural and functional homologue of human MCP-1. *J. Exp. Med.* **185:** 99–109.

65. Schaber, B., G. Bruchelt, J. Meyle, B. Jeschke, R. Handgretinger, D. Niethammer, P. Mayer, G. Rassner, and G. Fierlbeck. 1994. Chemotactic activity of substances derived from antibody-loaded tumor cells on granulocytes. *Immunology Lett.* **41:** 67–71.

66. Schall, T. J. 1991. Biology of the RANTES/SIS cytokine family. *Cytokine* **3:** 165–183.

67. Singh, R. K., K. Berry, K. Matsushima, K. Yasumoto, and I. J. Fidler. 1993. Synergism between human monocyte chemotactic and activating factor and bacterial products for activation of tumoricidal properties in murine macrophages. *J. Immunol.* **151:** 2786–2793.

68. Singh, R. K., M. Gutman, R. Radinsky, C. D. Bucana, and I. J. Fidler. 1994. Expression of interleukin 8 correlates with the metastatic potential of human melanoma cells in nude mice. *Cancer Res.* **54:** 3242–3247.

69. Strieter, R. M., P. J. Polverini, D. A. Arenberg, A. Walz, G. Opdenakker, J. Van Damme, and S. L. Kunkel. 1995. Role of C-X-C chemokines as regulators of angiogenesis in lung cancer. *J. Leukoc. Biol.* **57:** 752–762.

70. Takeshima, H., J.-I. Kuratsu, M. Takeya, T. Yoshimura, and Y. Ushio. 1994. Expression and localization of messenger RNA and protein for monocyte chemoattractant protein-1 in human malignant glioma. *J. Neurosurg.* **80:** 1056–1062.

71. Taub, D. D., J. R. Ortaldo, S. M. Turcovski-Corrales, M. L. Key, D. L. Longo, and

W. J. Murphy. 1996. β Chemokines costimulate lymphocyte cytolysis, proliferation, and lymphokine production. *J. Leukoc. Biol.* **59:** 81–89.

72. Taub, D. D., T. J. Sayers, C. R. D. Carter, and J. R. Ortaldo. 1995. α and β chemokines induce NK cell migration and enhance NK-mediated cytolysis. *J. Immunol.* **155:** 3877–3888.

73. Thirion, S., G. Nys, P. Fiten, S. Masure, J. Van Damme, and G. Opdenakker. 1994. Mouse macrophage derived monocyte chemotactic protein-3: cDNA cloning and identification as MARC/FIC. *Biochem. Biophys. Res. Commun.* **201:** 493–499.

74. Van Coillie, E., P. Fiten, H. Nomiyama, Y. Sakaki, R. Miura, O. Yoshie, J. Van Damme, and G. Opdenakker. 1997. The human MCP-2 gene (SCYA8): cloning, sequence analysis, tissue expression and assignment to the C-C chemokine gene contig on chromosome 17q11.2. *Genomics* **40:** 323–331.

75. Van Coillie, E., G. Froyen, H. Nomiyama, R. Miura, P. Fiten, I. Van Aelst, J. Van Damme, and G. Opdenakker. 1997. Human monocyte chemotactic protein-2 (MCP-2): cDNA cloning and related expression of mRNA in mesenchymal cells. *Biochem. Biophys. Res. Commun.* **231:** 726–730.

76. Van Damme, J., and R. Conings. 1995. Assays for chemotaxis, in *Cytokines. A Practical Approach* (Balkwill, F. R., ed.), IRL Press, Oxford, pp. 215–224.

77. Van Damme, J., B. Decock, R. Bertini, R. Conings, J.-P. Lenaerts, W. Put, G. Opdenakker, and A. Mantovani. 1991. Production and identification of natural monocyte chemotactic protein from virally infected murine fibroblasts: relationship with the product of the mouse competence (JE) gene. *Eur. J. Biochem.* **199:** 223–229.

78. Van Damme, J., B. Decock, R. Conings, J.-P. Lenaerts, G. Opdenakker, and A. Billiau. 1989. The chemotactic activity for granulocytes produced by virally infected fibroblasts is identical to monocyte-derived interleukin 8. *Eur. J. Immunol.* **19:** 1189–1194.

79. Van Damme, J., G. Opdenakker, R. J. Simpson, M. R. Rubira, S. Cayphas, A. Vink, A. Billiau, and J. Van Snick. 1987. Identification of the human 26-kDa protein, interferon β2 (IFN-β2), as a B cell hybridoma/plasmacytoma growth factor induced by interleukin 1 and tumor necrosis factor. *J. Exp. Med.* **165:** 914–919.

80. Van Damme, J., P. Proost, J.-P. Lenaerts, and G. Opdenakker. 1992. Structural and functional identification of two human, monocyte chemotactic proteins (MCP-2 and MCP-3) belonging to the chemokine family. *J. Exp. Med.* **176:** 59–65.

81. Van Damme, J., P. Proost, W. Put, S. Arens, J.-P. Lenaerts, R. Conings, G. Opdenakker, H. Heremans, and A. Billiau. 1994. Induction of monocyte chemotactic proteins MCP-1 and MCP-2 in human fibroblasts and leukocytes by cytokines and cytokine inducers: chemical synthesis of MCP-2 and development of a specific RIA. *J. Immunol.* **152:** 5495–5502.

82. Van Damme, J., J. Van Beeumen, G. Opdenakker, and A. Billiau. 1988. A novel NH$_2$-terminal sequence-characterized human monokine possessing neutrophil chemotactic, skin-reactive and granulocytosis-promoting activity. *J. Exp. Med.* **167:** 1364–1376.

83. Van Roy, N., G. Laureys, N. C. Cheng, P. Willem, G. Opdenakker, R. Versteeg, and F. Speleman. 1994. 1;17 Translocations and other chromosome 17 rearrangements in human primary neuroblastoma tumors and cell lines. *Genes, Chromosomes Cancer* **10:** 103–114.

84. Wakabayashi, H., P. G. Cavanaugh, and G. L. Nicolson. 1995. Purification and identification of mouse lung microvessel endothelial cell-derived chemoattractant for lung-metastasizing murine RAW117 large-cell lymphoma cells: identification as mouse monocyte chemotactic protein 1. *Cancer Res.* **55:** 4458–4464.

85. Wuyts, A., A. Haelens, P. Proost, J.-P. Lenaerts, R. Conings, G. Opdenakker, and J. Van Damme. 1996. Identification of mouse granulocyte chemotactic protein-2 from fibroblasts and epithelial cells: functional comparison with natural KC and macrophage inflammatory protein-2. *J. Immunol.* **157:** 1736–1743.

86. Xu, L. L., M. K. Warren, W. L. Rose, W. Gong, and J. M. Wang. 1996. Human recombinant monocyte chemotactic protein and other C-C chemokines bind and induce directional migration of dendritic cells *in vitro*. *J. Leukoc. Biol.* **60:** 365–371.

87. Yamamura, Y., T. Hattori, K. Obaru, K. Sakai, N. Asou, K. Takatsuki, Y. Ohmoto, H. Nomiyama, and K. Shimada. 1989. Synthesis of a novel cytokine and its gene (LD78) expressions in hematopoietic fresh tumor cells and cell lines. *J. Clin. Invest.* **84:** 1707–1712.

88. Zachariae, C. O. C., K. Thestrup-Pedersen, and K. Matsushima. 1991. Expression and secretion of leukocyte chemotactic cytokines by normal human melanocytes and melanoma cells. *J. Invest. Dermatol.* **97:** 593–599.

89. Zullo, J. N., B. H. Cochran, A. S. Huang, and C. D. Stiles. 1985. Platelet-derived growth factor and double-stranded ribonucleic acids stimulate expression of the same genes in 3T3 cells. *Cell* **43:** 793–800.

III

Modulation of Host Responses to Cancer

5

Natural Killer Cell–Chemokine Interactions
*Biologic Effects on Natural Killer Cell Trafficking and Cytolysis**

Dennis D. Taub

1. INTRODUCTION

The process of inflammation and immune recognition involve a complex series of events that result in an accumulation of specific leukocyte subsets at the site of tissue alteration or damage. These processes involve activation of cellular components and release of reactive mediators, changes in vascular endothelium, and penetration of the basement membrane, as well as chemotaxis of specific leukocyte subsets to the site of injury and infiltration into the tissue site *(1–4)*. While these extravasating leukocytes are critical for host defense, leading to clearance of the inciting factors such as infectious agents, it should also be appreciated that leukocyte recruitment may also contribute to the pathogenesis of an underlying disease. The maintenance of leukocyte recruitment during inflammation requires a "delicate" communication between infiltrating leukocytes and the endothelium *(1–5)*. These signals are mediated via the generation of several early response cytokines (such as interleukin-1 [IL-1] and tumor necrosis factor-α [TNF-α]), the expression of surface adhesion molecules, and the production of chemotactic molecules. All these processes, in one way or another, have been shown to be involved in the localization of neutrophils, monocytes, macrophages, eosinophils, basophils, T- and B-lymphocytes, and natural killer (NK) cells to inflammatory sites. In many disease states, this recruitment appears to be selective in that neutrophils are typically present in sites of acute inflammation whereas macrophages and lymphocytes are typically present at sites of chronic inflammation or at the later stages of disease. Likewise, in viral infections *(6,7)* and during the rejection of allografts *(8)*, NK cells selectively accumulate in the inflammatory site, in many cases before T-cell infiltration. However, over the many years of study, little is still known about the specific signaling network(s) by which quiescent and cytokine-activated NK cells are recruited to a compromised tissue site at the appropriate time. This chapter focuses attention on the role of a specific family of chemoattractants called *chemokines*, which appear to have potent effects on both NK cell trafficking and effector functions.

---

*The content of this publication does not necessarily reflect the views or policies of the Department of Health and Human Services, nor does mention of trade names, commercial products, or organizations imply endorsement by the U.S. Government.

From: *Chemokines and Cancer*
Edited by: B. J. Rollins © Humana Press Inc., Totowa, NJ

1.1. An Overview of NK Cells

NK cells compromise a heterogeneous population of CD3⁻CD56⁺CD16⁺ large granular lymphocytes, approx 5–10% of peripheral blood mononuclear cells, that are known to participate in both homeostatic and inflammatory host defense functions *(9–12)*. These cells spontaneously lyse a variety of parasites, fungi, bacteria, virally infected cells, and certain transformed cell populations, and are considered to play a role in the early protection against microbial infections and tumor cell development in a host before the development of specific immunity *(9–12)*. NK cells are mostly found circulating in the blood; however, under certain inflammatory conditions or in response to the administration of a biologic response modifier (BRM) such as IL-2, interferon-γ (IFN-γ), and/or poly I-C, these cells preferentially traffic to several organ sites, including the lung interstitium, intestinal mucosa, liver, spleen, and the peritoneal cavity *(9–14)*. This organ-specific trafficking is believed to be owing to the local release of various cytokines and other inflammatory mediators. Moreover, considerable evidence has accumulated to demonstrate that the cytokine-induced augmentation of organ-associated NK cell function can contribute to nonspecific antimetastatic responses observed in a number of immunotherapy studies *(13,14)*. Moreover, the ability of NK cells to secrete various cytokines including IFN-γ, TNF, and granulocyte-macrophage colony-stimulating factor (GM-CSF) is believed to play a central role in the regulation of both the immune response and hematopoiesis *(14)*. Indeed, studies within several experimental immunodeficient animal models have clearly demonstrated the importance of IFN-γ production by infiltrating NK cells in preventing overwhelming infection from several obligate intracellular pathogens *(15)*. Additionally, the production of both IFN-γ and TNF-α by NK cells appears to play a role in the pathogenesis of septic shock *(16)*.

In certain pathologic conditions, including viral and bacterial infections, NK cells selectively accumulate in infected tissue sites as well as in allograft infiltrates before graft rejection *(8,15)*. NK cells exhibit rapid migration in vitro *(17–19)*, express adhesion molecules that can recognize endothelial counterreceptors *(20–22)* or extracellular matrix proteins *(23)*, and are able to transmigrate actively across endothelial monolayers *(24,25)*. In fact, several studies have demonstrated that the migratory capacity of NK cells is greater than that of T-lymphocytes, supporting their presumed role as a first line of natural defense *(14)*. Similar to T-lymphocytes, cytokines have been shown to modulate the adhesive as well as chemotactic activities of NK cells, including IL-2, IL-4, IFN-γ, lymphotoxin, IL-12, IL-15, and TNF-α *(13,27–31)*. IL-2, TNF-α, IL-12, and IFN-γ have been shown to increase human and murine NK cell:endothelial cell interactions, whereas IL-4 has been shown to inhibit NK cell adhesion to some endothelial cell monolayers *(13,26,27)*. This adhesive activity appears to be activation dependent because cytokine-stimulated NK cells typically exhibit greater adhesion to various adhesive ligands than quiescent NK cells. The majority of NK cells and NK cell subpopulations have been shown to express a variety of adhesion molecules and selectins, including L-selectin (CD62L), Sialyl-Lewis X, CD57, LFA-1, Mac-1, p150,95, VLA-4, VLA-5, integrin α4β7, CD31, ICAM-1, VCAM-1, and MadCAM-1 *(14)*. Cytokine-activated NK cells have also been shown to express VLA-1, VLA-2, and VLA-6 *(14)*.

Many of these adhesive ligands have been shown to play a role in NK cell adhesion to and extravasation through the endothelial barrier. In addition to modulating NK cell adhesion, cytokines have also been shown to stimulate the random locomotion (chemokinesis) or chemotaxis *(13,18–20,24,28–30)* of NK cells in vitro.

In the mid-1980s, several laboratories described NK cell migration through nitrocellulose filters in response to activated serum, formyl-methionine-leucine-proline (fMLP), a potent granulocyte chemoattractant, and casein *(14)*. However, the recent characterization of the chemokine superfamily of chemoattractant cytokines has elucidated the more specific molecular mechanisms underlying the selective recruitment of NK cells from the blood vessels to the tissues.

Another important activity of NK cells is their ability on activation with IL-2 and/or other cytokines to exhibit greater cytolytic potential in comparison to their quiescent counterparts. These cells, termed *lympokine-activated killer* (LAK) cells, have the ability to kill a variety of histologic types of fresh and explanted tumor cells as well as tumor cells cultured in vitro in a major histocompatibility complex (MHC)-unrestricted and antigen-nonspecific fashion *(9–12,14,31–34)*. LAK cells in conjunction with IL-2 have been used for the treatment of cancer patients with melanoma, renal cell carcinoma, colorectal cancer, and non-Hodgkin lymphoma *(35)*. Over the years, a number of NK trafficking studies have also shown that adoptively transferred, lymphokine-activated NK cells can selectively accumulate within cancer metastases that are established in organ parenchyma *(9–12,14,35)*. Despite the potent antitumor activity of LAK cells in vitro, researchers in the field were faced with two major problems: the substantial toxic side effects of concurrent LAK and IL-2 administration in cancer patients, and the inability of the infused LAK cells to infiltrate selectively to the sites of tumor growth, instead showing a restricted pattern of tissue distribution in vivo, namely to the lungs, liver, and spleen after systemic administration. These in vivo experiments support the hypothesis that cytokines and various BRM, directly and indirectly, regulate NK cell proliferation, trafficking patterns, and recruitment into both normal and tumor-associated organ parenchyma, and that NK cells must therefore be able to recognize and respond to specific physiologic signals that induce localization into tissue sites.

1.2. An Overview of Chemokines and Their Receptors

Because the previous chapters in this book have already described the chemokine subfamilies and their functions in great detail, only a brief overview of chemokines and chemokine biology is provided here. Over the past decade, a rapidly growing superfamily of small, soluble, structurally related molecules called *chemokines* has been identified and shown to promote selectively the rapid adhesion and chemotaxis of a variety of leukocyte subtypes both in vivo and in vitro *(36–42)*. Chemokines are a superfamily of peptides that have from 20 to 70% amino acid homology and are related by a conserved motif containing four cysteine residues *(36–42)*. Chemokines are produced by almost every cell type in the body in response to a number of inflammatory signals, in particular those that activate leukocyte-endothelial cell interactions. IL-8; growth-related oncogene-α (GRO-α), GRO-β, GRO-γ; neutrophil-activating peptide-2 (NAP-2); platelet factor 4 (PF4); epithelial cell–derived neutrophil-activating factor-78 (ENA-78); granulocyte chemotactic protein-2; interferon-γ-inducible protein-10

(IP-10); monokine induced by IFN-γ (MIG); and stem cell differentiation factor-1α (SDF-1α) and SDF-1β are members of the C-X-C or the chemokine α class of the family that have an amino acid between the first two cysteines. Monocyte chemoattractant protein-1 (MCP-1), MCP-2, MCP-3, macrophage inflammatory protein-1α (MIP-1α), MIP-1β, RANTES, and I-309 are included in the C-C or the chemokine β class of the family. Lymphotactin (Ltn) or ATAC is a member of the C or the chemokine γ class of the family (36–43), and neurotactin and fractolkine are members of the C-X-X-X-C or the chemokine δ class of the family. Each of these chemotactic cytokines induces the directional migration of several leukocytic and nonleukocytic cell types including neutrophils, monocytes, T- and B-lymphocytes, NK cells, basophils, eosinophils, mast cells, fibroblasts, neurons, tumor cells, glial cells, and smooth muscle cells. Besides cell migration, some of these cytokines also have been reported to induce respiratory burst, enzyme release, intracellular Ca^{2+} mobilization, shape changes, degranulation, and an increase in adherence of leukocytes to endothelium and matrix proteins (36–42). These molecules also appear to play important roles in cellular activation and leukocyte effector functions (44–47). These activities appear to be relevant as chemokines have been found in the tissues of a variety of disease states characterized by distinct leukocytic infiltrates, including rheumatoid arthritis, sepsis, atherosclerosis, asthma, psoriasis, ischemia/reperfusion injury, a variety of pulmonary disease states, and more recently in Kaposi's sarcoma and AIDS (36–42).

Critical to our understanding of chemokine biology is an understanding of the specific receptors on various cell types that mediate their effects. Since 1995, the chemokine receptor field has exploded with the isolation and cloning of more than 15 human and rodent C-C and C-X-C chemokine receptors (36–42,48). All these receptors are members of the rhodopsin or serpentine receptor superfamily and have the characteristic G protein–coupled seven hydrophobic spanning transmembrane regions. There is a great deal of similarity between the tertiary structures of chemokine receptors and other G protein–coupled receptors (such as those for C5a, platelet-activating factor [PAF], and fMLP), yet chemokine receptors initiate unique and specific cellular activities only in response to their specific chemokines. These receptors also exhibit varying degrees of homology, particularly within their transmembrane-spanning regions. Although other chapters this book give a greater analysis of the structure, distribution, and specificity of the various chemokine receptors, in this chapter, only 10 C-X-C and C-C chemokine receptors are discussed. These include CCR1 (ligands including MIP-1α, MIP-1β, RANTES, MCP-3), CCR2A and CCR2B (MCP-1, MCP-2, MCP-3, MCP-4, MCP-5), CCR3 (eotaxin, RANTES, MCP-3), CCR4 (MIP-1α, RANTES, MCP-1), CCR5 (MIP-1α, MIP-1β, RANTES) CXCR1 (IL-8), CXCR2 (IL-8, GRO-α, MIP-2, ENA-78, NAP-2), CXCR3 (IP-10, MIG), and CXCR4 (SDF-1α, SDF-1β). The genomic localization and organization of most of the genes for these receptors as well as many inactive isoforms and pseudogenes have also been established (48).

Signal transduction through these receptors generally results in a number of biochemical reactions, including intracellular Ca^{2+} accumulation, guanine nucleotide-binding (G) protein activation, cAMP generation, phospholipase C activity, phosphoinositol hydrolysis, arachidonic acid metabolism, production of inositol triphosphate, the activation of protein kinase C, serine/threonine kinases and phosphoinositol 3-kinase, and the rapid elevation of diacylglycerol (DAG) *(41,42,48)*. Chemokine-receptor interactions initiate a characteristic pattern of responses including shape change, chemotaxis, degranulation, and respiratory burst. The coupling of a G protein to these receptors is believed to be essential for the high-affinity binding of both C-X-C and C-C chemokines. In addition, the effector functions induced by chemokine agonists depend on the type of G protein that couples to the receptor. All chemokine receptors characterized so far contain one or more of the consensus sequences for G protein activation. Within in vitro chemotaxis assays, leukocyte migration is often attenuated ("desensitized") in response to high concentrations of chemokines yielding the typical "bell-shaped" dose response curves. In addition, prior exposure of a receptor to its activating ligand rapidly results in a similar state of hyporesponsiveness. This desensitization, which involves either G protein signaling or protein phosphorylation, depending on the type of desensitization *(48)*, may actually have a physiologic role by preventing the remobilization and departure of leukocytes on entering sites of inflammation where the chemokine concentrations are believed to be maximal.

Overall, G proteins are heterotrimers composed of three subunits; α, β, and γ. Each G protein is distinguished by its α-subunit and approx 20 α-subunits have been described *(48)*. In their nonactivated form, they bind GDP, then on ligand-receptor interaction, an exchange of GDP for GTP bound to the α-subunit takes place, resulting in the dissociation of the α-GTP from the β- and γ-subunits. Previous studies have shown that the *Bordetella pertussis*–derived toxin, pertussis toxin (PTx), is able to catalyze the transfer of ADP ribose from NAD^+ to the cysteine residue in the α-subunit of G-inhibitory, G_i. The activity of PTx results in the functional uncoupling of G_i from its associated receptor, resulting in the eventual activation of the adenylyl cyclase pathway. By contrast, the *Vibrio cholera*–derived toxin, cholera toxin (CTx), has ADP-ribosyl transferase activity that catalyzes the transfer of ADP ribose from NAD^+ to a residue in the α-subunit of G-stimulatory, G_s. This covalent modification of G_s results in the inhibition of GTPase activity, and consequently, the α-subunit is maintained in a permanently activated state. Both of these toxins are typically used to determine whether chemokine activities on various cell populations are being mediated through G protein–linked receptors. Whereas G_s, G_i, and G_0 are sensitive to bacterial toxins, the other G proteins, G_q and G_z, are not. However, more detailed analyses using radiolabeled GTP molecules have provided greater proof of a direct interaction between chemokine receptors and G proteins in the chemokine-treated cell populations. It is believed that the specificity of chemokine-leukocyte interactions may be mediated through the specific association of various G proteins with chemokine receptors expressed on the cell surface of a given cell population. Thus, both G protein signaling and G protein phosphorylation are crucial to the signal transduction by these chemokine ligands.

Although a plethora of articles has been published over the last 8 yr describing the effects of chemokines on granulocyte, monocyte, and T-lymphocyte trafficking, the biologic roles for C-X-C, C-C, and C chemokines on resting and lymphokine-activated NK cells have only recently been reported (Table 1). This chapter primarily focuses on the role of chemokines on several NK cell functions including NK cell migration and NK cell cytolytic/effector functions. It is my hope to provide a thorough review of all the published studies on chemokine–NK cell interactions as well to relate these various findings to NK cell activities in pathologic disease states.

Table 1
Chemokine Activities on Human and Murine NK Cells[a]

Chemokine	Subfamily	Chemotaxis	Adhesion	Degranulation	Cytotoxicity	Proliferation
IL-8	C-X-C	+	–	–	–	ND
GRO-α	C-X-C	+	ND	–	–	ND
GRO-β	C-X-C	+	ND	ND	–	ND
IP-10	C-X-C	+	+	+	+	+
PF4	C-X-C	–	–	–	–	–
SDF-1α	C-X-C	+	ND	ND	+	ND
SDF-1β	C-X-C	+	ND	ND	ND	ND
MIP-1α	C-C	+	+	+	+	+
MIP-1β	C-C	+	+	+	+	+
RANTES	C-C	+	+	+	+	+
MCP-1	C-C	+	+	+	+	+
MCP-2	C-C	+	N D	+	+	ND
MCP-3	C-C	+	ND	+	+	ND
Ltn	C	+	–	+	+	ND

[a]This table represents various published data as well as unpublished data by the author's and other laboratories. +, positive results observed; –, negative results observed; ND, not determined.

2. REGULATION OF NK CELL MIGRATION

Similar to all leukocytes and lymphocytes, NK cell trafficking from the blood or lymph into inflammatory tissues requires a coordinated series of signals generated within the tissue lesion facilitating interactions between the circulating NK cell and the vascular endothelial cell barrier *(1–5,9,10)*. The early release of IL-1 and TNF-α is believed to prime the local vascular endothelial bed to express various cell adhesion molecules, selectins, and addressins initiating the primary adhesive interactions between these large granular lymphocytes and endothelial cells. Responding circulating NK cells roll along this primed endothelial bed slowing their transit through the circulation. On interacting with a proadhesive molecule(s), these cells tightly adhere to and spread out along this endothelial cell layer. These primary adhesion events are believed to be prerequisites for the successful trafficking of all circulating lymphocytes into extravascular tissues. The subsequent steps leading to lymphocyte transendothelial migration (diapedesis) and the movement of cells through the extravascular space directionally toward the signaling tissue is dependent on the presence of additional adhesive interactions as well as leukocyte-specific chemotactic molecules *(41,42)*.

As chemoattractants go, a plethora of proteins and agents have been shown to induce lymphocyte migration over the years, including complement components (e.g., C5a), PAF, eicosanoids (e.g., prostaglandin E_2, leukotriene B_4), bacterial-derived peptides (e.g., fMLP), endotoxin, growth factors (e.g., growth hormone), cytokines (e.g., IL-1α, TNF-α, IFN-γ), and neuroendocrine hormones (e.g., opioids). Many of these chemoattractants not only induce lymphocyte migration but also facilitate lymphocyte adhesion to endothelial cells and purified adhesive ligands *(36–42)*. This enhanced adhesiveness occurs within seconds of stimulation and, as with migration, is highly concentration dependent. Many of these chemotactic molecules also induce inflammatory infiltrates on injection in vivo *(41,42)*. Injections of the cytokines IL-1α, TNF-α, and IFN-γ have been shown to induce neutrophil, monocyte, and lymphocyte migration into the local injection site *(41,42)*. The subtype of leukocytes that appears in inflammatory infiltrates can differ markedly, depending on the identity of the inflammatory irritant as well as the duration of irritation. The chemotactic factors responsible for these differences are likely to be cell type–specific (selective) chemoattractants and/or chemoattractant receptors. Thus, although most of the previously cited chemotactic mediators facilitate leukocyte trafficking, their lack of subset specificity has brought their relevance in selective leukocyte recruitment into question. However, with the characterization of various proteins of the chemokine superfamily, the most specific and potent lymphocyte chemoattractants have now been identified.

Since the late 1980s, many of the C-C chemokines, including MIP-1α, MIP-1β, RANTES, MCP-1, MCP-2, MCP-3, MCP-4, C10, and eotaxin, as well as the C-X-C chemokines IL-8, GRO-α, IP-10, MIG, SDF-1α, and SDF-1β, and the C chemokine Ltn have been shown to induce significant human and murine T-lymphocyte migration and adhesion both in vitro and in vivo *(36–42,49–60)*. Depending on the laboratory, various C-C chemokines also possess the ability to mediate preferentially the directional migration of preactivated and quiescent human $CD4^+$ vs $CD8^+$, $CD26^+$ vs $CD26^-$, and/or $CD45RA^+$ (naive) vs $CD29^+$ (memory) T-cells in vitro *(41,42,49–60)*.

Several factors influence this chemokine-mediated T-lymphocyte migration, including the T-cell activation state, the memory-naive status, the presence of adhesive ligands, the differences in levels and signaling through both promiscuous and specific chemokine receptors on the lymphocyte cell surface, variations in the responsiveness of individual T-cells and their subsets, the T-cell donor, and (perhaps analogous to basophils and eosinophils) a need for cytokine priming. Some, if not all, of these factors may also contribute to the observed T-cell subset differences reported by these various laboratories. The one feature all these studies have in common is a strict dose-dependent migration in response to chemokines with optimal activity being observed between 0.1 and 10 n*M* in microchemotaxis chambers. However, higher chemokine doses (>10 n*M*) appear to be required to induce human T-cell transendothelial migration *(41,42)*. Furthermore, in vitro T-cell migration in response to a given chemokine required the presence of specific extracellular matrix proteins to facilitate optimal movement *(41,42)*. This adhesive ligand requirement appears to make sense since migration and adhesion are often coordinated. It is believed that this selective ability of C, C-C, and certain C-X-C chemokines to promote T-cell subset migration may play a critical role in sorting out various T-cell subsets toward certain inflammatory sites as well as into different lymphoid compartments.

Given this background on lymphocytes, the locomotive activity of NK cells is particularly interesting, as only a few of these agents have been reported to modulate the migratory activity of NK cells in vitro. Previous studies, from several laboratories, have revealed that NK cells migrate in response to a variety of stimuli, including activated serum, casein, fMLP, IL-2, IL-12, IFN-γ, DAG, and phorbol esters *(14,18,19)*. In many cases, NK cell migration through chemotaxis filters is increased only after cytokine activation *(14,33)*. IL-2, IFN-γ, transforming growth factor-β, and TNF-α increase both the chemotaxis (directional migration in response to a chemoattractant gradient) and chemokinesis (random migration owing to cellular activation) of human NK cells *(14,29,30)*. Cultured cytokine-stimulated NK cells, in many cases, exhibit poor chemotaxis in response to these cytokines; however, an increase in NK cell chemokinesis has been observed. More recent studies have reported that IL-12 and IL-15 are also highly chemokinetic (not chemotactic) for long-term cultured IL-2-activated NK cells (IANK) *(26,27)*. While these mediators facilitate NK cell trafficking, their lack of specificity and apparent activation-dependent activities have brought their relevance to the selective accumulation of NK cells into tumor tissues or in various organs postcytokine and post-BRM administration into question.

Several laboratories have demonstrated that the lymphokines TNF-α, IL-12, and IL-15 directly induce chemokine production by various leukocytes and stromal cell populations, suggesting that any in vivo migratory effects mediated by these molecules may be indirect through the production of these chemotactic mediators *([61,62]*, Taub, D., unpublished data). In addition, NK cells have been shown to produce MIP-1α, RANTES, MCP-1, IP-10, and IL-8 in response to various cytokines and/or activation stimuli (Taub, D., unpublished data). Recent studies examining murine NK cells demonstrated the expression of Ltn by immunohistologic and Northern blot analyses post-IL-2 activation *(59)*. Although the precise role of chemokine production by NK cells has not been fully investigated, it seems likely that since NK cells are found in the early infiltrates of certain inflammatory conditions, chemokine production by NK cells may mediate the subsequent infiltration of specific T-cells into the area.

The initial study describing chemokine effects on NK cells was reported by Maghazachi and colleagues in 1993 *(63)*. In this study, IL-8 was found to induce the chemokinesis of IANK cells in modified Boyden chambers. The bacterial toxins, PTx or CTx, inhibited this IL-8-induced chemokinetic response, suggesting a role for G proteins in IL-8 signal transduction in these IANK cells. This effect was found to be caused by the ability of this chemokine to activate the G protein in IANK cell membranes. Pretreatment of these IANK cell membranes with IL-8 did not affect PTx- or CTx-dependent ADP ribosylation but did result in the disappearance of G_o (but not G_i or G_s), suggesting that the IL-8 receptors expressed on IANK cells are coupled to G_o. These findings were confirmed by the ability of IL-8 to enhance the binding of GTP-$γ^{35}$S to IANK cell membranes, further demonstrating a role for the coupling of G proteins to IL-8 receptors in IANK cells. However, my laboratory has been unable to demonstrate significant human NK cell chemotaxis or chemokinesis in response to IL-8 despite the fact that purified human NK cells can express >2400 CXCR2 receptors per cell *(64)*. Based on the studies with T-lymphocytes, it seems quite possible that, depending on the activation status of the NK cell, CXCR2 may or may not be coupled to the necessary G proteins needed to facilitate this migrational event.

Many chemokine investigators have had difficulty demonstrating the ability of lymphocytes to migrate in response to the C-X-C chemokine, IP-10. Early results by my laboratory *(51)* demonstrated that primed but not resting T-lymphocytes migrate in response to IP-10. Subsequently, I and my colleagues reported that IP-10 and MIG are potent chemoattractants for human NK cells in vitro *(64)*. However, these studies were considered controversial as several laboratories were unable to demonstrate any T- or NK cell migration in response to these chemokines. More recently, with the cloning of the IP-10/MIG receptor, CXCR3, four independent laboratories have clearly demonstrated that CXCR3 is expressed on both resting and activated T- and NK cells and that IP-10 is a potent chemoattractant for both of these populations *(51,60,64,65)*. Maghazachi and coworkers *(66)* have also recently reported that IANK and C-C chemokine–activated NK (CHAK) cells are highly responsive to IP-10. Thus, as C-X-C chemokines go, only IL-8, IP-10, and MIG have been reported to have any chemotactic effects on NK cells. However, I have also recently found that human NK cells and NK cell clones also migrate in response to SDF-1α and SDF-1β and express significant levels of the SDF-1 receptor, CXCR4, on their cell surface (Taub, D., unpublished data).

In 1995 my laboratory reported that MIP-1α, MIP-1β, RANTES, MCP-1, MCP-2, MCP-3, and IP-10, but not IL-8 and PF4, induced the migration of quiescent NK cells in vitro *(64)*. MIP-1α and IP-10 were found to be the most potent NK chemotactic agents, exhibiting chemotactic activity at concentrations as low as 0.1 nM. Although the other C-C chemokines also induce NK cell migration, these responses are often less efficacious and less potent than MIP-1α-induced migratory responses and are highly donor dependent. Subsequently, Loetscher and coworkers *(55)* have confirmed my C-C chemokine findings through the use of human NK cell clones. Additional studies by Maghazachi and colleagues *(68,69)* have also demonstrated the ability of NK and IANK cells to migrate directionally in response to MIP-1α, RANTES, and MCP-1; however, these investigators failed to observe any response to MIP-1β. Furthermore, these investigators found that only RANTES and MCP-1, but not MIP-1α, were also able to induce the chemokinesis of IANK cells *(68)*. Note, however, that during this same time period, several laboratories published articles describing the migratory effects of a number of C-C chemokines, including MIP-1α, MIP-1β, RANTES, MCP-1, MCP-2, and MCP-3, on human NK cells *(55,57,69)*. As for receptor expression on human NK cells, expression of both specific and shared C-C chemokine receptors on the surface of these lymphocytes is supported, for the most part, by the use of both radiolabeled chemokine binding studies and calcium mobilization studies using purified human NK cells and NK cell clones *(55,64,70)*.

In the majority of these studies, pretreatment of NK cells with PTx and/or CTx abolished the majority of the C-C chemokine–specific migratory responses, suggesting the use of classical chemokine receptors coupled to G_0. However, Maghazachi and coworkers *(68,69,71)* have gone much further with the precise association of specific G proteins with chemokine receptors on human NK cells. In their studies, MCP-1- and RANTES-, but not MIP-1α-induced chemotaxis and GTP binding of IANK cells was inhibited by PTx whereas MCP-1 RANTES- and MIP-1α induced migration, and GTP binding were inhibited by the addition of CTx. Through the permeabilization of IANK cells with streptolysin O and using monoclonal anti–G protein antibodies, these investigators found that anti-G_s, and anti-G_0, and anti-G_x inhibited the migration of IANK cells to MIP-1α, RANTES, and MCP-1 but that anti-G_i inhibited only RANTES- and MCP-1- but not MIP-1α-induced migration of these same NK populations. Similarly, anti-G_s, anti-G_0, and anti-G_x also inhibited the GTP binding and GTPase activity in IANK cells in the presence of MIP-1α, RANTES, and MCP-1 but, again, anti-G_i blocked only RANTES- and MCP-1-mediated GTP binding and GTPase activity. These studies suggested that MCP-1 and RANTES receptors on the surface of NK cells are promiscuously coupled to multiple G proteins in IANK membranes and that this coupling is different from MIP-1α receptors, which seem to be coupled to G_s, G_0, and G_x

but not to G_i. Overall, these studies suggest that different G proteins are engaged on NK cells and IANK cells by different C-C chemokines and that the activation state of an NK cell may contribute to this differential association. Once specific G protein and chemokine receptor associations are determined, we may be able to manipulate specifically chemokine-mediated migration of NK cells.

Finally, Ltn, a member of the C chemokine subfamily that possesses only two of the four characteristic cysteines of the chemokine superfamily, has recently been shown to chemoattract freshly isolated and IL-2-activated human and murine NK cells and human NK cell clones in vitro *(59,66,72)*. Ltn mediates the migration of quiescent NK and IANK as well as NK cells pretreated with C-C chemokines for 7 d, called CHAK cells, at concentrations similar to those observed with C-C chemokines (between 0.01 and 10 ng/mL). Similarly, Ltn also induces significant calcium mobilization in human IANK cells *(66)*. Furthermore, injections of Ltn into the peritoneum of mice resulted in the selective recruitment of lymphocytes within a 24-h period *(59)*. Phenotypic analysis of the cellular infiltrate showed that a large proportion of these cells were T-lymphocytes and NK cells. This activity was found to be specific as the cellular influx was blocked by the administration of anti-Ltn monoclonal antibody. These in vivo Ltn results are quite important because very few agents have ever been shown to induce directly NK cell recruitment in vivo. Similar to the C-C chemokine studies by Maghazachi and coworkers *(66)*, the Ltn receptors on human NK cells also appear to mediate their chemotaxis and calcium mobilization through coupling with G_i, G_0, and G_q in IANK cells and to G_i and G_q in CHAK cells. This differential coupling of various G proteins to Ltn receptors on IANK vs CHAK cell populations is believed to be responsible for the distinct biologic effects of Ltn on IANK vs CHAK cells.

The migration of quiescent NK cells required precoating of polycarbonate filters with various extracellular matrix proteins to facilitate chemokine-mediated migration, suggesting that chemokines may activate these lymphocytes to adhere better to these matrix proteins via their integrin molecules, promoting migration, or that the chemokines are binding directly to the matrix proteins, resulting in a haptotactic chemokine:matrix gradient that promotes migration *(64)*. While quiescent NK cells also migrate in response to chemokines on uncoated filters (albeit weakly), a direct chemokine:NK cell interaction independent of matrix proteins suggests the presence of a direct chemotactic effect in the migration observed. Thus, many studies would suggest that prior activation of NK cells with IL-2 and/or another cytokine may be important to facilitate optimal migration. However, in vivo, infused IANK or LAK cells fail to infiltrate selectively to the sites of tumor growth or into inflammatory sites, but rather distribute into selective organs, namely the lungs, liver, and spleen *(9–12,14)*. Most likely, the interaction of quiescent circulating NK cells via their adhesive molecules with their corresponding ligands on endothelial cells along with a cytokine signal provides the necessary signal for optimal chemokine responsiveness.

3. CHEMOKINES AND NK CELL EFFECTOR FUNCTIONS

An important functional attribute of NK cells is their ability to lyse spontaneously a broad range of virally infected targets or tumor cells in a non-MHC-restricted fashion. Although the mechanisms and molecular bases of NK cell target recognition and interactions between NK cells and their targets are not fully understood, NK-mediated cytolysis of target cells is believed to involve several steps occurring in sequence as follows:

1. Recognition of target cells by an unknown mechanism
2. Conjugate formation between NK and target cells, probably involving various cell adhesion molecules on both effector and target cells
3. NK cell activation, leading to the mobilization and release of cytoplasmic granules (degranulation)
4. Injury or lysis of target cells mediated by granule components.

The NK cell is a selective killer cell that does not harm "self" but eliminates NK-susceptible targets without a need for antigen processing or presentation by MHC molecules *(9–12,73)*. Various cytokines, including IL-2, IFN-γ, IL-12, and IL-15, have been shown to modulate NK activity in nonlymphoid organs *(9–12,35)*. Subsequent studies have demonstrated that organ-associated NK cells contribute to the antimetastatic responses in a number of immunotherapy systems *(9–13,35)*. Mechanisms by which administered cytokines promote NK cell activity within various organs are believed to include the proliferation of resident NK cells after administration of a BRM; the redistribution of NK cells from the spleen to the liver; and/or the recruitment of NK cells from the bone marrow and the resulting subsequent rapid increase in the hepatic localization of these newly recruited cells. Although all these mechanisms most likely contribute, in one way or another, to the observed effects within a number of human immunotherapy trails and experimental rodent models, several investigators have hypothesized that bone marrow recruitment and subsequent localization in organs (such as the liver and lung) is the principal pathway for the observed increase in NK cell activity postcytokine and post-BRM administration. However, the precise mechanism(s) by which this recruitment occurs is still unknown.

Several cytokines including IL-2 and, to a lesser extent, IL-12, TNF-α, and IFN-γ have been shown to augment directly NK cell–mediated cytolysis in vitro *(9,14,27,33)*. These cytokines appear to stimulate and/or costimulate directly NK cell activation and proliferation, priming these lymphocytes into becoming more effective killer cells by promoting not only granule formation and production but also by potentiating conjugate formation and subsequent degranulation. Similarly, chemokines have also been reported to induce similar effects on the enzyme production, granule release, conjugate formation, and tumor cell cytolysis by monocytes, macrophages, and neutrophils *(36–42)*. Recent studies by my laboratory have demonstrated that many C-C chemokines, including MIP-1α, MIP-1β, RANTES, MCP-1, and MCP-3, also enhance human and murine NK cell– and cytotoxic T-lymphocyte (CTL)-mediated killing of susceptible target cells *(45,64)*. As with the chemotaxis studies described previously, many of the C-C chemokines also enhanced NK cell–mediated cytolysis of NK-sensitive target cells in a dose-dependent fashion (1–100 n*M*). Similarly, the C-X-C chemokines, IP-10 and MIG, but not IL-8 or PF4, were also found to induce an increase in NK cell–mediated cytolysis of K562 cells in vitro *(64)*. This chemokine-mediated effect on NK cell cytotoxicity required the presence of NK-sensitive target cells since NK-insensitive tumor cells fail to be lysed in the presence or absence of chemokines. Thus, these findings would suggest that the chemokine-mediated enhancement of NK cytotoxicity is not being mediated through a unique nonspecific cytotoxic pathway but rather by potentiating the ongoing normal response.

Interestingly, while all these C-C chemokines were capable of augmenting quiescent and IFN-γ or IL-2-primed NK-mediated killing of tumor cells, they were quite ineffective, in my hands, at enhancing LAK- or antibody-dependent cell-mediated cytotoxicity (ADCC)-specific cytolytic responses. The fact that chemokines failed to modulate ADCC- and LAK-mediated cytolysis was not surprising because LAK and ADCC responses are quite potent forms of cytotoxicity that are often difficult to augment even with additional IL-2 or IFN-γ. Although this statement appears to contradict the previous discussion of enhanced chemotactic responsiveness of IANK, these findings are not mutually exclusive. The previously cited trafficking studies required extended culturing of the isolated NK cells, in some cases up to 10 d, with IL-2 prior to observing any chemotactic effects by C-C chemokine on NK cells *(14,28,57,60)*. However, in the LAK cytotoxicity studies by my laboratory *(64)*, the isolated NK cells were only cultured for 24 h with IL-2 or IFN-γ prior to their examination with C-C chemokines in chromium release assays. Thus, it would appear that the extent and stage of NK cells' activation may affect their chemokine responsiveness. In general, the more active the cells are for cytotoxic function, the less responsive they are to the cytotoxicity-enhancing effects of chemokines.

Additional studies by Schall and colleagues *(74)* support cytotoxic findings on the cytotoxic-enhancing effects of chemokines demonstrating that pretreatment of CD56[+] but not CD4[+] or CD8[+] lymphocytes with C-C chemokines enhanced their cytotoxic activity toward K562 or Raji target cells. Pretreatment of NK cells for 7 d with any of the C-C chemokines or IL-8 (at 10 ng/mL) induced the generation of killer cells that lysed K562 and Raji cells. Furthermore, these investigators also found that C-C chemokines induced the proliferation of CD56[+] cells. However, in contrast to previous studies by some of these same investigators with T-lymphocytes *(44)*, this chemokine-mediated proliferation required the presence of other cell types such as CD4[+] or CD8[+] lymphocytes, suggesting that various T-cell–derived factors may be necessary for this activation. This hypothesis was confirmed by the use of antibodies to IL-2 and IFN-γ but not IL-1β, TNF-α, IL-8, or GM-CSF, which were found to inhibit RANTES-induced proliferation of nylon-wood column nonadherent cells. These results suggest that RANTES and most likely other C-C chemokines prime CD56[+] lymphocytes to become more responsive to various activation stimuli. However, more detailed studies are needed to determine precise mechanism(s) by which chemokines are modulating cell-mediated cytotoxicity and proliferation.

Previous studies have revealed that LFA-1 and ICAM-1 are critical accessory adhesion molecules for NK:tumor cell conjugate formation. Antibodies specific for these molecules typically block NK-mediated adhesion to K562 cells and subsequent cytolysis *(14,20,64)*. Chemokine effects on NK cytolysis also required β2 integrin–mediated conjugation between the lymphocytes and the target cell populations since antibodies to LFA-1, ICAM-1, and CD18 all blocked both normal and chemokine-mediated cytolysis of K562 cells *(64)*. These results support the previous statement that the chemokines are most likely only costimulating normal NK responses and not mediating unique conjugate-independent killing mechanisms (nonspecific killing).

There are many possible mechanisms for this chemokine-mediated enhancement of CTL and NK cell cytolysis, including increases in cellular degranulation, effector:target cell conjugate formation, or Fas/Fas-ligand/TNF expression. Granule exocytosis is believed to be an important mechanism in CTL- and NK-mediated killing *(9–12)*. Previous studies with neutrophils, basophils, eosinophils, mast cells, and monocytes have demonstrated the ability of chemokines to induce cellular degranulation *(41,42)*. Similarly, CTL clones incubated with various C-C chemokines (10–100 n*M*) were found to degranulate and release granule-derived serine esterases within 30 min of incubation *(45)*. Analogous to the CTL studies described previously, my laboratory has also demonstrated that human NK cells degranulate in response to high concentrations of C-C chemokines (10–250 n*M*) *(64)*. These findings have subsequently been substantiated by Loetscher and colleagues *(55)*, who have also demonstrated the ability of C-C but not C-X-C (including IL-8 or IP-10) chemokines to mediate the release of the granule components granzyme A and *N*-acetyl β-D-glucosaminidase from cloned and purified NK cells. With regard to IP-10, my laboratory, in collaboration with Dr. John Ortaldo *(64)*, has demonstrated that IP-10 also mediated NK cell degranulation and promoted greater degranulation in the presence of immobilized fibronectin or K562 cells. Similar to other chemokine functions, chemokine-induced degranulation also required G protein coupling postreceptor ligation since PTx and CTx treatment inhibited chemokine-induced granule release *(45,55,64)*. These results suggest that C-C chemokines as well as IP-10 may mediate enhanced CTL- and NK-mediated cytolysis via degranulation. At this point, one may ask, How do chemokines facilitate migration and degranulation on the same cells? Well, it seems possible that through a coordinated series of signals, CTL and NK cells migrate from regions of low chemokine concentrations to regions of higher ligand concentrations. On entry into the site(s) of chemokine production, it also seems likely that the CTL and NK cells are promoting migration; however, the cells desensitized to additional chemokine signals may now be stimulated by the chemokines to perform other functions such as adhesion, degranulation, and/or cytolysis.

While the mechanism by which chemokines enhance NK cell–mediated killing is unknown, one potential mechanism by which chemokines enhance cytolytic activity may be an increase in the ability of NK cells to adhere to their tumor cell targets. As described previously, NK cells require various adhesion molecules and integrin receptors to bind to NK-sensitive target cells and mediate lysis. Cell-cell contact is necessary for specific immunologic recognition by NK cells of virally infected or transformed cells *(9–12)*. Immunologic mediators such as IFN-γ, IL-2, IL-1, and TNF-α have been shown to promote these functions *(9–12)*. Chemokines, in addition to activating the chemotactic machinery of leukocytes, also selectively modulate the expression and affinity of adhesion molecules on migrating cells including T-lymphocytes *(41,42)*. A change in the expression or avidity of adhesion molecules on the leukocyte cell surface can profoundly alter the migratory and functional behavior of the effector cells. Previous and current studies from my laboratory have demonstrated that chemokines augment lymphocyte adhesion to endothelium and specific adhesion ligands (i.e., ICAM-1, VCAM-1, fibronectin, etc.) by altering the affinity of their adhesion molecules *(41,42)*. Thus, one may postulate that chemokines may alter NK:tumor cell conjugate formation by altering the avidity of adhesion molecule interactions between the NK cell and the tumor target cell, permitting a more efficacious and potent killing response.

However, the role of chemokines in promoting T cell or NK:tumor conjugate formation is currently under investigation. The role of adhesion molecules is strongly supported by the fact that NK-mediated lysis of K562 cells and degranulation in the presence of MIP-1α was enhanced in the presence of fibronectin and VCAM-1, suggesting that enhancement of cell adhesion and adhesion molecule presentation by chemokines may facilitate or potentiate NK cell cytotoxic activity *(64)*. In addition, I have recently found, using an adherent NK-sensitive melanoma line, that C-C chemokines and IP-10 facilitate NK cell adhesion to tumor cell monolayers within 15 min, suggesting that the chemokines are promoting NK:target cell conjugation (Taub, D., unpublished data). Another possible mechanism for chemokine-induced modulation of tumor cell lysis is provided by data demonstrating that chemokines induce NK cell degranulation *(45,64)*. Granule exocytosis is an important mechanism in NK cell–mediated killing *(9–12)*. Serine esterases, granzymes, and perforins have been shown to be present in NK cell granules and to play an essential role in tumor cell killing in vitro. Although the mechanism(s) of chemokine-induced granule release remains to be defined, it is speculated that as NK cells enter sites of chemokine production, they are induced to release granule contents on conjugation with NK-sensitive tumor cells or in the presence of various adhesion molecules. However, the role of additional factor(s) in these responses remains to be determined.

4. NK CELL TRAFFICKING AND CANCER: ANY RELEVANCE?

Immunohistologic analysis of leukocytic infiltrates in many human tumors indicates that they are composed mainly of macrophages and CD4+ and CD8+ T-lymphocytes with minor elements of neutrophils, B-lymphocytes, eosinophils, and NK cells *(14,35,76,77)*. This poor representation of NK cells in tumor infiltrates has raised many questions about the importance of their role as antitumor effector cells. However, because NK cells are believed to be a first line of defense against tumors, it may not be unusual for the tumor infiltrates of established tumors to lack these cytolytic cells. A number of reports in experimental rodent models have demonstrated NK cell infiltration only at the early stages of tumor growth and formation, not at the later stages in the tumor lesion *(14,76,77)*. Similarly, during viral infections or allograft rejections, infiltrating NK cells precede T-cell entry into the tissue lesions; however, at later time periods, NK cells were not found in these infiltrates. One possible reason for the absence of NK cells in tumor lesions is the fact that NK cells have shorter life spans than other lymphoid cells and macrophages. Although the half-life of an NK cell has not been clearly defined, it has recently been suggested that NK cells survive only a few days in culture and a few weeks in vivo whereas T-lymphocytes and macrophages may survive much longer *(9–12)*. Perhaps this is one reason that NK cells and the short-lived neutrophils and eosinophils are poorly represented within tumor infiltrates. However, it is also possible that certain tumors are not producing the proper chemoattractants to facilitate leukocyte entry.

Over the past 15 yr, several immunotherapy studies have demonstrated that the systemic infusion of cytokines induced significant changes in the phenotypes of cells within the tumor infiltrate *(78)*. Since IL-2 had been shown to exert profound effects on NK cell activation and proliferation *(9–12)*, it was the hope that systemic IL-2 administration would promote the activation, proliferation, and subsequent trafficking of circulating NK cells into established tumor lesions. Unfortunately, although a substantial increase in the number of circulating CD56+ CD16+ lymphocytes was observed, few

NK cells were observed within the intratumoral infiltrates of treated patients *(14,35,79, 80)*. Similarly, systemic infusion protocols using IL-1β, GM-CSF, IFN-γ, and/or TNF-α have also failed to promote increased NK cell trafficking into tumors *(35,78)*.

More recently, cytokine gene transfection into tumors or antigen-presenting cells has led to a more controlled means of introducing specific cytokines into the tumor microenvironment. In these studies, implantation of a cytokine-transfected tumor cell in a host permitted the secretion of high levels of cytokine locally in the tumor area, thus inducing a strong inflammatory response. In contrast to the systemic IL-2 infusion studies, significant lymphocytic infiltrates consisting of both CD4+ and CD8+ T-cells and GM1+ CD56+ NK cells were typically observed in tissue deposits bearing certain IL-2 transfected tumor cells *(78,81)*. In some studies, this tumor cell rejection was highly dependent on the presence of CD8+ T-cells and NK cells *(78)*. However, in other IL-2-transduced tumor models, poor cellular infiltration and poor tumor rejection were observed *(14,35,78)*. In many of these gene-transduced tumor cell studies, the leukocytic infiltrate in the tumor tissue is often quite variable and is highly dependent on a number of factors including the type of tumor utilized, the immunogenicity of the tumor, expression of MHC molecules and T-cell costimulatory molecules on the tumor, the level of tumor vascularization and access, the cytokine being expressed, and the level of cytokine secretion *(78)*. For example, certain IFN-γ-transduced tumor cells induce significant T-cell infiltration with few NK cells and neutrophils whereas IL-4-transduced tumors result in a significant eosinophil and macrophage infiltration with few to no lymphocytes and NK cells *(14,83)*.

Since the early 1980s, the adoptive transfer of LAK cells or tumor-infiltrating lymphocytes (TILs) has been performed in a series of cancer patients, resulting in a low but significant proportion of clinical responses, especially in those with renal cell carcinoma and melanoma *(35)*. Critical to the activity of these systemically transferred effector cells is their localization to tumor sites. However, for the most part, the proportion of LAK and TIL cells capable of penetrating tumor tissues is quite small, consistent with several early lymphocyte trafficking studies demonstrating that highly activated T- and mononuclear cells migrate poorly into peripheral tissues and tend to localize in various organs and lymphatic tissues *(35)*.

Overall, the biologic significance of NK cells as antitumor effector cells remains unproven. Their potent tumoricidal activities in vitro suggest that these cells would be capable of fighting established tumors in vivo. Furthermore, the incidence of cancers is higher in animals in which NK cells are depleted or nonfunctional. However, owing to their poor showing in multiple cytokine infusion and adoptive transfer studies in various cancer patients, and until more clearly defined biologic and molecular mechanisms involved in NK cell trafficking are defined, the use of various BRMs and cytokines in cancer patients, with the ultimate goal of specifically targeting NK cells to tumor sites, should be initiated with great caution. Perhaps with a greater definition of chemokine effects on NK cells, we may be able to specifically recruit quiescent and activated NK and LAK cells into tumor lesions and thus facilitate tumor rejection.

Unfortunately, the recent studies of C-C chemokine-transfected tumor cells suggest that this may be "easier said than done" since only modest effects on mouse survival were observed in response to these implanted tumors, despite the fact that significant monocytic and lymphocytic infiltration was observed within the lesions *(84,85)*. Thus, simply getting these various immune cells into the tumors may not be the only problem we are facing in the immune intervention.

By contrast, adoptive transfer of activated NK cells may have a role in certain clinical settings. Abundant preclinical data support a role for these cells in enhancing hematopoietic and immune reconstitution after bone marrow transplantation *(82)*.

5. CONCLUSION

For years NK cells have been considered invaluable tools for the study of lymphocyte biology and cytotoxicity as well as for the immunotherapy of neoplastic diseases. However, the majority of these studies have been performed within in vitro culture systems and highly controlled in vivo immunotherapy models. Thus, despite the highly supportive laboratory-based studies published on the relevance of NK cells to cancer treatment, the biologic and therapeutic relevance of these cells in cancer has not yet been defined. This chapter summarized the recent findings of chemokines and various cytokines on NK cell chemotaxis and trafficking. In addition to chemotaxis, several other biologic NK cell activities including adhesion, degranulation, proliferation, and cytotoxicity have been shown to be modulated by chemokines. At present, it appears that many of the C-C chemokines exert both unique and overlapping activities on human NK and IANK cells. Perhaps by promoting certain chemokine production within the tumor microenvironment or the chemokine responsiveness of NK or LAK cells in combination with another immunotherapeutic agent (e.g., IL-2 or IL-12), one may be able to enhance NK cell effector activities as well as their trafficking into tumors. Thus, once more detailed studies defining the role of chemokines on NK cell trafficking and effector functions are performed and described, it may be possible to orient effectively NK and LAK cells into tumors.

ACKNOWLEDGMENTS

The author thanks Drs. Dan Longo and Bill Murphy for review of the manuscript. The author also would like to thank Tracy Oppel for her excellent assistance in the preparation of this manuscript.

REFERENCES

1. Butcher, E. C. 1991. Leukocyte-endothelial cell recognition: three (or more) steps to specificity and diversity. *Cell* **67:** 1033.
2. Springer, T. A. 1994. Traffic signals for lymphocyte recirculation and leukocyte emigration: the multistep paradigm. *Cell* **76:** 301.
3. Springer, T. A. 1995. Traffic signals on endothelium for lymphocyte recirculation and leukocyte emigration. *Annu. Rev. Physiol.* **57:** 827.
4. Shimizu, Y., W. Newman, Y. Tanaka, and S. Shaw. 1992. Lymphocyte interactions with endothelial cells. *Immunol. Today* **13:** 106.
5. Butcher, E. C., and L. J. Picker. 1996. Lymphocyte homing and homeostasis. *Science* **272:** 60.
6. McIntyre, K. W., and R. M. Welsh. 1986. Accumulation of natural killer and cytotoxic T large granular lymphocytes in the liver during virus infection. *J. Exp. Med.* **164:** 1667.
7. Natuk, R. J., and R. M. Welsh. 1987. Accumulation and chemotaxis of natural killer/large granular lymphocytes at sites of virus replication. *J. Immunol.* **138:** 877.
8. Nemlander, A. , E. Saksela, and P. Hayrj. 1983. Are natural killer cells involved in allograft rejection? *Eur. J. Immunol.* **13:** 348.

9. Herberman, R. B., and J. R. Ortaldo. 1981. NK cells: their role in defense against disease. *Science* **214:** 24.

10. Robertson, M. J., and J. Ritz. 1990. Biology and clinical relevance of human natural killer cells. *Blood* **76:** 2421.

11. Trinchieri, G. 1989. Biology of natural killer cells, in *Advances in Immunology, vol. 47* (Dixon, F. J., ed.), Academic, San Diego, p. 187.

12. Whiteside, T. L., and R. B. Herberman. 1994. Role of human natural killer cells in health and disease. *Clin. Diag. Lab. Immunol.* **1:** 125.

13. Pilaro, A. M., D. D. Taub, K. L. McCormick, H. M. Williams, T. J. Sayers, W. E. Fogler, and R. H. Wiltrout. 1994. TNF-α is a principal cytokine involved in the recruitment of NK cells to liver parenchyma. *J. Immunol.* **153:** 333–342.

14. Allavena, P., S. Sozzani, and A. Mantovani. 1997. Molecules involved in trafficking of NK cells and dendritic cells: implications for tumour immunotherapy, in *Adhesion Molecules and Chemokines in Lymphocyte Trafficking*. Harwood Academic, Germany, p. 201.

15. Holmberg, L. A., K. A. Springer, and K. A. Ault. 1981. Natural killer activity in the peritoneal exudate of mice infected with listeria monocytogenes. *J. Immunol.* **127:** 1792.

16. Glimpel, G. R., D. W. Niesel, M. Asuncion, and K. D. Klimpel. 1988. Natural killer cell activation and interferon production by peripheral blood lymphocytes after exposure to bacteria. *Infect. Immun.* **56:** 1436–1441.

17. Bottazzi, B., M. Introna, P. Allavena, A. Villa, and A. Mantovani. 1985. In vitro migration of human large granular lymphocytes. *J. Immunol.* **134:** 2316.

18. Pohajdak, B., J. Gomez, F. W. Orr, N. Khalik, M. Talgoy, and A. H. Greenberg. 1986. Chemotaxis of large granular lymphocytes. *J. Immunol.* **136:** 278.

19. Polentarutti, N., B. Bottazzi, C. Balotta, A. Erroi, and A. Mantovani. 1986. Modulation of the locomotory capacity of human large granular lymphocytes. *Cell Immunol.* **101:** 204.

20. Somersalo, K., O. Carpen, and E. Saksela. 1994. Stimulated natural killer cells secrete factors with chemotactic activity, including NAP-1 IL-8, which supports VLA-4- and VLA-5-mediated migration of T lymphocytes. *Eur. J. Immunol.* **24:** 2957.

21. Allavena, P., C. Paganin, I. Martin Padura, G. Peri, M. Gaboli, E. Dejana, P. C. Marchisio, and A. Mantovani. 1991. Molecules and structures involved in the adhesion of natural killer cells to vascular endothelium. *J. Exp. Med.* **173:** 439.

22. Gismondi, A., S. Morrone, M. J. Humphries, M. Piccoli, L. Frati, and A. Santoni. 1991. Human natural killer cells express VLA-4 and VLA-5, which mediate their adhesion to fibronectin. *J. Immunol.* **146:** 384.

23. Somersalo, K., and E. Sakela. 1991. Fibronectin facilitates the migration of human natural killer cells. *Eur. J. Immunol.* **21:** 35.

24. Bianchi, G., M. Sironi, E. Ghibaudi, C. Selvaggini, M. Elices, P. Allavena, and A. Mantovani. 1993. Migration of natural killer cells across endothelial cell monolayers. *J. Immunol.* **151:** 5135.

25. Aronson, F. R., P. Libby, E. P. Brandon, M. W. Janicka, and J. W. Mier. 1988. IL-2 rapidly induces natural killer cell adhesion to human endothelial cells: a potential mechanism for endothelial injury. *J. Immunol.* **141:** 158.

26. Rabinovich, H., R. B. Herberman, and T. Whiteside. 1993. Differential effects of IL-12 and IL-2 in expression and function of cellular adhesion molecules on purified NK cells. *Cell Immunol.* **152:** 481.

27. Allavena, P., C. Paganin, D. Zhou, G. Bianchi, S. Sozzani, and A. Mantovani. 1994. Interleukin-12 is chemotactic for natural killer cells and stimulates their interaction with vascular endothelium. *Blood* **84(7):** 2261–2268.

28. Maghazachi, A. A., and A. Al-Aoukaty. 1993. Guanine nucleotide binding proteins mediate the chemotactic signal of transforming growth factor-1 in rat IL-2-activated natural killer cells. *Int. Immunol.* **5:** 825–832.

29. Maghazachi, A. A., and A. Al-Aoukaty. 1993. Transforming growth factor-1 is chemotactic for interleukin-2-activated natural killer cells. *Nat. Immunity* **12:** 57–61.

30. Maghazachi, A. A. 1991. Tumor necrosis factor-α is chemokinetic for lymphokine-activated natural killer cells: regulation by cyclic adenosine monophosphate. *J. Leuk. Biol.* **49:** 302–308.

31. Robertson, M. J., M. A. Caligiuri, T. J. Manley, H. Levine, and J. Ritz. 1990. Human natural killer cell adhesion molecules: differential expression after activation and participation in cytolysis. *J. Immunol.* **145:** 3194.

32. Maenpoaa, A., J. Jaakelainen, O. Carpen, M. Patarroyo, and T. Timonen. 1993. Expression of integrins and other adhesion molecules on NK cells: impact of IL-2 on short- and long-term cultures. *Int. J. Cancer* **53:** 850.

33. Ortaldo, J. R., A. Mason, and R. Overton. 1986. Lymphokine-activated killer (LAK) cells: analysis of progenitors and effectors. *J. Exp. Med.* **164:** 1193.

34. Pirelli, A., P. Allavena, and A. Mantovani. 1988. Activated adherent large granular lymphocytes/natural killer (LGL/NK) cells change their migratory behaviour. *Immunology* **65:** 651.

35. Rosenberg, S. A. 1992. Karnofsky Memorial Lecture. The immunotherapy and gene therapy of cancer. *J. Clin. Oncol.* **10:** 180.

36. Baggiolini, M., B. Dewald, and B. Moser. 1994. Interleukin-8 and related chemotactic cytokines—CXC and CC chemokines. *Adv. Immunol.* **55:** 97.

37. Oppenheim, J. J., J. M. Wang, O. Chertov, D. D. Taub, and A. Ben-Baruch. 1996. The role of chemokines in transplantation, in *Transplantation Biology: Cellular and Molecular Aspects* (Tilney, N. L., et al., eds.), Lippincott-Raven, Philadelphia, p. 21.1.

38. Schall, T. J., and K. B. Bacon. 1994. Chemokines, leukocyte trafficking, and inflammation. *Curr. Opin. Immunol.* **6:** 865.

39. Tanaka, Y., D. H. Adams, and S. Shaw. 1993. Proteoglycans on endothelial cells present adhesion-inducing cytokines to leukocytes. *Immunol. Today* **14:** 111.

40. Taub, D. D., and J. J. Oppenheim. 1994. Chemokines, inflammation and the immune system. *Ther. Immunol.* **1:** 229.

41. Taub, D. D., and W. J. Murphy. Chemokines as mediators of adhesion and migration, in *Adhesion Molecules and Lymphocyte Trafficking* (Hamann, A., ed.), Harwood Academic, Switzerland.

42. Taub, D. D. 1996. Chemokines-leukocyte interactions: the voodoo that they do so well. *Cytokine Growth Factor Rev.* **7(4):** 355–376.

43. Kelner, G. S., J. Kennedy, K. Bacon, S. Kleynsteuber, D. A. Largaespada, N. A. Jenkins, N. G. Copeland, J. F. Bazan, K. W. Moore, T. J. Schall, and A. Zlotnik. 1994. Lymphotactin: a cytokine that represents a new class of chemokines. *Science* **266:** 1395.

44. Bacon, K. B., B. A. Premack, P. Gardner, and T. J. Schall. 1995. Activation of dual T cell signaling pathways by the chemokine RANTES. *Science* **269:** 1727.

45. Taub, D. D., J. R. Ortaldo, S. M. Turcovski-Corrales, M. L. Key, D. L. Longo, and W. J. Murphy. 1996. β Chemokines costimulate lymphocyte cytolysis, proliferation, and lymphokine production. *J. Leuk. Biol.* **59:** 81.

46. Taub, D. D., S. M. Turcovski-Corrales, M. L. Key, D. L. Longo, and W. J. Murphy. 1996. Chemokines and T lymphocytes: α and β chemokines costimulate human T lymphocyte proliferation and lymphokine production in vitro. *J. Immunol.* **156:** 2095.

47. Murphy, W. J., Z.-G. Tian, O. Asai, S. Funakoshi, P. Rotter, M. Henry, R. M. Strieter, S. L. Kunkel, D. L. Longo, and D. D. Taub. 1996. Chemokines and T lymphocyte activation. II. Facilitation of human T cell trafficking in severe combined immunodeficiency mice. *J. Immunol.* **156:** 2104.

48. Murphy, P. M. 1994. The molecular biology of leukocyte chemoattractant receptors. *Annu. Rev. Immunol.* **12:** 593.

49. Taub, D. D., A. R. Lloyd, K. Conlon, J. M. Wang, J. R. Ortaldo, A. Harada, K. Matsushima,

D. J. Kelvin, and J. J. Oppenheim. 1993. Recombinant human interferon-inducible protein 10 is a chemoattractant for human monocytes and T lymphocytes and promotes T cell adhesion to endothelial cells. *J. Exp. Med.* **177:** 1809.

50. Taub, D. D., K. Conlon, A. R. Lloyd, J. J. Oppenheim, and D. J. Kelvin. 1993. Preferential migration of activated CD4$^+$ and CD4$^+$ T cells in response to MIP-1α and MIP-1β. *Science* **260:** 355.

51. Taub, D. D., A. S. R. Lloyd, K. Conlon, J. M. Wang, J. R. Ortaldo, A. Harada, K. Matsushima, D. J. Kelvin, and J. J. Oppenheim. 1993. Recombinant human interferon-inducible protein 10 is a chemoattractant for human monocytes and T lymphocytes and promotes T cell adhesion to endothelial cells. *J. Exp. Med.* **177:** 1809.

52. Tanaka, Y., D. H. Adams, S. Hubscher, H. Hirano, U. Siebenlist, and S. Shaw. 1993. T-cell adhesion induced by proteoglycan-immobilized cytokine MIP-1. *Nature* **361:** 81.

53. Taub, D. D., P. Proost, W. J. Murphy, M. Anver, D. L. Longo, J. Van Damme, and J. J. Oppenheim. 1995. Monocyte chemotactic protein-1 (MCP-1), -2, and -3 are chemotactic for human T lymphocytes. *J. Clin. Invest.* **95:** 1370.

54. Murphy, W. J., D. D. Taub, M. Anver, K. Conlon, J. J. Oppenheim, D. J. Kelvin, and D. L. Longo. 1994. Human RANTES induces the migration of human T lymphocytes into the peripheral tissues of mice with severe combined immune deficiency. *Eur. J. Immunol.* **24(8):** 1823.

55. Loetscher, P., M. Seitz, I. Clark-Lewis, M. Baggiolini, and B. Moser. 1996. Activation of NK cells by CC chemokines: chemotaxis, Ca^{2+} mobilization, and enzyme release. *J. Immunol.* **156:** 322–327.

56. Loetscher, P., M. Seitz, I. Clark-Lewis, M. Baggiolini, and B. Moser. 1994. Monocyte chemotactic proteins MCP-1, MCP-2, and MCP-3 are major attractants for human CD4$^+$ and CD8$^+$ T lymphocytes. *FASEB J.* **8:** 1055.

57. Allavena, P., G. Bianchi, D. Zhou, J. Van Damme, P. Jilek, S. Sozzani, and A. Mantovani. 1994. Induction of natural killer cell migration by monocyte chemotactic protein-1, -2, and -3. *Eur. J. Immunol.* **24:** 3233–3236.

58. Carr, M. W., S. J. Roth, E. Luther, S. S. Rose, and T. A. Springer. 1994. Monocyte chemoattractant protein 1 acts as a T-lymphocyte chemoattractant. *Proc. Natl. Acad. Sci. USA* **91:** 3652.

59. Hedrick, J. A., V. Saylor, D. Figueroa, L. Mizoue, Y. Xu, S. Menon, J. Abrams, T. Handel, and A. Zlotnick. 1997. Lymphotactin is produced by NK cells and attracts both NK cells and T cells in vivo. *J. Immunol.* **158:** 1533–1540.

60. Loetscher, A., B. Gerber, P. Loetscher, S. A. Jones, L. Piali, I. Clark-Lewis, M. Baggiolini, and B. Moser. 1996. Chemokine receptor specific for IP-10 and Mig: structure, function, and expression in activated T-lymphocytes. *J. Exp. Med.* **184:** 963–969.

61. Bluman, E. M., K. J. Bartynski, B. R. Avalos, and M. A. Caligiuri. 1996. Human natural killer cells produce abundant macrophage inflammatory protein-1 in response to monocyte-derived cytokines. *J. Clin. Invest.* **97:** 2722–2727.

62. Taub, D. Unpublished data.

63. Sebok, K., D. Woodside, A. Al-Aoukaty, A. D. Ho, S. Gluck, and A. A. Maghazachi. 1993. IL-8 induces the locomotion of human IL-2-activated natural killer cells: involvement of a guanine nucleotide binding (G$_0$) protein. *J. Immunol.* **150:** 1524–1534.

64. Taub, D. D., T. Sayers, C. Carter, and J. R. Ortaldo. 1995. Chemokines induce NK cell migration and enhance NK cell cytolytic activity via cellular degranulation. *J. Immunol.* **155:** 3877.

65. Taub, D. D., D. L. Longo, and W. J. Murphy. 1996. Human IP-10 induces mononuclear cell infiltration in mice and promotes the migration of human T lymphocytes into the peripheral tissues of huPBL-SCID mice. *Blood* **87:** 1423.

66. Maghazachi, A. A., B. S. Skalhegg, B. Rolstad, and A. Al-Aoukaty. 1997. Interferon-

inducible protein-10 and lymphotactin induce the chemotaxis and mobilization of intracellular calcium in natural killer cells through pertussis toxin-sensitive and -insensitive heterotrimeric G-proteins. *FASEB J.* **11:** 765–774.

67. Taub, D. Unpublished data.

68. Maghazachi, A. A., A. Al-Aoukaty, and T. J. Schall. 1994. C-C chemokines induce the chemotaxis of NK and IL-2-activated NK cells: role of G proteins. *J. Immunol.* **153:** 4969–4977.

69. Maghazachi, A. A., T. J. Schall, and A. Al-Aoukaty. Differential coupling of CC chemokine receptors to multiple heterotrimeric G proteins in human interleukin-2-activated natural killer cells. *Blood.* **87:** 4255–4260.

70. Polentarutti, N., et al. 1997. IL-2 regulated expression of the monocyte chemotactic protein-1 receptor (CC CKR2) in human NK cells: characterization of a predominant 3.4 Kb transcript containing CC CKR2A and CC CKR2B sequences. *J. Immunol.* **158:** 2689–2694.

71. Maghazachi, A. A., and A. Al-Aoukaty. 1994. G_s is the major G protein involved in interleukin-2-activated natural killer (IANK) cell-mediated cytotoxicity: successful introduction of anti-G protein antibodies inside streptolysin O-permeabilized IANK cells. *J. Biol. Chem.* **269:** 6796–6802.

72. Bianchi, G., S. Sozzani, A. Zlotnik, A. Mantovani, and P. Allavena. 1996. Migratory response of human natural killer cells to lymphotactin. *Eur. J. Immunol.* **26:** 3238–3241.

73. Frey, J. L., T. Bino, R. R. S. Kantor, D. M. Segal, S. L. Giardina, J. Roder, S. Anderson, and J. R. Ortaldo. 1991. Mechanism of target cell recognition by natural killer cells: characterization of a novel triggering molecule restricted to CD3⁻ large granular lymphocytes. *J. Exp. Med.* **174:** 1527.

74. Maghazachi, A. A., A. Al-Aoukaty, and T. J. Schall. 1996. CC chemokines induce the generation of killer cells from CD56⁺ cells. *Eur. J. Immunol.* **26:** 315–319.

75. Taub, D. Unpublished data.

76. Allavena, P., and A. Mantovani. 1994. Therapeutic strategies targeted to tumor-associated leukocytes in human tumors, in *Tumor-Associated Leukocytes: Pathophysiology and Therapeutic Applications* (Mantovani, A., ed.), R. G. Landes, Austin, p. 90.

77. Kurosawa, S., G. Matsuzaki, M. Harada, T. Ando, and K. Nomoto. 1993. Early appearance and activation of natural killer cells in tumor-infiltrating lymphoid cells during tumor development. *Eur. J. Immunol.* **23:** 1029.

78. Pardoll, D. M. 1995. Paracrine cytokine adjuvants in cancer immunotherapy. *Annu. Rev. Immunol.* **13:** 399.

79. Velotti, F., A. Stoppacciaro, L. Ruc, A. Tubsaro, A. Pettinato, S. Morrone, T. Napolitano, P. C. Bossola, C. R. Franks, P. Palmer, et al. 1991. Local activation of immune response in bladder cancer patients treated with intraarterial infusion of recombinant interleukin-2. *Cancer Res.* **51:** 2456.

80. Cohen, P. J., M. T. Lotze, J. R. Roberts, S. A. Rosenberg, and E. S. Jaffe. 1987. The immunopathology of sequential tumor biopsies in patients treated with interleukin-2: correlation of response with T-cell infiltration and HLA-DR expression. *Am. J. Pathol.* **129:** 208.

81. Gansbacher, B., K. Zier, B. Daniels, K. Cronin, R. Bannerji, and E. Gilboa. 1990. Interleukin 2 gene transfer into tumor cells abrogates tumorigenicity and induces protective immunity. *J. Exp. Med.* **172:** 1217.

82. Murphy, W. J., and D. L. Longo. 1997. The potential role of NK cells in the separation of graft-versus-tumor effects from graft-versus-host disease after allogeneic bone marrow transplantation. *Immunol. Rev.* **157:** 167–176.

83. Gansbacher, B., R. Bannerji, B. Daniels, K. Zier, K. Cronin, and E. Gilboa. 1990. Retroviral vector-mediated gamma-interferon gene transfer into tumor cells generates potent and long lasting antitumor immunity. *Cancer Res.* **50:** 7820.

84. Dilloo, D., K. Bacon, W. Holden, W. Zhong, S. Burdach, A. Zlotnik, and M. Brenner. 1996. Combined chemokine and cytokine gene transfer enhances antitumor immunity. *Nat. Med.* **2(10):** 1090–1095.

85. Tannenbaum, C. S., N. Wicker, D. Armstrong, R. Tubbs, J. Finke, R. M. Bukowski, and T. A. Hamilton. 1996. Cytokine and chemokine expression in tumors of mice receiving systemic therapy with IL-12. *J. Immunol.* **156:** 693–699.

6

Tumor Infiltration by Monocytes and the Antitumor Effects of Monocyte Chemoattractant Protein-1

Barrett J. Rollins, Howard A. Fine,
Long Gu, Kenzo Soejima, and Susan Tseng

1. A HISTORY OF MONONUCLEAR CELL INFILTRATION IN CANCER

Mononuclear cell infiltration is a common feature of many types of human cancers. In fact, its occurrence is considered so unremarkable that there are no systematic studies describing the prevalence or intensity of infiltrates by tumor type or stage. Instead, it is generally asserted that intense infiltrates are associated with certain tumor types, such as medullary carcinoma of the breast and malignant melanoma (1,2), and that most other cancers are also infiltrated to differing extents. Even without an "epidemiology" of tumor-related inflammatory infiltrates, tumor biologists have extensively focused on this phenomenon for more than 100 yr.

Leukocyte infiltration in cancer has been appreciated since the beginning of microscopic analyses of human tumors, but controversy surrounded the question of its origin and the causal relationship in which it stands to carcinogenesis. Virchow (3) first described the association of inflammatory cells with human tumors and inferred that cancers arose from transformed connective tissue elements (including leukocytes) at sites of chronic inflammation. Later, Waldeyer (4) argued more persuasively for homotypic tissue sources for malignancy, e.g., carcinomas derived from transformed epithelial cells. Nonetheless, he and others asserted that the infiltrative component was an integral and causal part of the tumor.

Not until the early 1900s could some of these issues be resolved through the analysis of transplantable tumors in animals. Jensen (5) used a murine tumor to demonstrate that tumor tissue in the recipient animal was derived from injected tumor cells rather than the host. Bashford (6) used Jensen's tumor and other models to show that donor stroma contaminating the injected tumor dies after inoculation, and thus the stroma surrounding and infiltrating the mature tumor in the recipient was derived from the recipient host rather than the donor tumor. This stroma was examined in detail by Russell (7), who coined the term *stromal reaction* to describe the collection of mononuclear cells, fibroblasts, and connective tissue elements elicited by a transplanted tumor in a susceptible host. A more thorough analysis of the stromal reaction in transplanted murine tumors was provided by Da Fano (8). In fully developed tumors, he described an infiltration by "lymphocytes" and large numbers of the "quiescent wandering cells" of Maximow, which have a monocyte-like morphology and were later shown to stain for nonspecific esterase *(9)*. Similar observations were made by Wade *(10)*, in his analysis of transplantable sarcomas in dogs.

In susceptible animals, i.e., those that did not reject tumors, Russell was careful to point out that the character of the stromal response could vary among different tumor types. Notably, however, the characteristic stromal reaction was tumor-type specific and remained constant during subsequent passage of the tumor in different animals. For example, tumors that elicited highly cellular stromal reactions always did so. This led Russell to postulate, for the first time, that tumors might have specific "chemotactic" properties that elicit a characteristic stromal reaction. (A similar chemotactic property was suggested to account for capillary ingrowth both by Russell and Ehrlich, anticipating the recent interest in tumor angiogenesis by 75 yr *[11]*.) Still, the general consensus was that the stromal reaction was necessary to support malignant growth. Thus, in immunized animals that rejected tumors, the mechanism of resistance was believed to be the inability of the tumor to induce the development of a properly organized stroma *(7,8)*.

During the first half of the twentieth century, as most of these studies were being performed, there was little precision in identifying leukocytes involved in tumor infiltration. However, by the 1950s, stains based on nonspecific esterase activity demonstrated that the "resting wandering cells" surrounding and invading solid tumors were macrophages, and significant numbers could be found in association with human cancers *(9)*. The number of macrophages in these tumors was found to vary widely, and based on enzymatic profiles it could be shown that some of the macrophages associated with tumors were derived from blood monocytes *(12)*. Electron microscopic examination of human tumors confirmed the presence of lymphocytes, macrophages, and plasma cells as common elements in the stroma of human malignancies *(1,2,13)*.

2. QUANTITATION OF MACROPHAGE INFILTRATES AND THEIR FUNCTION

Despite these historical observations, there has been ongoing controversy about whether or not macrophages comprise a significant proportion of the cellular population of human cancers. Simple morphologic assessment by light microscopic examination of conventionally stained sections may underestimate the number of macrophages. For example, an analysis of 52 breast cancer specimens identified an average of 22 CD45+ cells per high-power field, 78% of which were classified as monocytes based on nonspecific esterase activity or surface marker staining *(14)*. However, most of these cells had a spindle morphology and would have been scored as fibroblasts without the staining information. Interestingly, these cells appeared mostly in stroma surrounding the tumors and vastly outnumbered any associated T-lymphocyte infiltration. Macrophages can also commonly be mistaken for lymphocytes in conventional analyses.

In another study of 45 tumors of various types, nearly all were associated with stromal infiltrates containing a high proportion of CD16+/CD11c+ cells *(15)*. These cells were most likely to be monocytes and not natural killer (NK) cells because they had nonspecific esterase activity. In many cases, these cells comprised 50–70% of the total cellular population. These results are certainly consistent with some experimental models in which macrophages can account for 25–50% of the entire cellular content of syngeneic tumors in rodents *(16)*. Infiltrates varied with tumor type and were most common in renal cell carcinoma, melanoma, and colorectal carcinomas, although CD16⁻/CD11c⁺ cells of similar appearance were also very common in breast and lung carcinomas. Expression of CD16 may be related to the activation or maturation status of the monocytes and may explain why other investigators see lower proportions of CD16⁺ cells in tumor infiltrates (although technical differences may also account for the discrepancy) *(17)*. This suggests that some straightforward immunohistochemical analyses may also underestimate the true proportion of macrophages in tumors.

Macrophages have also been identified in human cancers by disrupting tumor tissue and plating cells in tissue culture *(18)*. In 27 tumors examined in one such study, the proportion of macrophages ranged from 0 to 30%, and this procedure routinely identified a higher proportion of macrophages in the tumor than that predicted by light microscopy. Interestingly, all tumors that were known to have metastasized had fewer than 10% macrophages, suggesting the possibility that local macrophage infiltration might suppress this phenomenon. However, nonmetastatic tumors were found to have the full range of macrophage infiltration. Still, the low proportion of macrophages cultured from metastatic tumors is reminiscent of a rodent model in which the proportion of macrophage infiltration in tumors correlated inversely with the presence of metastases *(19)*.

These latter observations led to the presumption that macrophage infiltration reflected the host's attempt to reject the tumor, rather than support it. Several studies have attempted to test this hypothesis by correlating macrophage content with clinical outcome, but the results have been decidedly mixed. For example, retrospective analyses of infiltrating ductal breast cancers suggested that a plasma cell infiltrate *(20)* or a lymphoid infiltrate *(21)* correlated with long-term survival. In the latter case, sinus histiocytic reactions in draining lymph nodes was also associated with improved survival *(21)*. However, another breast cancer study demonstrated no such correlation *(22)*. In esophageal carcinomas, the extent of inflammatory cell infiltration, primarily macrophages, plasma cells, and eosinophils, correlated with postsurgical survival *(23)*. Lymphocytic infiltration also portended improved survival in childhood neuroblastoma *(24)*, but no prognostic information could be attributed to infiltrates in a study of ovarian cancer *(25)*.

These contradictory results could be a reflection of the dual role played by infiltrating cells, in particular macrophages. On the one hand, their cytocidal capacity immediately suggests a mechanism for direct antitumor activity, and a variety of experimental models have generated evidence consistent with this idea. For example, Fidler *(26)* demonstrated several years ago that activated syngeneic macrophages could reduce the incidence of pulmonary metastases in the murine B16 melanoma model. Similar results have been found in other models, some of which may be partially T-lymphocyte dependent *(27,28)*.

On the other hand, it has been appreciated that an immune effector response can also enhance tumor cell growth. Prehn *(29)* demonstrated that mixing a small number of sensitized spleen cells with a tumor inoculum enhanced tumor growth, whereas a larger proportion of spleen cells inhibited growth. This biphasic influence of macrophages on tumor growth has more recently been advanced by Mantovani and colleagues *(30)* (*see* Chapter 3). One straightforward mechanism for enhanced tumor growth, which has been recognized experimentally since the 1920s *(31)*, is that macrophages secrete growth-promoting substances, i.e., growth factors. In addition, however, macrophages may also secrete angiogenic factors, thereby contributing indirectly to tumor growth. A recent analysis of 101 breast cancers demonstrated a striking correlation between macrophage index (proportion of CD68[+] cells) and vascular grade (areas of CD31 positivity) *(32)*. In this carefully performed study there was also a strong association between macrophage index and decreased survival.

The foregoing summary indicates that monocyte/macrophage infiltration can comprise a significant proportion of the cellular component of many human malignancies and might influence their clinical behavior in complex ways. However, this simple statement raises more questions than it answers: What is the signal that attracts monocytes to these tumors? Why do some cancers attract monocytes and others do not? And, perhaps most important, do the infiltrating monocytes and macrophages have any predictable effect on cancer behavior? One would like to think that macrophages are involved in the host's antitumor response, but as pointed out previously, in some cases macrophages clearly contribute more to the well-being of the tumor than the host. And, of course, the fact remains that even well-infiltrated malignancies kill people. As R. Evans, one of the pioneers in this field, once wrote, "It is difficult to envisage that tumor macrophages, or any other infiltrating host cells, may be cytotoxic when in general terms syngeneic tumors continue to grow and overwhelm the host" *(16)*.

To address these questions in a rigorous way, one would like to be able to alter the macrophage content of experimental tumors and to assess the resulting changes in biologic behavior. The ability of chemokines to attract specific types of leukocytes in vivo may provide the potential for manipulating tumor macrophage content in vivo. Engineering alterations of chemokine expression may permit one to address the question, Do macrophages influence tumor behavior and, if so, in what direction? A great deal of effort has focused on monocyte chemoattractant protein-1 (MCP-1), which is a major monocyte chemotactic factor in a variety of inflammatory conditions. Furthermore, MCP-1 is expressed by many human tumor cell types. The remainder of this chapter discusses the properties of MCP-1 in vitro and in vivo, and presents data that may link MCP-1 expression to monocyte/macrophage function, which, in turn, may influence the behavior of cancers in vivo.

3. MCP-1 AS A TUMOR-DERIVED CHEMOATTRACTANT FOR MONOCYTES

The search for tumor-derived monocyte chemoattractants coincided temporally with the more general search for leukocyte-specific chemotactic factors that resulted in the discovery of chemokines. In the early 1980s, Mantovani and colleagues *(33)* demonstrated that tumor cells in culture secreted monocyte-specific chemoattractant activity that correlated with the extent of monocyte infiltration when these cells formed tumors in vivo. This observation indicated the possibility that infiltrating monocytes were attracted by the tumors themselves rather than by an associated T-cell-dependent immune response, and suggested the existence of a tumor-derived chemotactic factor, as anticipated by Russell *(7)*. A similar correlation was found for human ovarian cancer explants *(34)*.

These observations, and the postulated existence of a tumor-derived chemoattractant for monocytes, occurred at about the same time that several groups isolated a novel

Table 1
Tumors and Tumor Cells That Secrete MCP-1

Glioblastoma cell lines *(36)*
Primary glioblastomas *(82)*
Malignant ependymoma *(82)*
Myelomonocytic leukemia cell lines (THP-1 *[37]*; HL-60 *[83]*)
Fibrosarcoma cell line *(45)*
Mammary carcinoma cell line (rat) *(66)*
Osteosarcoma cell lines *(39,84)*
Ovarian carcinomas (primary) *(85)*
Melanoma cell lines *(39)*
Rhabdomyosarcoma cell lines *(39)*
Renal cell carcinoma cell lines (murine; RENCA) *(86)*
Lung cancer cell line (Calu-3) *(87)*
Primary melanoma *(88)*
Malignant fibrous histiocytoma explants *(89)*

monocyte-specific chemotactic factor. The primate form, called smooth muscle cell chemotactic factor, was purified from the medium of baboon aortic smooth muscle cells in culture *(35)*. However, the human version was isolated independently, by two groups, from malignant cell lines: MCP-1 from gliomas, and monocyte chemotactic and activating factor from myelomonocytic leukemia cells *(36,37)*. Later, it became clear that at least part of the activity ascribed to a tumor-derived monocyte chemotactic factor was due to MCP-1 *(38,39)*.

The murine version of MCP-1 had been described several years earlier as the product of a gene whose expression is induced rapidly after the exposure of murine fibroblasts to platelet-derived growth factor *(40–42)*. Human MCP-1 is 76 amino acids in length, and the first 76 amino acids of murine MCP-1 are very similar to the human version. However, murine MCP-1 differs from its human counterpart by the presence of an additional 49 amino acids at the C-terminus that are highly substituted with sialylated O-linked carbohydrate *(43)*. This glycosylated extension does not affect monocyte chemoattractant activity in vitro, since human and murine MCP-1 have identical biologic specific activities in Boyden chamber monocyte chemotaxis assays. It remains to be determined whether or not the C-terminal domain has a distinctive function in vivo that may be lacking in the human form or supplied *in trans* by another molecule.

The identification and cloning of MCP-1 provided an opportunity to screen tumors for their expression of a bona fide monocyte-specific chemoattractant. Table 1 lists several types of cell lines, tumor explants, and primary tumor tissues that express MCP-1. Although the list appears to be extensive, MCP-1 expression is not a universal property of tumor cells since there are many tumor types that do not express MCP-1, e.g., prostate carcinoma and many lung cancers *(44)*.

4. IN VIVO ACTIVITIES OF MCP-1

What is lacking from lists such as the one presented in Table 1 is proof that MCP-1 is responsible for whatever monocytic infiltrate may be associated with these tumors in vivo. Thus, another opportunity afforded by the cloning of MCP-1 is the ability to manipulate its expression in experimental tumor models. However, the first question that must be addressed is, Do MCP-1's in vitro chemoattractant properties accurately predict its in vivo functions? This has been an important issue to settle because of controversy in the literature about the effects of injecting MCP-1 into rodents. For example, whereas some groups describe elicitation of a mild mononuclear cell infiltrate, others report no such response even after injection of very high concentrations of MCP-1 *(43,45)*.

One reason for the discrepancy may involve technical problems inherent in delivering chemokines by injection. MCP-1 might have a relatively short half-life in vivo so that a single injection could have a very limited biologic effect. Hence, another way to test the effects of MCP-1 in vivo is through transgenic expression. This has been attempted by several investigators, with some interesting and unexpected results. One of the first attempts at transgenic MCP-1 expression was a model in which murine MCP-1 was expressed under the control of the mouse mammary tumor virus long terminal repeat (MMTV-LTR) *(46)*. The MMTV-LTR is a powerful promoter capable of directing transgene expression in a variety of organs including salivary gland, breast, gonads, and, to a lesser extent, lung, spleen, and kidney. MMTV-MCP-1 mice were constructed with the expectation that in any organ in which MCP-1 was expressed, a significant monocytic infiltrate would be observed. MMTV-MCP-1 mice could be shown to express high levels of biologically active MCP-1 in selected organs consistent with the known expression patterns of the MMTV-LTR. However, no monocytic infiltrates were ever observed in any organ of any mouse at any age.

The absence of inflammatory infiltration in this model was ascribed to the high level of MCP-1 found in the serum of these transgenic mice. Serum concentrations were essentially as high as those that induce optimal chemoattractant responses in vitro, and therefore it was suggested that receptors for MCP-1 on circulating monocytes might be desensitized. Consistent with this explanation was the observation that these transgenic mice were more susceptible to lethal infection by intracellular pathogens that require an intact monocyte response for their eradication, such as *Listeria monocytogenes* and *Mycobacterium tuberculosis*. In other words, the transgenic mice behaved as if they suffered from a general depression of monocyte activity. (A similar impairment of neutrophil responses to local interleukin-8 [IL-8] was observed in transgenic mice expressing systemic IL-8 *[47]* or in rabbits injected intravenously with IL-8 *[48,49]*.) However, it should be pointed out that an alternative explanation might be that MCP-1 stimulates a Th2 response at the expense of Th1, which would be necessary in order for the animals to handle these infections. There are, in fact, some indications that Th2 responses can be stimulated by MCP-1 *(50,51)*.

These observations suggest that systemic and high-level expression of MCP-1 does not produce monocyte infiltration and that it may instead have a suppressive effect. Therefore, to examine the effect of local expression of MCP-1, several investigators have examined other transgenic models in which MCP-1 expression is under the control of promoters with more highly tissue-restricted activity. For example, when controlled by the myelin basic protein promoter (MBP-MCP-1 mice), MCP-1 produced a mild perivascular monocyte accumulation in the central nervous system (CNS) that could be markedly enhanced by systemic administration of lipopolysaccharide (LPS). Similarly, lck promoter-driven expression resulted in an increased proportion of monocytes in the thymus *(52)*. When expressed under the control of a surfactant promoter, human MCP-1 did not produce an increase in monocytes in lung parenchyma, but these transgenic mice did have more monocytes in their bronchoalveolar lavage fluid *(53)*. Expression in the skin by a keratin 14 promoter produced mice with increased numbers of Langerhans-like dendritic cells in the skin, but no overt monocytic infiltration *(54)*. However, these mice did display an abnormally vigorous response to contact-hypersensitivity reagents. Although some groups find that MCP-1 has no chemoattractant activity for dendritic cells in vitro *(55)*, others ascribe this property to MCP-1 *(56)*. Thus, in this transgenic model, it is possible that MCP-1 itself attracted Langerhans cells to the skin, or that it secondarily induced the expression of an authentic dendritic cell attractant.

In another model, murine MCP-1 was expressed under the control of a rat insulin promoter (RIP-MCP-1 transgenic mice) *(57)*. From birth these mice displayed a mononuclear insulitis consisting almost entirely of F4/80$^+$ monocytes with very small numbers of CD4$^+$, CD8$^+$, or B220$^+$ cells. (Although B220 is also expressed on NK cell surfaces, these are unlikely to be NK cells because they were not stained by the NK marker, NK1.1.) Notably, despite an impressive infiltrate, these mice never became diabetic, suggesting that MCP-1 can attract monocytes efficiently but cannot activate them to engage in tissue destruction.

In the aggregate, then, it appears that some of the in vitro chemoattractant properties of MCP-1 can be recapitulated in vivo, but only when expressed in a specific manner, namely at relatively low levels in anatomically confined areas. Such a requirement is perhaps not surprising since this is the way that MCP-1 is expressed naturally. These rules for chemokine action in vivo were emphasized by mating the RIP-MCP-1 mice to the MMTV-MCP-1 mice. Offspring that inherited both transgenes expressed as much MCP-1 in the pancreas as offspring from a control mating involving only the RIP-MCP-1 transgene. In spite of islet cell expression, the double transgenic mice had essentially no insulitis, indicating that the high levels of systemic MCP-1 produced by the MMTV-MCP-1 transgene were able to prevent the locally expressed RIP-MCP-1 transgene from eliciting an infiltrate.

Note, however, that based on analysis of transgenic models, there are some discrepancies between in vitro and in vivo activities. For example, although MCP-1 is a potent chemoattractant for memory T-lymphocytes and NK cells in vitro, these cells are not prominent components of the in vivo infiltrates elicited by transgenic MCP-1. One reason may be that MCP-1 is not really an efficient T- or NK cell chemoattractant in vivo. Another may be that the microenvironment of the brain, thymus, or islets of Langerhans may not be optimal for lymphocyte or NK cell diapedesis. However, an even more likely possibility is based on the observation that the expression of many chemokine receptors, including one of MCP-1's receptors, CCR2, is tightly regulated in T-lymphocytes *(58–60)*. It may be that in the absence of T-cell activation in these transgenic models, there are no populations of T-lymphocytes expressing CCR2, and therefore capable of responding to MCP-1.

In terms of monocyte activation, early analyses indicated that MCP-1 could activate the respiratory burst in human monocytes in vitro, although this is, at best, merely a surrogate for functional monocyte activation *(61)*. In fact, as described previously, it appears that MCP-1 alone is insufficient to induce monocyte activation as assessed by tissue destruction in the infiltrative transgenic models. MCP-1 was also shown to stimu-late the ability of human monocytes to suppress the growth of various human tumor cell lines in vitro *(37)*. However, this was a cytostatic rather than cytocidal effect.

5. ANTITUMOR EFFECTS OF MCP-1 IN VIVO

With clear-cut data indicating the ability of MCP-1 to attract monocytes in vivo, one can now ask, Does MCP-1 play a role in the host response to cancer? In some of the first experiments to address this question, Chinese hamster ovary (CHO) cells were engineered to express either human or murine MCP-1 *(62)*. The expression system used in these studies involved coexpression with dihydrofolate reductase (DHFR) in a $DHFR^{-/-}$ cell *(63)*. This permitted coamplification of the *MCP-1* gene along with *DHFR* when cells were exposed to increasing concentrations of methotrexate. Ultimately, sev-eral cell lines were created that expressed varying levels of MCP-1.

When CHO cells expressing any level of human or murine MCP-1 were injected subcutaneously into nude mice, no tumors formed. This is in contrast to control, nonexpressing cells selected to the same level of methotrexate resistance, which pro-duced large tumors within 2 to 3 wk of injection. Suppression of tumor growth occurred even with inocula up to 2×10^7 cells, and it occurred despite the fact that MCP-1 expression had no effect on cell growth rate in vitro or on the ability of cells to form colonies in soft agar. This suggested that the mechanism of tumor suppression might be host derived, perhaps through MCP-1-mediated recruitment of mononuclear cells. Consistent with this idea, histologic examination of inoculation sites 24 h after injec-tion demonstrated an intense monocyte-rich infiltrate in association with MCP-1-expressing cells but not with non-MCP-1 expressers. Examination of these sites 2 to 3 wk after injection showed no evidence for any residual tumor cells.

The notion that tumor rejection in this system occurred because of MCP-1 secretion and recruitment of inflammatory cells would imply that the effect is not cell autono-mous. This was proven by coinjecting MCP-1-expressing CHO cells with a number of non-MCP-1-expressing cells that would ordinarily give rise to a tumor. The presence of MCP-1 expressers was able to suppress tumor formation. The same experiment was also performed by coinjecting MCP-1-expressing CHO cells with a heterologous cell type, namely HeLa cells. Again MCP-1-expressing cells were capable of suppressing tumor formation by HeLa cells.

Although a direct demonstration that tumor suppression was due to MCP-1 was not provided in these experiments, e.g., by neutralizing the effect with anti-MCP-1 anti-bodies, other evidence suggests that this was, indeed, the mechanism. First, all the CHO cell clones used in these experiments were identical except for the engineered expression of MCP-1, suggesting that MCP-1 was responsible for their differences in tumorigenicity. Second, the availability of CHO clones expressing varying amounts of MCP-1 permitted the establishment of a dose response for the tumor-suppressive effect. Thus, when high-level MCP-1 expressers were coinjected with nonexpressing CHO or HeLa cells, tumor formation was completely suppressed. However, when the same number of low-level MCP-1 expressers was coinjected, tumor formation was delayed by 7–10 d (compared to coinjection with nonexpressers), after which tumors began to grow. This indicates that the degree of tumor suppression in vivo is proportional to the amount of MCP-1 expressed by coinjecting cells, further supporting the notion that MCP-1 itself is responsible for this effect.

A similar connection between MCP-1 and host response to cancer has been inferred by correlating the amount of MCP-1 expressed by different clones of sarcoma cell lines with macrophage infiltration and growth rate in vivo *(64)*. One of the Rous sarcoma virus (RSV)-induced sarcoma clones expressed high levels of MCP-1 whereas the other expressed almost none. The former showed nearly twice the number of tumor-associated macrophages compared with the latter, and the tumors formed by these cells appeared later and grew more slowly.

These results suggest that MCP-1-mediated macrophage infiltration into tumors occurs in immunocompetent animals as well as in athymic mice. This was demonstrated directly by engineering MCP-1 expression in a B16 murine melanoma–derived cell line that does not ordinarily express MCP-1 *(65)*. A clone expressing MCP-1 formed a tumor with double the proportion of macrophages and a slower growth rate compared to nonexpressing tumors. Again, this difference occurred despite identical growth rates in vitro for expressing and nonexpressing clones. Interestingly, however, despite forming slower-growing tumors, the MCP-1-expressing cells actually had a higher tumor-forming efficiency at low inocula (i.e., 10^2 cells/site). This phenomenon is considered to be supportive evidence for the tumor-promoting role of macrophages. As in the work of Prehn *(52)*, at low inocula, the growth factors provided by infiltrating macrophages can promote the clonogenic growth of individual tumor cells. However, with continued growth and macrophage recruitment, the antitumor activities of macrophages supervene.

Another correlative study was performed in the rat by comparing the behavior of 9L glioblastoma, Ad-2 mammary carcinoma, and MT-P malignant fibrous histiocytoma cell lines that express high, intermediate, and undetectable levels of MCP-1, respectively *(66)*. As in other systems, the degree of macrophage infiltration into tumors derived from these cell lines was proportional to the amount of MCP-1 they expressed. In addition, the investigators were able to distinguish blood monocyte–derived infiltrating macrophages (TRPM-3[+] and/or ED-3[+]) from resident tissue macrophages (ED2[+] and Ki-M2R[+]). The MCP-1-expressing tumors were infiltrated predominantly with monocyte-derived macrophages. To demonstrate the role of MCP-1 in this system, non-MCP-1-expressing MT-P cells were engineered to express rat MCP-1, and several clones were isolated that demonstrated different levels of expression. Again, the degree of macrophage infiltration was proportional to the amount of MCP-1 expressed by the cells that comprised the tumor, and the phenotype of the infiltrating cells indicated that they were derived from blood monocytes. As expected, the growth rate of tumors was inversely proportional to the amount of MCP-1 the tumors' cells expressed.

In a model of metastatic disease, CT26 colon carcinoma cells from Balb/c mice were engineered to express MCP-1 and injected intravenously in syngeneic hosts. Despite homing to the lungs in similar numbers, the MCP-1-expressing cells formed fewer lung metastases than their non-MCP-1-expressing counterparts *(67)*. The mechanism was ascribed to macrophage cytocidal effects since the MCP-1 expressers were more susceptible to syngeneic macrophage-mediated cytolysis in vitro (in the presence of LPS) than nonexpressers. However, this effect was not directly demonstrated in vivo.

In primary human tumors, a correlation has been established between MCP-1 expression and monocyte infiltration. Twenty epithelial ovarian tumors were examined for MCP-1 expression by *in situ* hybridization, and the degree of infiltration was determined by immunohistochemical analysis of paraffin sections *(68)*. In this case, the number of epithelial cells expressing MCP-1 significantly correlated with the number of CD68+ macrophages, which comprised the majority of the infiltrate, and CD8+ T-lymphocytes, which were present in lower numbers. This finding is further indirect support for the role of MCP-1 in attracting inflammatory cells to "real" human cancers in vivo.

It has also been suggested that MCP-1 expression may relate to the pattern of infiltration into tumors by macrophages. As noted previously, many tumors display predominantly peritumoral macrophage infiltration although a significant proportion also have intratumoral infiltration. In an analysis of four human cancers with varying levels of MCP-1 expression, it was found that high amounts of MCP-1 expression were associated with intratumoral macrophage infiltration when cells were injected into nude mice *(69)*. Although only a small number of tumor cells were investigated, and each cell type differs by more than just MCP-1 expression, the number of intratumoral macrophages could be reduced to non-MCP-1-expressing control levels by administration of anti-MCP-1 antibodies.

Obviously, in nude mouse models, all antitumor effects are immunologically nonspecific. Therefore, as expected, the effects are completely local, so that injection of MCP-1-expressing cells into one flank of a mouse will not prevent formation of a tumor by non-MCP-1-expressing cells injected into the contralateral flank. Even in immunocompetent animals, as described in the previously cited studies, there were no direct tests of the ability of MCP-1 to effect systemic resistance to tumor growth. Nonetheless, given the ability of MCP-1 to attract T-lymphocytes in vitro, it might be expected that it could potentially enhance immunologically specific antitumor responses. This has been tested in a rat glioblastoma model *(70)*. The murine *MCP-1* gene was transduced into rat 9L glioma cells that expressed no detectable MCP-1. (This was presumably a different clone from the 9L clone used by Yamashira et al. *[66]*, which did express MCP-1.) These cells or appropriate controls were γ-irradiated to make them unable to proliferate and used to immunize immunocompetent Fisher rats. Two weeks later, immunized and control rats were challenged with varying inocula of wild-type 9L cells. As shown in Figure 1, sc challenge with 5×10^7 wild-type 9L cells produced rapidly growing tumors in nonimmunized rats. In response to the same challenge, there was a slight delay in tumor growth in rats that had been immunized with wild-type 9L cells that had not undergone genetic manipulation, suggesting that 9L cells are somewhat inherently immunogenic. There was an even greater tumor delay in rats that had been immunized with G418-resistant 9L cells, perhaps reflecting an "adjuvant" effect of the expression of bacterial neomycin phosphotransferase. However, the only rats to remain tumor free were those that had been immunized with 9L cells expressing MCP-1.

Although these results indicate that the expression of MCP-1 enhances systemic antitumor immunity, there are some limitations. For example, at lower inocula some animals immunized with G418-resistant 9L cells were able to suppress tumor growth completely. Thus, in this system, it appears that, at best, MCP-1 was able to enhance a

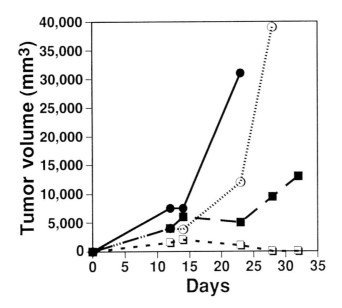

Fig. 1. Effect of MCP-1 on tumor vaccination in rats. Rats were immunized with irradiated 9L glioblastoma cells (○), irradiated G418-resistant 9L cells (■), or irradiated MCP-1-expressing 9L cells (□). Two weeks later, immunized and nonimmunized (●) rats were inoculated subcutaneously with 5×10^7 wild-type 9L cells, and tumor volumes were monitored.

weak but somewhat effective response to these immunogenic cells. It remains to be seen whether MCP-1 can render a nonimmunogenic cell visible to the immune system. Another limitation of this system is that intracranial injection of 9L cells resulted in tumor growth and the demise of the animals regardless of immunization status. This may simply indicate that memory T-lymphocytes were unable to enter the CNS until the blood-brain barrier had been disrupted by a tumor mass that was too large to suppress.

6. MECHANISMS OF MCP-1 ANTITUMOR EFFECTS

There is now a preponderance of evidence that MCP-1 can contribute to host antitumor activity, but there are strikingly few data on the mechanism. Efficacy in nude mouse models indicates that the effect of MCP-1 is not T-lymphocyte dependent, but there are no data to indicate what the effector cell might be (i.e., monocyte *vs* NK cell) or whether MCP-1 is necessary for effector cells to suppress tumor growth. In other words, MCP-1 might attract effector cells as it attracts monocytes in transgenic models, but it may not be required to activate antitumor function. What few data there are can be summarized as follows.

In an early study, the addition of MCP-1 to purified human monocytes in tissue culture enhanced their ability to inhibit DNA synthesis in six malignant human cell lines *(37)*. These included colon and breast carcinoma lines as well as melanoma, rhabdomyosarcoma, and leiomyosarcoma lines. The effect was clearly cytostatic and occurred with an ED_{50} of approx 0.3 nM, consistent with MCP-1's K_d for its receptor on monocytes.

By contrast, the ability of MCP-1 to enhance the tumoricidal effects of monocytes in vitro has been documented *(71)*. Elicited peritoneal macrophages from C3H mice were incubated with radiolabeled syngeneic murine melanoma cells (K-1735) at an effector:target ratio of 10:1. In the presence of 1 μg/mL of LPS, macrophages were able to lyse melanoma cells engineered to express human MCP-1, but not parental or control cells. (LPS plus interferon-γ induced lysis regardless of MCP-1 expression status.) The addition of LPS and human MCP-1 to cultures of macrophages induced lysis of non-MCP-1-expressing melanoma cells, indicating that MCP-1 secretion by the engineered cells was responsible for activating macrophage antitumor activity. Identical results were obtained in another mouse strain (Balb/c) using syngeneic colon carcinoma cell lines and murine MCP-1 *(67)*. These tantalizing data suggest the possibility of synergistic effects between MCP-1 and other agents to induce macrophage tumoricidal activity. However, the relevance of this precise effect has yet to be demonstrated in vivo.

An alternative approach to using MCP-1 was demonstrated by transfecting an MCP-1 cDNA into small-cell lung cancer cell lines that express P-glycoprotein *(72)*. As in other systems, MCP-1 did not alter the growth rate of these cells in vitro, but in this model, MCP-1 expressers formed tumors in nude mice with the same efficiency and growth rate as control cells. However, the tumor-suppressive effects of systemically administered anti-P-glycoprotein antibody were much greater against the MCP-1-expressing cells. This suggests that even when MCP-1-mediated macrophage attraction is insufficient to produce tumor cell death, the presence of MCP-1 can enhance antibody-dependent cellular cytotoxicity. (The MCP-1 effect is probably related to macrophage elicitation in vivo since the addition of recombinant MCP-1 to mixed macrophage/tumor cell cultures in vitro did not enhance cytotoxicity.)

Finally, there is the demonstration cited previously that MCP-1 can enhance immunologically specific antitumor responses *(70)*. This could simply be a result of the ability of MCP-1 to attract macrophages (or dendritic cells) to a tumor. Enhanced antigen presentation or T-lymphocyte costimulation could be due to other local influences.

7. THE MCP-1/MALIGNANCY PARADOX

An ironic observation that tumor models have not yet addressed is that most of the original isolates of MCP-1 actually came from malignant cells *(36,37)*. One is forced to ask the following question: If MCP-1 were truly a potent antitumor cytokine, then why does its expression occur so commonly and at such high levels in biologically successful tumors? One possible explanation comes from observations on the MMTV-MCP-1 transgenic mouse model described previously. In this mouse, high levels of MCP-1 expression were suggested to desensitize MCP-1 receptors on circulating monocytes, thereby rendering them incapable of responding to local chemoattraction or activation signals. It is conceivable that high levels of MCP-1 expression by some malignant cells may do the same thing. In other words, MCP-1 expression would provide a selective advantage for tumors based on its ability to disarm components of natural or acquired immunity that would normally protect the host from tumor growth.

This model predicts that abnormalities in monocyte/macrophage function might be observed in tumor-bearing patients or animals. Of course, depression of cell-mediated immunity has long been recognized in patients with nonhematologic malignancies, but one of the more interesting examples in the context of MCP-1 involves gliomas. It has been reported that lymphocytes from patients with nonmetastatic gliomas have decreased proliferative responses in vitro to autochthonous tumor cells, and that this suppression was due to a circulating cationic protein *(73)*. One is put in mind of MCP-1 because of its frequent expression in gliomas *(36,74)* and because of its unusually high p*I*.

Other data speak more directly to problems in monocyte/macrophage migration. Boetcher and Leonard *(75)* showed that about 50% of cancer patients who were otherwise healthy at the time of testing showed diminished monocyte chemotaxis in vitro in response to lymphocyte-derived chemotactic factors. Similar observations were made by Snyderman et al. *(76)*, who pointed out that the chemotactic response returned to normal after surgical resection of the tumor. This suggests that the suppressive factor is generated by the tumor itself, and is consistent with the observation that some tumor cell lines secrete a substance that inhibits monocyte chemotaxis in vitro *(77)*. To examine this phenomenon in humans in vivo, skin can be abraded and the local accumulation of leukocytes at the abrasion site can be quantified. In this model, one study demonstrated that cancer patients showed a 50% reduction in the number of elicited monocytes *(78)*, and another showed that the proportion of monocytes infiltrating the abrasion site correlated with Karnofsky performance status *(79)*.

Animal models also provide evidence for tumor-mediated suppression of host responses. Implantation of syngeneic tumors in mice reduces the number of macrophages elicited by ip injection of phytohemagglutinin (PHA) or peptone *(76,80)*. North et al. *(81)* has demonstrated that several syngeneic murine tumors produce a circulating factor in vivo that increases host susceptibility to *L. monocytogenes* and *Yersinia pestis* *(81)*. Interestingly, lethally irradiated tumors produce this effect just as well as proliferating tumors, suggesting that the effect is not based on increasing tumor load *per se*. Furthermore, this factor appears to prevent monocyte emigration from the blood into local inflammatory foci. In many respects, this model behaves like the MMTV-MCP-1 transgenic mice described previously. Whether the factor is MCP-1 itself or not, it lends support to the notion that tumor-derived chemoattractants could act to depress host chemoattractant responses to tumor sites. In this way, expression of factors such as MCP-1 would actually be advantageous to the tumor, and might explain the high frequency of MCP-1 expression in human malignancies.

8. CONCLUSION

Most of the studies catalogued herein indicate that, when administered in the proper manner, MCP-1 can suppress tumor growth in vivo. How it accomplishes this is still not well understood. For example: Does MCP-1 actually stimulate macrophage antitumor cell activity and, if so, how? Or does MCP-1 merely get macrophages to the right place at the right time? Are other signals then necessary to elicit cytotoxicity? Are the T-lymphocyte-dependent aspects of MCP-1's activity a reflection of MCP-1's activity on T-cells, or is this a fortunate but indirect result of macrophage recruitment and/or activation?

These questions must be answered before MCP-1 or MCP-1 analogs can be considered in a therapeutic context. In many studies, the MCP-1 effect is relatively weak, and tumors can still grow despite the expression of significant levels of MCP-1. In this case, it may be reasonable to consider combination cytokine therapy. For example, if the role of MCP-1 is attraction without activation, then perhaps the addition of macrophage colony-stimulating factor could contribute to more vigorous tumor cell cytotoxicity. In the vaccine approach, granulocyte-macrophage colony-stimulating factor (GM-CSF) has been shown to be helpful in eliciting systemic antitumor immunity, and the combination of MCP-1 with GM-CSF may prove to be even more efficacious.

At the same time, there is some evidence that MCP-1 expression by tumors might disarm components of natural or acquired immunity that would normally protect the host from tumor growth. This hypothesis will be amenable to testing by the use of MCP-1-deficient animals, and cell lines derived therefrom, that are constructed by gene targeting. These knockouts will also be used to answer questions about the possible role of MCP-1 in immune surveillance. Armed with this information, we will have a better understanding of monocyte-based host responses to malignancy, whether or not they directly involve MCP-1.

REFERENCES

1. Underwood, J. C. E. 1974. Lymphoreticular infiltration in human tumors: prognostic and biological implications: a review. *Br. J. Cancer* **30:** 538–548.
2. Underwood, J. C. E., and I. Carr. 1972. The ultrastructure of the lymphoreticular cells in non-lymphoid human neoplasms. *Virchows Arch. Abt. B Zellpath.* **12:** 39–50.
3. Virchow, R. 1863. *Die krankhaften Geschwulste. Dreißig Vorlesungen, gehalten während des Wintersemesters 1872–1863 an der Universität zu Berlin.* Vorlesungen uber Pathologie, Verlag von August Hirschwald, Berlin.
4. Waldeyer, H. W. G. 1872. Die entwicklung der carcinome. *Virchows Arch. Path. Anat.* 55–67.
5. Jensen, C. O. 1903. Experimentelle untersuchungen über krebs bei mäusen. *Zentralbl. f. Bakt. Parasit. Infekt.* **I Abt. Originale. 34:** 122–143.
6. Bashford, E. F. 1905. The growth of cancer under natural and experimental conditions. In: E. F. Bashford, J. A. Murray, and W. Cramer (eds.), *Scientific Reports on the Investigations of the ICRF*, No. 2 part II. Imperial Cancer Research Fund, London.
7. Russell, B. R. G. 1908. The nature of resistance to the inoculation of cancer. *Third Sci. Rep. ICRF* **3:** 341–358.
8. Da Fano, C. 1911. A cytological analysis of the reaction in animals resistant to implanted carcinomata. *Fifth Sci. Rep. ICRF* **5:** 57–75.
9. Monis, B., and Weinberg, T. 1960. Cytochemical study of esterase activity of human neoplasms and stromal macrophages. *Cancer* **14:** 369–377.
10. Wade, H. 1980. An experimental investigation of infective sarcoma of the dog, with a consideration of its relationship to cancer. *J. Pathol. Bacteriol.* **12:** 384–425.
11. Ehrlich, P. 1907. Experimentelle studien an mäustumoren. *Zeitschr. f. Krebsforschung* **5:** 59–81.
12. Burg, G., and Braun-Falco, O. 1972. The cellular stromal reaction in malignant melanoma: a cytochemical investigation. *Arch. Derm. Forsch.* **245:** 318–333.
13. Carr, I., and J. C. E. Underwood. 1974. The ultrastructure of the local cellular reaction to neoplasia. *Int. Rev. Cytol.* **37:** 329–347.
14. Göttlinger, H. G., P. Rieber, J. M. Gokel, K. J. Lohe, and G. Riethmüller. 1985. Infiltrating mononuclear cells in human breast carcinoma: predominance of T4[+] monocytic cells in the tumor stroma. *Int. J. Cancer* **35:** 199–205.
15. van Ravenswaay Claasen, H. H., P. M. Kluin, and G. J. Fleuren. 1992. Tumor infiltrating cells in human cancer: on the possible role of CD16[+] macrophages in antitumor cytotoxicity. *Lab. Invest.* **67:** 166–174.
16. Evans, R. 1972. Macrophages in syngeneic animal tumors. *Transplantation* **14:** 468–473.

17. Cohen, P. J., M. T. Lotze, J. R. Roberts, S. A. Rosenberg, and E. S. Jaffe. 1987. The immunopathology of sequential tumor biopsies in patients treated with interleukin-2: correlation of response with T-cell infiltration and HLA-DR expression. *Am. J. Pathol.* **129:** 208–216.

18. Gauci, C. L., and P. Alexander. 1975. The macrophage content of some human tumors. *Cancer Lett.* **1:** 29–32.

19. Eccles, S. A., and P. Alexander. 1974. Macrophage content of tumors in relation to metastatic spread and host immune reaction. *Nature* **250:** 667–669.

20. Berg, J. W. 1959. Inflammation and prognosis in breast cancer: a search for host resistance. *Cancer* **12:** 714–720.

21. Black, M. M., S. R. Opler, and F. D. Speer. 1955. Survival in breast cancer cases in relation to the structure of the primary tumor and regional lymph nodes. *Surg. Gynecol. Obstet.* **100:** 543–551.

22. Champion, H. R., I. W. J. Wallace, and R. J. Prescott. 1972. Histology in breast cancer diagnosis. *Br. J. Cancer* **26:** 129–138.

23. Takahashi, K. 1961. Squamous cell carcinoma of the esophagus: stromal inflammatory cell infiltration as a prognostic factor. *Cancer* **14:** 921–933.

24. Lauder, I., and W. Aherne. 1972. The significance of lymphocytic infiltrate in neuroblastoma. *Br. J. Cancer* **26:** 321–330.

25. Barber, H. R. K., S. C. Sommers, R. Snyder, and T. H. Kwon. 1975. Histologic and nuclear grading and stromal reactions as indices for prognosis in ovarian cancer. *Am. J. Obstet. Gynecol.* **121:** 795–807.

26. Fidler, I. J. 1974. Inhibition of pulmonary metastasis by intravenous injection of specifically activated macrophages. *Cancer Res.* **34:** 1074–1078.

27. Dullens, H. F. J., and W. Den Otter. 1974. Therapy with allogeneic immune peritoneal cells. *Cancer Res.* **34:** 1726–1730.

28. Keller, R. 1976. Promotion of tumor growth in vivo by antimacrophage agents. *J. Natl. Cancer Inst.* **57:** 1355–1361.

29. Prehn, R. T. 1972. The immune reaction as a stimulator of tumor growth. *Science* **176:** 170, 171.

30. Mantovani, A., B. Bottazzi, F. Colotta, S. Sozzani, and L. Ruco. 1992. The origin and function of tumor-associated macrophages. *Immunol. Today* **13:** 265–270.

31. Carrel, A. 1922. Growth-promoting function of leukocytes. *J. Exp. Med.* **36:** 385–391.

32. Leek, R. D., C. E. Lewis, R. Whitehouse, M. Greenall, J. Clarke, and A. L. Harris. 1996. Association of macrophage infiltration with angiogenesis and prognosis in invasive breast carcinoma. *Cancer Res.* **56:** 4625–4629.

33. Bottazzi, B., N. Polentarutti, R. Acero, A. Balsari, D. Boraschi, P. Ghezzi, M. Salmona, and A. Mantovani. 1983. Regulation of the macrophage content of neoplasms by chemoattractants. *Science* **220:** 210–212.

34. Bottazzi, B., P. Ghezzi, G. Tarboletti, M. Salmona, N. Colombo, C. Bonazzi, C. Mangioni, and A. Mantovani. 1985. Tumor-derived chemotactic factor(s) from human ovarian carcinoma: evidence for a role in the regulation of macrophage content of neoplastic tissues. *Int. J. Cancer* **36:** 167–173.

35. Valente, A. J., D. T. Graves, C. E. Vialle-Valentin, R. Delgado, and C. J. Schwartz. 1988. Purification of a monocyte chemotactic factor secreted by nonhuman primate vascular cells in culture. *Biochemistry* **27:** 4162–4168.

36. Yoshimura, T., E. A. Robinson, S. Tanaka, E. Appella, J. I. Kuratsu, and E. J. Leonard. 1989. Purification and amino acid analysis of two human glioma-derived monocyte chemoattractants. *J. Exp. Med.* **169:** 1449–1459.

37. Matsushima, K., C. G. Larsen, G. C. DuBois, and J. J. Oppenheim. 1989. Purification and characterization of a novel monocyte chemotactic and activating factor produced by a human myelomonocytic cell line. *J. Exp. Med.* **169:** 1485–1490.

38. Bottazzi, B., F. Colotta, A. Sica, N. Nobili, and A. Mantovani. 1990. A chemoattractant expressed in human sarcoma cells (tumor-derived chemotactic factor, TDCF) is identical to monocyte chemoattractant protein-1/monocyte chemotactic and activating factor (MCP-1/MCAF). *Int. J. Cancer* **45:** 795–797.

39. Graves, D. T., Y. L. Jiang, M. J. Williamson, and A. J. Valente. 1989. Identification of monocyte chemotactic activity produced by malignant cells. *Science* **245:** 1490–1493.

40. Cochran, B. H., A. C. Reffel, and C. D. Stiles. 1983. Molecular cloning of gene sequences regulated by platelet-derived growth factor. *Cell* **33:** 939–947.

41. Rollins, B. J., E. D. Morrison, and C. D. Stiles. 1988. Cloning and expression of *JE*, a gene inducible by platelet-derived growth factor and whose product has cytokine-like properties. *Proc. Natl. Acad. Sci. USA* **85:** 3738–3742.

42. Rollins, B. J., P. Stier, T. E. Ernst, and G. G. Wong. 1989. The human homologue of the *JE* gene encodes a monocyte secretory protein. *Mol. Cell. Biol.* **9:** 4687–4695.

43. Ernst, C. A., Y. J. Zhang, P. R. Hancock, B. J. Rutledge, C. L. Corless, and B. J. Rollins. 1994. Biochemical and biological characterization of murine MCP-1: identification of two functional domains. *J. Immunol.* **152:** 3541–3549.

44. Mazzucchelli, L., P. Loetscher, A. Kappeler, M. Uguccioni, M. Baggiolini, J. A. Laissue, and C. Mueller. 1996. Monocyte chemoattractant protein-1 gene expression in prostatic hyperplasia and prostate adenocarcinoma. *Am. J. Pathol.* **149(2):** 501–509.

45. Zachariae, C. O. C., A. O. Anderson, H. L. Thompson, E. Appella, A. Mantovani, J. J. Oppenheim, and K. Matsushima. 1990. Properties of monocyte chemotactic and activating factor (MCAF) purified from a human fibrosarcoma cell line. *J. Exp. Med.* **171:** 2177–2182.

46. Rutledge, B. J., H. Rayburn, R. Rosenberg, R. J. North, R. P. Gladue, C. L. Corless, and B. J. Rollins. 1995. High level monocyte chemoattractant protein-1 expression in transgenic mice increases their susceptibility to intracellular pathogens. *J. Immunol.* **155:** 4838–4843.

47. Simonet, W. S., T. M. Hughes, H. Q. Nguyen, L. D. Trebasky, D. M. Danilenko, and E. S. Medlock. 1994. Long-term impairment of neutrophil migration in mice overexpressing human interleukin-8. *J. Clin. Invest.* **94:** 1310–1319.

48. Hechtman, D. H., M. I. Cybulsky, H. J. Fuchs, J. B. Baker, and M. A. Gimbrone. 1991. Intravascular IL-8: inhibitor of polymorphonuclear leukocyte accumulation at sites of acute inflammation. *J. Immunol.* **147:** 883–892.

49. Ley, K., J. B. Baker, M. I. Cybulsky, M. A. Gimbrone, and F. W. Luscinskas. 1993. Intravenous interleukin-8 inhibits granulocyte emigration from rabbit mesenteric vessels without altering L-selectin expression or leukocyte rolling. *J. Immunol.* **151:** 6347–6357.

50. Karpus, W. J., N. W. Lukacs, K. J. Kennedy, W. S. Smith, S. D. Hurst, and T. A. Barrett. 1997. Differential CC chemokine-induced enhancement of T helper cell cytokine production. *J. Immunol.* **158:** 4129–4136.

51. Chensue, S. W., K. S. Warmington, J. H. Ruth, P. S. Sanghi, P. Lincoln, and S. L. Kunkel. 1996. Role of monocyte chemoattractant protein-1 (MCP-1) in Th1 (mycobacterial) and Th2 (schistosomal) antigen-induced granuloma formation: relationship to local inflammation, Th cell expression, and IL-12 production. *J. Immunol.* **157:** 4602–4608.

52. Fuentes, M. E., S. K. Durham, M. R. Swerdel, A. C. Lewin, D. S. Barton, J. R. Megill, R. Bravo, and S. A. Lira. 1995. Controlled recruitment of monocytes/macrophages to specific organs through transgenic expression of MCP-1. *J. Immunol.* **155:** 5769–5776.

53. Gunn, M. D., N. A. Nelken, X. Liao, and L. T. Williams. 1997. Monocyte chemoattractant protein-1 is sufficient for the chemotaxis of monocytes and lymphocytes in transgenic mice but requires an additional stimulus for inflammatory activation. *J. Immunol.* **158:** 376–383.

54. Nakamura, K., I. R. Williams, and T. S. Kupper. 1995. Keratinocyte-derived monocyte

chemoattractant protein 1 (MCP-1): analysis in a transgenic model demonstrates MCP-1 can recruit dendritic and Langerhans cells to skin. *J. Invest. Dermatol.* **105:** 635–643.

55. Sozzani, S., F. Sallusto, W. Luini, D. Zhou, L. Piemonti, P. Allavena, J. Van Damme, S. Valitutti, A. Lanzavecchia, and A. Mantovani. 1995. Migration of dendritic cells in response to formyl peptides, C5a, and a distinct set of chemokines. *J. Immunol.* **155:** 3292–3295.

56. Xu, L. L., M. K. Warren, W. L. Rose, W. Gong, and J. M. Wang. 1996. Human recombinant monocyte chemotactic protein and other C-C chemokines bind and induce directional migration of dendritic cells in vitro. *J. Leuk. Biol.* **60(3):** 365–371.

57. Grewal, I. S., B. J. Rutledge, J. A. Fiorillo, L. Gu, R. P. Gladue, R. A. Flavell, and B. J. Rollins. 1997. Transgenic monocyte chemoattractant protein-1 (MCP-1) in pancreatic islets produces monocyte-rich insulitis without diabetes: abrogation by a second transgene expressing systemic MCP-1. *J. Immunol.* **159:** 401–408.

58. Olin, S., G. LaRosa, J. J. Campbell, H. Smith-Heath, N. Kassam, X. Shi, L. Zeng, E. C. Buthcher, and C. R. Mackay. 1996. Expression of monocyte chemoattractant protein-1 and interleukin-8 receptors on subsets of T cells: correlation with transendothelial chemotactic potential. *Eur. J. Immunol.* **26:** 640–647.

59. Loetscher, P., M. Seitz, I. Clark-Lewis, M. Baggiolini, and B. Moser. 1996. Activation of NK cells by CC chemokines: chemotaxis, Ca2$^+$ mobilization, and enzyme release. *J. Immunol.* **156:** 322–327.

60. Tangirala, R. K., K. Murao, and O. Quehenberger. 1997. Regulation of expression of the human monocyte chemotactic protein-1 receptor (hCCR2) by cytokines. *J. Biol. Chem.* **272:** 8050–8056.

61. Rollins, B. J., A. Walz, and M. Baggiolini. 1991. Recombinant human MCP-1/JE induces chemotaxis, calcium flux, and the respiratory burst in human monocytes. *Blood* **78:** 1112–1116.

62. Rollins, B. J., and M. E. Sunday. 1991. Suppression of tumor formation *in vivo* by expression of the *JE* gene in malignant cells. *Mol. Cell. Biol.* **11:** 3125–3131.

63. Kaufman, R. J., P. Murtha, and M. Davies. 1987. Translational efficiency of polycistronic mRNAs and their utilization to express heterologous genes in mammalian cells. *EMBO J.* **6:** 187–193.

64. Walter, S., B. Bottazzi, D. Govoni, F. Colotta, and A. Mantovani. 1991. Macrophage infiltration and growth of sarcoma clones expressing different amounts of monocyte chemotactic protein/JE. *Int. J. Cancer* **49:** 431–435.

65. Bottazzi, B., S. Walter, D. Govoni, F. Colotta, and A. Mantovani. 1992. Monocyte chemotactic cytokine gene transfer modulates macrophage infiltration, growth, and susceptibility to IL-2 therapy of a murine melanoma. *J. Immunol.* **148:** 1280–1285.

66. Yamashira, S., M. Takeya, T. Nishi, J. Kuratsu, T. Yoshimura, Y. Ushio, and K. Takahashi. 1994. Tumor derived monocyte chemoattractant protein-1 induces intratumoral infiltration of monocyte-derived macrophage subpopulation in transplanted rat tumors. *Am. J. Pathol.* **145:** 856–867.

67. Huang, S., R. K. Singh, K. Xie, M. Gutman, K. K. Berry, C. D. Bucana, I. J. Fidler, and M. Bar-Eli. 1994. Expression of the JE/MCP-1 gene suppresses metastatic potential in murine colon carcinoma cells. *Cancer Immunol. Immunother.* **39:** 231–238.

68. Negus, R. P., G. W. Stamp, J. Hadley, and F. R. Balkwill. 1997. Quantitative assessment of the leukocyte infiltrate in ovarian cancer and its relationship to the expression of C-C chemokines. *Am. J. Pathol.* **150:** 1723–1734.

69. Zhang, L., A. Khayat, H. Cheng, and D. T. Graves. 1997. The pattern of monocyte recruitment in tumors is modulated by MCP-1 expression and influences the rate of tumor growth. *Lab. Invest.* **76:** 579–590.

70. Manome, Y., P. Y. Wen, A. Hershowitz, T. Tanaka, B. J. Rollins, D. W. Kufe, and

H. A. Fine. 1995. Monocyte chemoattractant protein-1 (MCP-1) gene transduction: an effective tumor vaccine strategy for non-intracranial tumors. *Cancer Immunol. Immunother.* **41:** 227–235.

71. Singh, R. K., K. Berry, K. Matsushima, K. Yasumoto, and I. J. Fidler. 1993. Synergism between human monocyte chemotactic and activating factor and bacterial products for activation of tumoricidal properties in murine macrophages. *J. Immunol.* **151:** 2786–2793.

72. Nishioka, Y., S. Yano, F. Fujiki, N. Mukaida, K. Matsushima, T. Tsuruo, and S. Sone. 1997. Combined therapy of multidrug-resistant human lung cancer with anti-P-glycoprotein antibody and monocyte chemoattractant protein-1 gene transduction: the possibility of immunological overcoming of multidrug resistance. *Int. J. Cancer* **71:** 170–177.

73. Brooks, W. H., M. G. Netsky, D. E. Normansell, and D. A. Horwitz. 1972. Depressed cell-mediated immunity in patients with primary intracranial tumors: characterization of a humoral immunosuppressive factor. *J. Exp. Med.* **136:** 1631–1647.

74. Kuratsu, J., K. Yoshizato, T. Yoshimura, E. J. Leonard, H. Takeshima, and Y. Ushio. 1993. Quantitative study of monocyte chemoattractant protein-1 (MCP-1) in cerebrospinal fluid and cyst fluid from patients with malignant glioma. *J. Natl. Cancer Inst.* **85:** 1836–1839.

75. Boetcher, D. A., and E. J. Leonard. 1974. Abnormal monocyte chemotactic response in cancer patients. *J. Natl. Cancer Inst.* **52:** 1091–1099.

76. Snyderman, R., M. C. Pike, L. Meadows, G. Hemstreet, and S. Wells. 1975. Depression of monocyte chemotaxis by neoplasia. *Clin. Res.* **34:** 297A.

77. Normann, S. J., and E. Sorkin. 1977. Inhibition of macrophage chemotaxis by neoplastic and other rapidly proliferating cells *in vitro. Cancer Res.* **37:** 705–711.

78. Goldsmith, H. S., A. G. Levin, and C. M. Southam. 1965. A study of cellular responses in cancer patients by qualitative and quantitative Rebuck tests. *Surg. Forum* **16:** 102–104.

79. Dizon, Q. S., and C. M. Southam. 1963. Abnormal cellular response to skin abrasion in cancer patients. *Cancer* **16:** 1288–1292.

80. Snyderman, R., M. C. Pike, B. L. Blaylock, and P. Weinstein. 1976. Effects of neoplasms on inflammation: depression of macrophage accumulation after tumor implantation. *J. Immunol.* **116:** 585–589.

81. North, R. J., D. P. Kirstein, and R. L. Tuttle. 1976. Subversion of host defense mechanisms by murine tumors. I. A circulating factor that suppresses macrophage-mediated resistance to infection. *J. Exp. Med.* **143:** 559–573.

82. Takeshima, H., J. Kuratsu, M. Takeya, T. Yoshimura, and Y. Ushio. 1994. Expression and localization of messenger RNA and protein for monocyte chemoattractant protein-1 in human malignant glioma. *J. Neurosurg.* **80:** 1056–1062.

83. Furutani, Y., H. Nomura, M. Notake, Y. Oyamada, T. Fukui, M. Yamada, C. G. Larsen, J. J. Oppenheim, and K. Matsushima. 1989. Cloning and sequencing of the cDNA for human monocyte chemotactic and activating factor (MCAF). *Biochem. Biophys. Res. Commun.* **159:** 249–255.

84. Van Damme, J., B. Decock, J. P. Lenaerts, R. Conings, R. Bertini, A. Montovani, and A. Billau. 1989. Identification by sequence analysis of chemotactic factors for monocytes produced by normal and transformed cells stimulated with virus, double-stranded RNA or cytokine. *Eur. J. Immunol.* **19:** 2367–2373.

85. Negus, R. P., G. W. Stamp, M. G. Relf, F. Burke, S. T. Malik, S. Bernasconi, P. Allavena, S. Sozzani, A. Mantovani, and F. R. Balkwill. 1995. The detection and localization of monocyte chemoattractant protein-1 (MCP-1) in human ovarian cancer. *J. Clin. Invest.* **95:** 2391–2396.

86. Sonouchi, K., T. A. Hamilton, C. S. Tannenbaum, R. R. Tubbs, R. Bukowski, and J. H. Finke. 1994. Chemokine gene expression in the murine renal cell carcinoma, RENCA, following treatment *in vivo* with Interferon-α and Interleukin-2. *Am. J. Pathol.* **144:** 747–755.

87. Melani, C., S. M. Pupa, A. Stoppacciaro, S. Menard, M. I. Colnaghi, G. Parmiani, and M. P. Colombo. 1995. An in vivo model to compare human leukocyte infiltration in carcinoma xenografts producing different chemokines. *Int. J. Cancer* **62:** 572–578.
88. Graves, D. T., R. Barnhill, T. Galanopoulos, and H. N. Antoniades. 1992. Expression of monocyte chemotactic protein-1 in human melanoma in vivo. *Am. J. Pathol.* **140:** 9–14.
89. Takeya, M., T. Yoshimura, E. J. Leonard, T. Kato, H. Okabe, and K. Takahashi. 1991. Production of monocyte chemoattractant protein-1 by malignant fibrous histiocytoma: relation to the origin of histiocyte-like cells. *Exp. Mol. Pathol.* **54:** 61–71.

7

Interactions Between Chemokines and Other Cytokines in Host Response to Tumor

Thomas A. Hamilton, Charles S. Tannenbaum,
James Finke, and Ronald Bukowski

1. INTRODUCTION: CHEMOKINE FUNCTIONS

This chapter focuses on interactions between chemokines and other cytokines that influence the nature of the host response to tumor. The basic structural and functional features of chemokines are presented in Chapters 1 and 2 in this volume, and a general discussion of these issues is therefore not provided here. The functional repertoire of the chemokine family is, however, known to encompass much beyond its ability to promote directed migration of leukocytes *(1–4)*. Since the cooperative potential of individual chemokines for modulating host response to tumor is likely to be heavily influenced by the functional potential of each molecule, it is appropriate to provide a brief overview of such activities.

As part of their ability to induce chemotactic function in target cells, many chemokines have been shown to modulate the avidity of the interaction between leukocyte adhesion ligands and their counterparts on endothelial cells. This finding provides further support for the importance of chemokines in controlling inflammatory leukocyte tissue infiltration *(5–8)*. Several chemokines have also been shown to either enhance or diminish the generation of new blood vessels *(9–17)*. Some chemokines are able to modulate the proliferative activity of selected hematopoietic progenitors and may thereby influence the size of different leukocyte populations *(18–20)*. Some tumors (melanomas) exhibit a requirement for a subset of C-X-C chemokines as growth factors *(21)*. Selected chemokines can modulate the effector functions of their target cells. For example, T-cell, macrophage, and natural killer (NK) cell cytotoxicity are enhanced by monocyte chemoattractant protein-1 (MCP-1) *(22–26)*, whereas interferon-γ-inducible protein-10 (IP-10) has been reported to enhance selectively the production of interferon-γ (IFN-γ) by Th1 cells. In this regard, macrophage inflammatory protein-1α (MIP-1α) and MCP-1 have been reported to modulate the nature of T-cell development by promoting Th1 or Th2 function, respectively *(27–30)*.

From: *Chemokines and Cancer*
Edited by: B. J. Rollins © Humana Press Inc., Totowa, NJ

2. PARTICIPATION OF CHEMOKINES IN HOST DEFENSE AGAINST TUMORS

2.1. Chemokines as Antitumor Agents

Multiple laboratories have examined the potential role of chemokines as mediators of antitumor activity *(31–48)*. Indeed, expression of transduced chemokine genes by tumor cells has been shown to promote an antitumor effect in multiple experimental settings *(31,34,40–43,45,46,48–50)*. C-C chemokines (MCP-1, TCA-3, MIP-1α, and RANTES), C-X-C chemokines (interleukin-8 [IL-8] and IP-10), and the single C chemotaxin lymphotactin (Ltn) have all been demonstrated to promote an antitumor response in this setting. The outcomes of these studies is not, however, uniformly positive or consistent. In fact, there is remarkable diversity in both the quality and quantity of the antitumor response. The variability is likely to derive from multiple sources. Certainly, the nature of the tumor model (e.g., immunogenicity) and the anatomic location of the tumor are likely to be important determinants. Another major source of variability is the immunocompetence of the host animal. However, even under circumstances in which these variables are held constant, individual chemokines are likely to have distinct consequences on the host–tumor relationship that will reflect the diverse functional potential of each chemokine. Possible contributions of individual functions are discussed next.

2.2. Antitumor Chemokine Activities

2.2.1. Chemotaxis

The most obvious functional contribution to be considered is chemotactic activity itself. Clearly the recruitment of immune effector cells into a tumor site is a critical requirement for the success of immune-mediated antitumor response, and chemokines are likely to play important roles in this process. The control of leukocyte trafficking both to and from a tumor site by chemokines could contribute to both the afferent and efferent aspects of the response.

Expression of a chemokine may not, however, represent an adequate independent signal to induce appropriate leukocytic tumor infiltration. The control of leukocytic tissue infiltration is clearly multifactorial and will be influenced by receptor expression on appropriate target cells and by the preparation of the tissue site. For example, the chemokines IP-10 and monokine-induced by IFN-γ (MIG) may have little chemotactic effect in the absence of accompanying T-cell activation that is associated with the expression of the IP-10/MIG receptor (CXCR3) *(51,52)*. By contrast, overexpression of a chemokine may produce target cell desensitization, thus reducing chemotactic response *(53)*. At the site of inflammation, leukocyte tissue infiltration will also depend on the appropriate expression of requisite cell adhesion receptors and ligand on endothelial cells and leukocytes, respectively *(5,54)*.

2.2.2. Growth Regulation

As mentioned briefly in the foregoing, chemokines exhibit activities in addition to chemotaxis that may be important determinants of the relationship between host and tumor. For example, the ability of certain chemokines to modulate cell growth may impact host–tumor interactions in a number of ways. Chemokines (especially C-X-C family members) have been linked with both enhancing and inhibiting cell growth; this kind of activity could thus have both beneficial and detrimental consequences for the host *(18–21,55)*. Indeed, growth-related oncogene-alpha and IL-8 have been identified as important growth factors for melanomas, an activity that appears to be mediated by the CXCR2 receptor *(21,55)*. Several chemokines have also been demonstrated to inhibit the growth of hematopoietic progenitor cells in the bone marrow *(18–20)*. This kind of activity has been implicated as important for determining the availability of different leukocyte populations in the circulation, which may be a contributing component of an antitumor response *(43)*. In hematopoietic tumors, such growth inhibitory activity could also provide a more direct impact.

2.2.3. Modulation of Leukocyte Development and Effector Function

Both C-C and C-X-C chemokines have been reported to modulate directly the activity of potential antitumor effector cells *(23–27,29,30,56,57)*. For example, MCP-1 (also termed macrophage chemotactic and activating factor) has been shown to enhance the activity of monocytes and macrophages, particularly with respect to antitumor activity, either alone or combined with other stimuli such as lipopolysaccharide *(56)*. More recently, several C-C chemokines have been reported to induce or enhance the effector functions of both T-lymphocytes and NK cells, which could be an important contribution when acting in a localized fashion *(23–26,57)*. In addition to modulating the effector functions of immune cells, MIP-1α, MCP-1, and IP-10 have been shown to modulate the nature of cytokine secretion patterns, reflecting alterations in T-cell differentiation *(29,30)*.

2.2.4. Angiogenesis

As mentioned previously, the role of chemokines in angiogenesis may have a significant impact on the host–tumor interaction *(9–17)*. Much recent attention has been focused on the importance of angiogenesis in tumor progression; in the absence of the active development of a vascular supply, many tumors either do not grow or are unable to metastasize *(58–60)*. In this regard, some C-X-C chemokines (e.g., IL-8, epithelial cell–derived neutrophil-activating factor-78) have been shown to have potent angiogenic activity whereas others (e.g., IP-10, platelet factor 4) are able to block this activity effectively *(9,13,15,16,61)*. The presence of a 3 amino acid motif (ELR) in the amino terminus of the mature chemokine peptide appears to be an important determinant of whether a chemokine is angiogenic (ELR⁺) or angiostatic (ELR⁻). These observations have collectively led to the hypothesis that the balance of angiogenic vs angiostatic C-X-C chemokines expressed at the tumor site may be an important determinant of tumor progression or regression *(9,13,61)*.

2.3. Chemokine Antitumor Function Involves Cooperation with Other Cytokines

The orchestration of immune-inflammatory responses is clearly a process in which multiple cell types and products participate. Thus, a requirement for cooperation among different components of the host immune system is obvious. Nevertheless, numerous studies of direct antitumor function of chemokines indicate that these agents are often insufficient by themselves to promote the execution of a fully effective antitumor response and, rather, depend on cooperation with other cytokines. Evidence from two kinds of experiments, in particular, support this concept and help define the functional nature of the cooperative activities.

2.3.1. Chemokines as Tumor Transgenes

The first example of cooperativity involves the antitumor response induced or promoted by chemokines expressed as transgenes in tumor cell lines *(31,34,40–43,45,46,48–50)*. Although some studies have concluded that chemokine expression can prevent tumor formation, several examples clearly demonstrate that the expression of chemokine alone either is insufficient to provide full protection or only does so in immunocompetent animals *(31,34,40,44,48,62)*. When the RANTES chemokine was expressed as a transgene in an immunogenic murine fibrosarcoma cell line, the ability to form tumors in vivo was abolished *(40)*. The effect was shown to be chemokine dependent and to require the participation of several different populations of host immune effector cell types, though the specific molecular nature of the cooperative activities was not clearly demonstrated. Similar findings have been reported in tumor cells transduced with other chemokine genes including MCP-1 and IP-10 *(31,44)*. Tumor cells expressing Ltn, the single member of the C family of chemokines, were infiltrated by T-lymphocytes, but tumor growth under these conditions was not interrupted. When mice bearing such tumors were also treated with IL-2 or granulocyte-macrophage colony-stimulating factor (GM-CSF), a marked T-cell-dependent antitumor activity was obtained *(48)*. Thus, under these particular circumstances, cooperation among chemokines and other components of the host immune response are readily demonstrable.

2.3.2. Chemokine Expression During Cytokine Therapy

The second example of cooperativity is evident in the role of individual chemokines in antitumor responses elicited by other cytokines either when used as transgenes or by local or systemic injection. For example, IL-4 has been demonstrated to be one of the more potent lymphokine products when used as a transgene for promoting specific antitumor response, and histologic evaluation of IL-4-expressing tumor sites reveals a heavy infiltration with eosinophils *(47,63)*. The recent identification of the chemokine eotaxin as a potent eosinophil-directed chemotaxin and its expression in tumor tissue from IL-4-secreting tumors suggests that this product plays an important cooperative role in the efficacy of IL-4 as an antitumor cytokine *(47)*.

A third example involves the use of IL-12 as a highly potent antitumor cytokine therapy in rodent tumor models even against well-established tumors *(64–69)*. The effect is T-cell and IFN-γ dependent *(66,70)*. Examination of tumor tissue for the expression of other cytokines has revealed a tight correlation between IL-12 treatment and the expression of the IFN-γ-inducible chemokine IP-10 *(68,69)*. Two features of this response may be causally linked with the expression of IP-10. First, IL-12 treatment results in a marked infiltration of tumor tissue by CD8[+] and CD4[+] T-lymphocytes *(64,68,69,71)*. Since IP-10 binds to a receptor expressed exclusively on activated T-cells, the lymphocytic infiltrate could be IP-10 dependent as well *(51)*. Indeed, the antitumor activity of IL-12 and the accompanying T-cell infiltrate are at least partially abrogated by cotreatment with neutralizing antibody to IP-10 *(72)*. Second, IL-12 exhibits antiangiogenic activity, which has been reported to be directly related to the expression of IP-10 *(10,12,14,17,73)*. Thus, in these two models, the dissection of the complex immune response to tumor suggests important roles for chemokines in cooperation with other cytokines.

2.4 Cytokine Activities That May Cooperate with Chemokines

There is currently little published experience regarding the effects of combining different cytokines in therapeutic protocols for the treatment of malignancy or other diseases. However, as the knowledge of cytokine function in vivo expands, the development of strategies using cytokine combinations is likely to be a fertile area. The range of functional contributions that various chemokines may make to a host antitumor response has been presented and discussed in the foregoing. In consideration of the cooperation among chemokines and other cytokines, the activities that could be provided by other cytokines should be complementary to those provided by one or more chemokines. The appropriate combination of such complementary functions should generate a comprehensive and efficacious response to the tumor challenge. The following discussion focuses on the activities provided by other cytokines that might complement chemotaxis-related chemokine function. A brief consideration of the cooperation with nonchemotaxis functions is also presented.

2.4.1. Complementing Chemotactic Function

The recruitment of leukocytes is likely to be the most frequent role played by chemokines in antitumor responses. This is supported by the available examples of chemokine function in antitumor activities described previously *(48,68)*. Chemotactic function will be a valuable activity in the context of both specific T-cell-mediated antitumor immunity and antitumor mechanisms of the innate immune system, such as NK cells and macrophages. A fully effective host antitumor response will depend on the generation of potent tumor-directed effector cells and a mechanism (chemotaxis) to direct such a response to the appropriate anatomic site (tumor). Thus, the most likely cytokines to cooperate with chemokines will be those that enhance the ability of the host to mount such a response.

Indeed, the failure of the host to mount an appropriate antitumor immune response is perhaps the most limiting feature of immunotherapy. The restricted immune response to tumor is likely to involve both the number of tumor-specific immune cells that can be produced and the quantity or quality of the state of activation achieved in such immune-cell populations. Contributing to this problem is the limited immunogenicity of many tumors and the well-documented ability of many tumors to promote an immunosuppressive environment. Recent experience examining the ability of different cytokines to induce the development of tumor-specific immunity when expressed as transgenes identifies these cytokines as potential targets to consider for use in cooperation with chemokines. Examples of the most potent agents identified through such studies include IFN-γ, IL-2, IL-4, GM-CSF, and IL-12 *(65,67,74–77)*. The capability of these agents to provide immune-mediated protection from and/or destruction of implanted tumors demonstrates their ability to overcome at least some of the limiting aspects of host-derived immune response. These cytokines are likely to modulate the afferent limb of the immune response by enhancing antigen presentation or the differentiation of T-lymphocytes into functionally distinct subsets. In addition, these cytokines can act on a variety of cell types that can function in a relatively antigen-independent fashion, including NK cells, macrophages, eosinophils, and neutrophils.

Although the use of such cytokines either systemically or by expression as transgenes in transplanted tumor cells has shown efficacy in animal models, phase I human trials have yet to yield appreciable success *(78–82)*. This failure could derive either from an inability to recruit appropriate cells to such sites or because the magnitude of the antitumor response is insufficient. Induction of localized chemokine expression at distant tumor sites could provide an important and complementary activity that could enhance this strategy. An alternative (though not mutually exclusive) approach involves the use of such tumor vaccines to promote the initial development of a specific antitumor response that could be amplified in vitro *(83–88)*. Populations of specific antitumor T-lymphocytes might then be utilized in adoptive-transfer protocols, and some efficacy of this approach in animal models and phase I human trials has been reported *(88,89)*. This may be an optimal setting in which to attempt cooperative strategies involving chemokines in which the ability to target the therapeutic agent (tumor-specific effector T-cells) could be enhanced significantly.

In addition to cytokines that help promote host immune response to the tumor, cytokines that upregulate the expression of leukocyte endothelial cell adhesion molecules would also be expected to cooperate with chemokines. Effector cell infiltration of the tumor depends on endothelial cell activation and the expression of adhesion ligands that are strongly inducible by cytokines such as tumor necrosis factor and IL-1 as well as IFN-γ *(5–8)*. Under circumstances in which a robust immune response to the tumor develops, it is likely, however, that appropriate upregulation of these cytokines and the associated alteration in endothelial cell function will occur.

2.4.2. Complementing Nonchemotactic Function

As previously stated, the efficacy of cytokine- and chemokine-mediated antitumor activities will be linked to their individual or cooperative ability to promote a specific immune response to the tumor, and this will include the process of chemotaxis. Chemokine functions that are not related to chemoattraction may, however, also cooperate in the overall ability of the host to eliminate the tumor. The ability of chemokines to promote leukocyte activation and/or differentiation, to inhibit angiogenesis, or to regulate proliferation may enhance their role in antitumor function. Indeed, for some chemokines, the nonchemotactic functions may predominate *(14,17)*. In such circumstances, appropriate (and perhaps requisite) chemotactic activity would be contributed as well or by other chemoattractants. A specific example is provided by treatment with IL-12 in which chemotaxis and inhibition of angiogenesis may both be important components of the successful response *(14,68,69,72)*. IL-12 promotes a strong Th1-type response that can markedly enhance the host's normal response to tumor *(64,66,90,91)*. IL-12-stimulated expression of IFN-γ will induce the T-cell-specific chemokines IP-10 and MIG, both of which can recruit activated T-cells, inhibit angiogenesis, and produce tumor necrosis. In this case, both chemotaxis and angiostasis combine and cooperate with IL-12 to promote the destruction of tumor.

3. CONCLUSION

Chemokines are now believed to be important participants in the orchestration of inflammatory processes. The functions provided by this family of cytokines will work cooperatively with those produced by other cytokines, and this is likely to be an important feature of host antitumor defense. Immunotherapy of cancer continues to exhibit significant potential but is of only limited clinical value at present. This process, when successful, involves the controlled development of an immune-mediated inflammatory response at the tumor site. This approach is limited by a number of factors, at least two of which are relevant to the current discussion. First, although antitumor immune response can be frequently demonstrated, the abundance of antitumor effector cells is often inadequate, especially when faced with tumor-induced immunosuppression. Second, appropriately activated cells must be effectively targeted to the tumor site. These two functions provide the opportunity for cooperative interaction among two or more cytokine reagents. The central importance of effector cell recruitment to the tumor site underscores the potential importance of chemokines in such function.

The activities of chemokines that are not strictly linked to leukocyte chemotaxis are, however, also likely to be important players in antitumor responses. The role of angiogenesis in tumor growth and metastasis is an issue currently receiving substantial attention. Although inhibition of angiogenesis is not sufficient as antitumor therapy alone, it may provide an important component of a multifactorial approach. The contribution of the non-ELR C-X-C chemokines in this area may also be of particular importance. Indeed, as these products can also serve to recruit activated T-cells, they are able to provide multiple functions that are mechanistically independent.

REFERENCES

1. Howard, O. M. Z., A. Ben-Baruch, and J. J. Oppenheim. 1996. Chemokines: progress toward identifying molecular targets for therapeutic agents. *Trends Biotechnol.* **14:** 46.
2. Negus, R. P. M. 1996. The chemokines: cytokines that direct leukocyte migration. *J. R. Soc. Med.* **89:** 312.
3. Rollins, B. J. 1997. Chemokines. *Blood* **90:** 909.
4. Baggiolini, M. 1998. Chemokines and leukocyte traffic. *Nature* **392:** 565.
5. Springer, T. A. 1994. Traffic signals for lymphocyte recirculation and leukocyte emigration: the multistep paradigm. *Cell* **76:** 301.
6. Lollo, B. A., K. W. H. Chan, E. M. Hanson, V. T. Moy, and A. A. Brian. 1993. Direct evidence for two affinity states for lymphocyte function associated antigen-1 on activated T cells. *J. Biol. Chem.* **268:** 21,693.
7. Diamond, M. S., and T. A. Springer. 1993. A subpopulation of Mac-1 (CD11b/CD18) molecules mediates neutrophil adhesion to ICAM-1 and fibrinogen. *J. Cell Biol.* **120:** 545.
8. Snyderman, R., and R. J. Uhing. 1992. Chemoattractant stimulus–response coupling, in *Inflammation: Basic Principles and Classical Correlates,* 2nd ed. Gallin, J. I., I. M. Goldstein, and R. Snyderman, eds.), *Raven,* New York, p. 421.
9. Strieter, R. M., P. J. Polverini, D. A. Arenberg, A. Walz, G. Opdenakker, J. Van Damme, and S. L. Kunkel. 1995. Role of C-X-C chemokines as regulators of angiogenesis in lung cancer. *J. Leuk. Biol.* **57:** 752.
10. Angiolillo, A. L., C. Sgadari, D. D. Taub, F. Liao, J. M. Farber, S. Maheshwari, H. K. Kleinman, G. H. Reaman, and G. Tosato. 1995. Human interferon inducible protein IP-10 is a potent inhibitor of angiogenesis in vivo. *J. Exp. Med.* **182:** 155.
11. Strieter, R. M., S. L. Kunkel, D. A. Arenberg, M. D. Burdick, and P. J. Polverini. 1995. Interferon gamma-inducible protein 10 (IP-10), a member of the C-X-C chemokine family, is an inhibitor of angiogenesis. *Biochem. Biophys. Res. Commun.* **210:** 51.
12. Luster, A. D., S. M. Greenberg, and P. Leder. 1995. The IP-10 chemokine binds to a specific cell surface heparan sulfate site shared with platelet factor 4 and inhibits endothelial cell proliferation. *J. Exp. Med.* **182:** 219.

13. Strieter, R. M., P. J. Polverini, D. A. Arenberg, and S. L. Kunkel. 1995. The role of CXC chemokines as regulators of angiogenesis. *Shock* **4:** 155.
14. Sgadari, C., A. L. Angiolillo, and G. Tosato. 1996. Inhibition of angiogenesis by interleukin-12 is mediated by the interferon-inducible protein 10. *Blood* **87:** 3877.
15. Arenberg, D. A., S. L. Kunkel, P. J. Polverini, M. Glass, M. D. Burdick, and R. M. Strieter. 1996. Inhibition of interleukin-8 reduces tumorigenesis of human non-small cell lung cancer in SCID mice. *J. Clin. Invest.* **97:** 2792.
16. Arenberg, D. A., S. L. Kunkel, P. J. Polverini, S. B. Morris, M. D. Burdick, M. C. Glass, D. T. Taub, M. D. Iannettoni, T. I. Whyte, and R. M. Strieter. 1996. Interferon-gamma-inducible protein 10 (IP-10) is an angiostatic factor that inhibits human non-small cell lung cancer (NSCLC) tumorigenesis and spontaneous metastases. *J. Exp. Med.* **184:** 981.
17. Sgadari, C., A. Angiolillo, B. W. Cherney, S. E. Pike, J. M. Farber, L. G. Koniaris, P. Vanguri, P. R. Burd, N. Sheik, G. Gupta, J. Teruya-Feldstein, and G. Tosato. 1996. Interferon inducible protein 10 identified as a mediator of tumor necrosis in vivo. *Proc. Natl. Acad. Sci. USA* **93:** 13,791.
18. Broxmeyer, H. E., B. Sherry, S. Cooper, L. Lu, R. Maze, M. P. Beckmann, A. Cerami, and P. Ralph. 1993. Comparative analysis of the human macrophage inflammatory protein family of cytokines (chemokines) on proliferation of human myeloid progenitor cells: interacting effects involving suppression, synergistic suppression, and blocking of suppression. *J. Immunol.* **150:** 3448.
19. Youn, B.-S., I.-K. Jang, H. E. Broxmeyer, S. Cooper, N. A. Jenkins, D. J. Gilbert, N. G. Copeland, T. A. Elick, M. J. Fraser, Jr., and B. S. Kwon. 1995. A novel chemokine, macrophage inflammatory protein-related protein-2, inhibits colony formation of bone marrow myeloid progenitors. *J. Immunol.* **155:** 2661.
20. Aronica, S. M., C. Mantel, R. Gonin, M. S. Marshall, A. Sarris, S. Cooper, N. Hague, X. F. Zhang, and H. E. Broxmeyer. 1995. Interferon-inducible protein 10 and macrophage inflammatory protein-1α inhibit growth factor stimulation of Raf-1 kinase activity and protein synthesis in a human growth factor-dependent hematopoietic cell line. *J. Biol. Chem.* **270:** 21,998.
21. Schadendorf, D., A. Moller, B. Algermissen, M. Worm, M. Sticherling, and B. M. Czarnetzki. 1993. IL-8 produced by human malignant melanoma cells in vitro is an essential autocrine growth factor. *J. Immunol.* **151:** 2667.
22. Singh, R. K., K. Berry, K. Matsushima, K. Yasumoto, and I. J. Fidler. 1993. Synergism between human monocyte chemotactic and activating factor and bacterial products for activation of tumoricidal properties in murine macrophages. *J. Immunol.* **151:** 2786.
23. Taub, D. D., T. J. Sayers, C. R. D. Carter, and J. R. Ortaldo. 1995. α and β chemokines induce NK cell migration and enhance NK-mediated cytolysis. *J. Immunol.* **155:** 3877.
24. Taub, D. D., J. R. Ortaldo, S. M. Turcovski-Corrales, M. L. Key, D. L. Longo, and W. J. Murphy. 1996. β Chemokines costimulate lymphocyte cytolysis, proliferation, and lymphokine production. *J. Leuk. Biol.* **59:** 81.
25. Taub, D. D., S. M. Turcovski-Corrales, M. L. Key, D. L. Longo, and W. J. Murphy. 1996. Chemokines and T lymphocyte activation. I. β chemokines costimulate human T lymphocyte activation in vitro. *J. Immunol.* **156:** 2095.
26. Maghazachi, A. A., A. Al-Aoukaty, and T. J. Schall. 1996. CC chemokines induce the generation of killer cells from CD56+ cells. *Eur. J. Immunol.* **26:** 315.
27. Chensue, S. W., K. S. Warmington, J. H. Ruth, P. S. Sanghi, P. Lincoln, and S. L. Kunkel. 1996. Role of monocyte chemoattractant protein-1 (MCP-1) in Th1 (mycobacterial) and Th2 (schistosomal) antigen-induced granuloma formation—relationship to local inflammation, Th cell expression, and IL-12 production. *J. Immunol.* **157:** 4602.
28. Karpus, W. J., and K. J. Kennedy. 1997. MIP-1α and MCP-1 differentially regulate acute and relapsing autoimmune encephalomyelitis as well as Th1/Th2 lymphocyte differentiation. *J. Leuk. Biol.* **62:** 681.

29. Karpus, W. J., N. W. Lukacs, K. J. Kennedy, W. S. Smith, S. D. Hurst, and T. A. Barrett. 1997. Differential CC chemokine-induced enhancement of T helper cell cytokine production. *J. Immunol.* **158:** 4129.

30. Gangur, V., F. E. Simons, and K. T. Hayglass. 1998. Human IP-10 selectively promotes dominance of polyclonally activated and environmental antigen-driven IFN-gamma over IL-4 responses. *FASEB J.* **12:** 705.

31. Luster, A. D., and P. Leder. 1993. IP-10, a C-X-C-chemokine, elicits a potent thymus-dependent antitumor response in vivo. *J. Exp. Med.* **178:** 1057.

32. Anderson, J. A., A. B. Lentsch, D. J. Hadjiminas, F. N. Miller, A. W. Martin, K. Nakagawa, and M. J. Edwards. 1996. The role of cytokines, adhesion molecules, and chemokines in interleukin-2-induced lymphocytic infiltration in C57BL/6 mice. *J. Clin. Invest.* **97:** 1952.

33. Cao, Y., C. Chen, J. A. Weatherbee, M. Tsang, and J. Folkman. 1995. gro-β, a CXC chemokine is an angiogenesis inhibitor that suppresses the growth of Lewis lung carcinoma in mice. *J. Exp. Med.* **182:** 2069.

34. Laning, J., H. Kawasaki, E. Tanaka, Y. Luo, and M. Dorf. 1994. Inhibition of in vivo tumor growth by the beta chemokine TCA3. *J. Immunol.* **153:** 4625.

35. Negus, R. P., and F. R. Balkwill. 1996. Cytokines in tumor growth, migration, and metastasis. *World J. Urol.* **14:** 157.

36. Negus, R. P., G. W. Stamp, M. G. Relf, F. Burke, S. T. Malik, S. Bernasconi, P. Allavena, S. Sozzani, A. Mantovani, and F. R. Balkwill. 1995. The detection and localization of monocyte chemoattractant protein-1 (MCP-1) in human ovarian cancer. *J. Clin. Invest.* **95:** 2391.

37. von Luettichau, I., P. J. Nelson, J. M. Pattison, M. van de Rijn, P. Huie, R. Warnke, C. J. Wiederman, R. A. Stahl, R. K. Sibley, and A. M. Krensky. 1996. RANTES expression in diseased and normal human tissues. *Cytokine* **8:** 89.

38. Wiltrout, R. H., T. A. Gregorio, R. G. Fenton, D. L. Longo, P. Ghosh, W. J. Murphy, and K. L. Komschlies. 1995. Cellular and molecular studies in the treatment of murine renal cancer. *Semin. Oncol.* **22:** 9.

39. Mazzucchelli, L., P. Loetscher, A. Kappeler, M. Uguccioni, M. Baggiolini, J. A. Laissue, and C. Mueller. 1996. Monocyte chemoattractant protein-1 gene expression in prostatic hyperplasia and prostate adenocarcinoma. *Am. J. Pathol.* **149:** 501.

40. Mule, J. J., M. Custer, B. Averbook, J. C. Yang, J. S. Weber, D. V. Goeddel, S. A. Rosenberg, and T. J. Schall. 1996. RANTES secretion by gene modified tumor cells results in loss of tumorigenicity in vivo: role of immune cell subpopulations. *Hum. Gene Ther.* **7:** 1545.

41. Huang, S., R. K. Singh, K. Xie, M. Gutman, K. K. Berry, C. D. Bucana, I. J. Fidler, and M. Bar-Eli. 1994. Expression of the *JE/MCP-1* gene suppresses metastatic potential in murine colon carcinoma cells. *Cancer Immunol. Immunother.* **39:** 231.

42. Huang, S., K. Xie, R. K. Singh, M. Gutman, and M. Bar-Eli. 1995. Suppression of tumor growth and metastasis of murine renal adenocarcinoma by syngeneic fibroblasts genetically engineered to secrete the JE/MCP-1 cytokine. *J. Interferon Cytokine Res.* **15:** 655.

43. Hoshino, Y., K. Hatake, T. Kasahara, Y. Takahashi, M. Ikeda, H. Tomizuka, T. Ohtsuki, M. Uwai, N. Mukaida, K. Matsushima, and Y. Miura. 1995. Monocyte chemoattractant protein-1 stimulates tumor necrosis and recruitment of macrophages into tumors in tumor-bearing nude mice: increased granulocyte and macrophage progenitors in murine bone marrow. *Exp. Hematol.* **23:** 1035.

44. Hirose, K., M. Hakozaki, Y. Nyunoya, Y. Kobayashi, K. Matsushita, T. Takenouchi, A. Mikata, N. Mukaida, and K. Matsushima. 1995. Chemokine gene transfection into tumour cells reduced tumorigenicity in nude mice in association with neutrophilic infiltration. *Br. J. Cancer* **72:** 708.

45. Manome, Y., P. Y. Wen, A. Hershowitz, T. Tanaka, B. J. Rollins, D. W. Kufe, and H. A. Fine. 1995. Monocyte chemoattractant protein-1 (MCP-1) gene transduction: an

effective tumor vaccine strategy for non-intracranial tumors. *Cancer Immunol. Immunother.* **41:** 227.

46. Rollins, B., and M. E. Sunday. 1991. Suppression of tumor formation in vivo by expression of the JE gene in malignant cells. *Mol. Cell. Biol.* **11:** 3125.

47. Rothenberg, M. E., A. D. Luster, and P. Leder. 1995. Murine eotaxin: an eosinophil chemoattractant inducible in endothelial cells and in interleukin 4-induced tumor suppression. *Proc. Natl. Acad. Sci. USA* **92:** 8960.

48. Dilloo, D., K. Bacon, W. Holden, W. Zhong, W. Burdach, A. Zlotnik, and M. Brenner. 1996. Combined chemokine and cytokine gene transfer enhances anti-tumor immunity. *Nat. Med.* **2:** 1090.

49. Gattass, C. R., L. B. King, A. D. Luster, and J. D. Ashwell. 1994. Constitutive expression of interferon gamma-inducible protein 10 in lymphoid organs and inducible expression in T cells and thymocytes. *J. Exp. Med.* **179:** 1373.

50. Mule, J. J., and S. A. Rosenberg. 1991. Combination cytokine therapy: experimental and clinical trials, in *Biological Therapy of Cancer.* (DeVita, V. T., S. Hellman, and S. A. Rosenberg, eds.), J. B. Lipincott, Philadelphia, p. 393.

51. Loetscher, M., B. Gerber, P. Loetscher, S. A. Jones, L. Piali, I. Clark-Lewis, M. Baggiolini, and B. Moser. 1996. Chemokine receptor specific for IP-10 and Mig: structure, function and expression in activated T lymphocytes. *J. Exp. Med.* **184:** 963.

52. Mackay, C. R. 1996. Chemokine receptors and T cell chemotaxis. *J. Exp. Med.* **184:** 799.

53. Rutledge, B. R., H. Rayburn, R. Rosenberg, R. J. North, R. P. Gladue, C. Corless, and B. J. Rollins. 1995. High level monocyte chemoattractant protein-1 expression in transgenic mice increases their susceptibility to intracellular pathogens. *J. Immunol.* **155:** 4838.

54. Butcher, E. C. 1991. Leukocyte-endothelial cell recognition: three (or more) steps to specificity and diversity. *Cell* **67:** 1033.

55. Norgauer, J., B. Metzner, and I. Schraufstatter. 1996. Expression and growth promoting function of the IL-8 receptor-β in human melanoma cells. *J. Immunol.* **156:** 1132.

56. Singh, R. K., and I. J. Fidler. 1993. Synergism between human recombinant monocyte chemotactic and activating factor and lipopolysaccharide for activation of antitumor properties in human blood monocytes. *Lymphokine Cytokine Res.* **12:** 285.

57. Murphy, W. J., Z. G. Tian, O. Asai, S. Funakoshi, P. Rotter, M. Henry, R. M. Strieter, S. L. Kunkel, D. L. Longo, and D. D. Taub. 1996. Chemokines and T lymphocyte activation. 2. Facilitation of human T cell trafficking in severe combined immunodeficiency mice. *J. Immunol.* **156:** 2104.

58. Folkman, J. 1996. Patterns and emerging mechanisms of the angiogenic switch during tumorigenesis. *Cell* **86:** 383.

59. D'Amore, P. A., and D. T. Shima. 1996. Tumor angiogenesis: a physiological process or genetically determined? *Cancer Metastasis Rev.* **15:** 205.

60. Folkman, J. 1995. Angiogenesis in cancer, vascular, rheumatoid and other disease. *Nat. Med.* **1:** 27.

61. Strieter, R. M., D. G. Remick, J. P. Lynch, R. N. Spengler, and S. L. Kunkel. 1989. Interleukin-2-induced tumor necrosis factor-alpha (TNF-α) gene expression in human alveolar macrophages and blood monocytes. *Am. Rev. Respir. Dis.* **139:** 335.

62. Burdach, S., N. Zessack, D. Dilloo, M. Shatsky, D. Thompson, and L. Levitt. 1991. Differential regulation of lymphokine production by distinct subunits of the T cell interleukin 2 receptor. *J. Clin. Invest.* **87:** 2114.

63. Golumbek, P. T., A. J. Lazenby, H. I. Levitsky, L. M. Jaffee, H. Karasuyama, M. Baker, and D. M. Pardoll. 1991. Treatment of established renal cancer by tumor cells engineered to secrete interleukin-4. *Science* **254:** 713.

64. Brunda, M. J., L. Luistro, R. R. Warrier, R. B. Wright, B. R. Hubbard, M. Murphy,

S. F. Wolf, and M. K. Gately. 1993. Antitumor and antimetastatic activity of interleukin 12 against murine tumors. *J. Exp. Med.* **178:** 1223.

65. Tahara, H., H. J. Zeh, III, W. J. Storkus, I. Pappo, S. C. Watkins, U. Gubler, S. F. Wolf, P. D. Robbins, and M. T. Lotze. 1994. Fibroblasts genetically engineered to secrete interleukin 12 can suppress tumor growth and induce antitumor immunity to a murine melanoma *in vivo. Cancer Res.* **54:** 182.

66. Nastala, C. L., H. D. Edington, T. G. McKinney, H. Tahara, M. A. Nalesnik, M. J. Brunda, M. K. Gately, S. F. Wolf, R. D. Schreiber, W. J. Storkus, and M. T. Lotze. 1994. Recombinant interleukin-12 (IL-12) administration induces tumor regression in association with interferon-gamma production. *J. Immunol.* **153:** 1697.

67. Tahara, H., L. Zitvogel, W. J. Storkus, H. J. Zeh, III, T. G. McKinney, R. D. Schreiber, U. Gubler, P. D. Robbins, and M. T. Lotze. 1995. Effective eradication of established murine tumors with IL-12 gene therapy using a polycistronic retroviral vector. *J. Immunol.* **154:** 6466.

68. Tannenbaum, C. S., N. Wicker, D. Armstrong, R. Tubbs, J. Finke, R. M. Bukowski, and T. A. Hamilton. 1996. Cytokine and chemokine expression in tumors of mice receiving systemic therapy with IL-12. *J. Immunol.* **156:** 693.

69. Dias, S., H. Thomas, and F. Balkwill. 1998. Multiple molecular and cellular changes associated with tumour stasis and regression during IL-12 therapy of a murine breast cancer model. *Int. J. Cancer* **75:** 151.

70. Brunda, M. J., L. Luistro, J. A. Hendrzak, M. Fountoulakis, G. Garotta, and M. K. Gately. 1995. Role of interferon-gamma in mediating the antitumor efficacy of interleukin-12. *J. Immunother.* **17:** 71.

71. Brunda, M. J., L. Luistro, L. Rumennik, R. B. Wright, M. Dvorozniak, A. Aglione, J. M. Wigginton, R. H. Wiltrout, J. A. Hendrzak, and A. V. Palleroni. 1996. Antitumor activity of interleukin 12 in preclinical models. *Cancer Chemother. Pharmacol.* **38(Suppl.):** S16.

72. Tannenbaum, C. S., R. Tubbs, D. Armstrong, J. H. Finke, R. M. Bukowski, and T. A. Hamilton. 1998. The CXC chemokines IP-10 and Mig are necessary for IL-12-mediated regression of the mouse RENCA tumor. *J. Immunol.* **161:** 927.

73. Voest, E. E., B. M. Kenyon, M. S. O'Reilly, G. Truitt, R. J. D'Amato, and J. Folkman. 1995. Inhibition of angiogenesis in vivo by Interleukin 12. *JNCI* **87:** 581.

74. Porgador, A., B. Gansbacher, R. Bannerji, E. Tzehoval, E. Gilboa, M. Feldman, and L. Eisenbach. 1993. Anti-metastatic vaccination of tumor-bearing mice with IL-2-gene-inserted tumor cells. *Int. J. Cancer* **53:** 471.

75. Porgador, A., R. Bannerji, Y. Watanabe, M. Feldman, E. Gilboa, and L. Eisenbach. 1993. Antimetastatic vaccination of tumor-bearing mice with two types of IFN-γ gene-inserted tumor cells. *J. Immunol.* **150:** 1458.

76. Dranoff, G., E. Jaffee, A. Lazenby, P. Golumbek, H. Levitsky, K. Brose, V. Jackson, H. Hamada, D. Pardoll, and R. C. Mulligan. 1993. Vaccination with irradiated tumor cells engineered to secrete murine granulocyte-macrophage colony stimulating factor stimulates potent, specific, and long lasting anti-tumor immunity. *Proc. Natl. Acad. Sci. USA* **90:** 3539.

77. Zitvogel, L., H. Tahara, P. D. Robbins, W. J. Storkus, M. R. Clarke, M. A. Nalesnik, and M. T. Lotze. 1995. Cancer immunotherapy of established tumors with IL-12: effective delivery by genetically engineered fibroblasts. *J. Immunol.* **155:** 1393.

78. Simmons, J. W., E. M. Jaffee, C. E. Weber, H. L. Levitsky, W. G. Nelson, M. A. Carducci, A. J. Lazenby, L. K. Cohen, C. C. Finn, S. M. Clift, K. M. Hauda, L. A. Beck, K. M. Leiferman, A. H. Owens, Jr., S. Piantadosi, G. Dranoff, R. C. Mulligan, D. M. Pardoll, and F. F. Marshall. 1997. Bioactivity of autologous irradiated renal cell carcinoma vaccines generated by ex-vivo granulocyte-macrophage-colony stimulating factor gene transfer. *Cancer Res.* **57:** 1537.

79. Gilboa, E. 1996. Immunotherapy of cancer with genetically modified tumor vaccines. *Semin. Oncol.* **23:** 101.

80. Vieweg, J., F. M. Rosenthal, R. Bannerji, W. D. Heston, W. R. Fair, B. Gansbacher, and E. Gilboa. 1994. Immunotherapy of prostate cancer in the Dunning rat model: use of cytokine gene modified tumor vaccines. *Cancer Res.* **54:** 1760.

81. Saito, S., R. Bannerji, B. Gansbacher, F. M. Rosenthal, P. Romanenko, W. D. Heston, W. R. Fair, and E. Gilboa. 1994. Immunotherapy of bladder cancer with cytokine gene-modified tumor vaccines. *Cancer Res.* **54:** 3516.

82. Jaffee, E. M., and D. M. Pardoll. 1995. Gene therapy: its potential applications in the treatment of renal-cell carcinoma. *Semin. Oncol.* **22:** 81.

83. Yoshizawa, H., A. E. Chang, and S. Shu. 1991. Specific adoptive immunotherapy mediated by tumor-draining lymph node cells sequentially activated with anti-CD3 and IL-2. *J. Immunol.* **147:** 729.

84. Kagamu, H., J. E. Touhalisky, G. E. Plautz, J. C. Krauss, and S. Shu. 1996. Isolation based on L-selectin expression of immune effector T cells derived from tumor-draining lymph nodes. *Cancer Res.* **56:** 4338.

85. Inoue, M., G. E. Plautz, and S. Shu. 1996. Treatment of intracranial tumors by systemic transfer of superantigen-activated tumor-draining lymph node T cells. *Cancer Res.* **56:** 4702.

86. Chang, A. E., and S. Shu. 1996. Current status of adoptive immunotherapy of cancer. *Crit. Rev. Oncol. Hematol.* **22:** 213.

87. Mitsuma, S., H. Yoshizawa, K. Ito, H. Moriyama, M. Wakabayashi, T. Chou, M. Arakwa, and S. Shu. 1994. Adoptive immunotherapy mediated by anti-TCR/IL-2 activated tumor-draining lymph node cells. *Immunology* **83:** 45.

88. Chang, A. E., A. Aruga, M. J. Cameron, V. K. Sondak, D. P. Normolle, B. A. Fox, and S. Y. Shu. 1997. Adoptive immunotherapy with vaccine-primed lymph node cells secondarily activated with anti-CD3 and interleukin-2. *J. Clin. Oncol.* **15:** 796.

89. Kagamu, H., and S. Shu. 1998. Purification of L-selectin (low) cells promotes the generation of highly potent CD4 antitumor effector T lymphocytes. *J. Immunol.* **160:** 3444.

90. Manetti, R., P. Parronchi, M. G. Giudizi, M.-P. Piccinni, E. Maggi, G. Trinchieri, and S. Romagnani. 1993. Natural killer cell stimulatory factor (interleukin 12 [IL-12]) induces T helper type 1 (Th1)-specific immune response and inhibits the development of IL-4-producing Th cells. *J. Exp. Med.* **177:** 1199.

91. Seder, R. A., A. Gazzinelli, A. Scher, and W. E. Paul. 1993. IL-12 acts directly on CD4+ T cells to enhance priming for IFNγ production and diminishes IL-4 inhibition of such priming. *Proc. Natl. Acad. Sci. USA* **90:** 10,188.

IV

Chemokines and Tumor Growth, Metastasis, and Angiogenesis

8

Chemokine Modulation of Tumor Cell Physiology*

Ji Ming Wang, Weipin Shen, Oleg Chertov, Jo Van Damme, and Joost J. Oppenheim

1. INTRODUCTION

Leukocyte infiltration into inflamed or injured tissues is regulated by a variety of cell-associated and soluble factors that mediate the communications between circulating leukocytes and vascular endothelial cells. Since the late 1980s, a superfamily of polypeptide leukocyte chemoattractants known as chemokines has been identified and demonstrated to selectively induce rapid endothelial cell adhesion and transmigration of leukocyte subpopulations *(1)*. Chemokines are produced by virtually every mammalian somatic cell type in response to inflammatory and immunologic stimuli, and have been detected in tissues of numerous disease states characterized by infiltration of distinct leukocyte subsets. Chemokines bind and activate cell-surface receptors that belong to the seven-transmembrane, G protein–coupled receptor superfamily *(2)*. Several chemokine receptors have been identified as fusion cofactors for human immunodeficiency virus. Chemokines have also been shown to play a critical role in the host interaction with malignant tumors via recruitment of immune cells into the tumor tissue, induction of angiogenesis or angiostasis, or through their direct effect on tumor cell migration and proliferation. As chemokine research is a rapidly expanding area, this chapter reviews the available information concerning the role of chemokines in tumor growth and metastasis.

2. THE ROLE OF CHEMOKINES IN MALIGNANCY

2.1. Malignant Tumors Are a Major Source of Chemokines

Many solid tumors of epithelial origin are infiltrated by a significant number of host immune cells, mainly of the mononuclear lineage. Analysis of a variety of malignant tumors, including carcinomas of the colon, lung, breast, and stomach, shows the presence of infiltrating mononuclear cells, particularly in the stroma *(3)*. Earlier efforts to identify the molecules responsible for the mononuclear cell infiltration in tumors led to the detection of a tumor-derived chemotactic factor (TDCF) in the culture media of a

---

* The content of this publication does not necessarily reflect the views or policies of the Department of Health and Human Services, nor does mention of trade names, commercial products, or organizations imply endorsement by the US Government.

From: *Chemokines and Cancer*
Edited by: B. J. Rollins © Humana Press Inc., Totowa, NJ

number of human and murine malignant tumor cell lines (*see* ref. *4* for a review), with the characteristic property of inducing directional migration of monocytes. The production of TDCF in vitro correlated with the level of macrophage content in tumors transplanted in vivo *(5)*. The C-C chemokine monocyte chemoattractant protein-1 (MCP-1) was later purified and identified as responsible for much of the TDCF activity from several human tumor cell supernatants, including glioma and fibrosarcoma lines *(6,7)*. Two C-C chemokines closely related to MCP-1, MCP-2, and MCP-3 were subsequently purified from the supernatant of a human osteosarcoma cell line *(8)*. These C-C chemokines are potent chemoattractants and activators of monocytes and T-lymphocytes in vitro *(1)*, and MCP-1, in particular, has been shown to be an important determinant of the monocyte infiltration in tumors *(9–11)*. With the availability of DNA probes and specific antichemokine antibodies, a number of C-C and C-X-C chemokines have been detected in tumor tissue. In a fine study by Negus et al. *(9)*, immunohistology and *in situ* hybridization of paraffin-embedded biopsies of epithelial ovarian tumors showed that the majority of the tumor-infiltrating host cells in tumor tissue are $CD68^+$ macrophages and $CD8^+/CD45RO^+$ T-lymphocytes. Among the C-C chemokines probed, MCP-1 was predominantly expressed in tumor epithelial areas and correlated with the number of infiltrating macrophages. Stromal cells expressed predominantly MCP-1 and macrophage inflammatory protein-1α (MIP-1α). A minority of stromal cells also expressed MIP-1β and RANTES, presumably accounting for the infiltration of tumor stroma by various subsets of T-lymphocytes *(9)*.

Although chemokines have been detected in several malignant tumors and have been implicated in determining the level of mononuclear infiltrate, the significance of the tumor infiltration by host cells has not been clarified. In addition to acting as a chemoattractant for monocytes, MCP-1 activates the respiratory burst and cytostatic activity of monocytes on tumor cell lines *(6)*. MCP-1 also synergizes with lipopolysaccharide (LPS) in inducing mouse macrophage cytotoxicity *(12)*. These observations suggest that MCP-1 may promote host antitumor responses. On the other hand, MCP-1 is a potent inducer of gelatinase and urokinase-type plasminogen activator (uPA), and concomitantly increases the cell-surface expression of the receptor for uPA. MCP-2 and MCP-3 also have these effects *(8)*. Thus, it is suggested *(13)* that these C-C chemokines may facilitate the monocyte-mediated digestion of extracellular matrix components in the course of monocyte recruitment. In tumor tissues, the release of proteolytic enzymes by MCP-1-stimulated infiltrating monocytes may provide a pathway for the invasion of tumor cells and therefore contribute to an augmented incidence of metastasis associated with inflammation *(4,13)*.

2.2. Effects of Chemokine Gene Transfer on the Growth of Malignant Tumors

It has been difficult to attribute antitumor effects to systemically administered chemokines. Therefore, investigators have resorted to gene therapy and vaccine approaches. The introduction of genes encoding diverse types of immunostimulatory molecules into tumor cells has resulted in enhancement of the antitumor immunity in the host *(14–16)*. The fact that chemokines attract and promote the effector functions of different leukocyte populations in vitro prompted numerous studies on the effects of transduction of chemokine genes into tumor cells on the biologic behavior of the tumors (Table 1).

Table 1
The Effect of Chemokine Gene Transduction on Tumor Growth and Metastasis

Chemokine gene	Tumor model	Animal	Injection site	Tumorigenicity and growth	Infiltrating cells	Immunity	Reference
mJE/MCP-1	CHO	Swiss nu/nu mice	sc	Lost tumorigenicity	Monocytes	Prevent tumor formation by parent tumor cells when coinjected	17
hMCP-1	B16 melanoma	C57BL6 and NCr nu/nu	im in hind limb or sc at inguinal region.	Retarded growth, increased tumorigenicity and lung metastasis at low tumor inocula	Monocytes	Unknown	18
mJE/MCP-1	9L glioblastoma	Fisher 344 rats	sc	Unchanged	Mainly monocytes	sc of irradiated MCP-1-expressing tumor cells provide protection against sc tumors	20
mJE/MCP-1	Adenocarcinoma (colon 26)	Balb/c	sc	Reduced tumorigenicity and lung metastases	Monocytes	mJE/MCP-1 synergizes with LPS to promote macrophage tumor killing	12
hMCP-1	Adenocarcinoma (colon 26)	Balb/c	Foot pad or hind leg	Same as parental tumor but increased lung metastases	Not known locally, increased vascularization in lung lesions	Unknown	19
hMCP-1	Myeloma	Balb/c nu/nu	ip	Retarded tumor growth	Macrophages and increased tumor necrosis	Unknown	53
mTCA3	IgG and IgA myelomas	Balb/c, C.B-17 SCID	sc	Complete regression in immune competent mice	Monocytes neutrophils	Long-term protection	23

(continued)

Table 1 (continued)

Chemokine gene	Tumor model	Animal	Injection site	Tumorigenicity and growth	Infiltrating cells	Immunity	Reference
mIP-10	Plasmacytoma J558 and mammary adenocarcinoma K485	Balb/c, Balb/c nu/nu, Swiss nu/nu, and FVB	sc lower abdominal quadrant	Reduced or no tumor formation in immune-competent mice, rapid tumor growth in nude mice	Monocytes lymphocytes, and neutrophils in imne competent mice; no infiltration in nude mice	Thymic-dependent immunity	21
mMIP-1α or hMIP-1α	Adenocarcinom (colon 26)	Balb/c	Footpad	Reduced tumorigenicity	Macrophages and neutrophils	Immune to parent tumor cells	24
hRANTES	mFibrosarcoma WP4	C57BL/6	sc	No tumor formation	T-cells and macrophages	Immune to parent tumor cells	22
hIL-8, hMIP-1α, mMIP-1α	CHO	Balb/c	sc lower abdominal quadrant	Reduced tumorigenicity	Neutrophils	Reduced tumorigenicity of co-injected parent cells	54
hIL-8	Melanoma SB-2	Balb/c nu/nu	sc scapular region	Increased tumor invasiveness, tumorigenicity and lung metastases	Not known	Increased collagenase (MMP-2) activity	28
hIP-10	Burkitt lymphoma	Balb/c nu/nu	sc	Reduced, tumorigenicity	Damaged vasculature in tumors	Unknown	26
mLtn + IL-2 or GM-CSF	Pre-B lymphoblastoid cells A20	Balb/c	sc Ltn+ and IL-2+ fibroblasts followed by tumor cells	Retarded tumor growth, inhibits preexisting tumors	CD4 and CD8 T-cells	CD4 and CD8 cell-mediated immunity	25

Basically, inoculation of tumor cells transfected with various chemokine genes caused tumor infiltration by host immune cell subsets that would migrate in vitro in response to the transfected chemokines. However, divergent results were obtained depending on the tumor models and whether human or murine chemokine genes were used. Based on its potent monocyte chemotactic/activating activity and its correlation with the macrophage content in in vivo tumors, JE/MCP-1 was the first and also the most extensively studied chemokine in gene transduction experiments *(17,18)*. Complete inhibition of tumorigenicity was achieved when Chinese hamster ovary (CHO) cells were transfected with the JE/MCP-1 gene and a macrophage-mediated tumoricidal host response was implicated *(17)*. Similarly, B16 melanoma cells transduced with MCP-1 gene showed growth retardation when injected in mice. Injection with lower numbers of transfected tumor cells resulted in increased tumorigenicity and lung metastases *(18)*. An increase in lung metastases was also observed with a murine colon adenocarcinoma cell line transfected with MCP-1, and was possibly owing to augmentation of neovascularization *(19)*. Manome et al. *(20)* reported that although JE/MCP-1 gene transduction into a rat glioblastoma 9L did not change the tumorigenicity, irradiated JE/MCP-1-expressing tumor cells provided protection against subcutaneously, but not intracranially, injected parental tumor cells. Histologic examination revealed the presence of infiltrating T-lymphocytes at the sites of sc tumors undergoing regression, suggesting the involvement of a T-cell-mediated immune response *(20)*.

Several other chemokine genes, such as interferon-γ-inducible protein-10 (IP-10) *(21)*, RANTES *(22)*, TCA3 *(23)*, and MIP-1α *(24)*, when transduced into tumor cells, not only consistently reduced tumorigenicity but also stimulated host immune response, which provided animals with long-term protection against tumor challenge. This is based on chemokine-induced indirect development of T-cell-dependent memory cells responsive to the tumor antigen. Dilloo et al. *(25)* have proposed a novel approach called *attraction-expansion* for chemokine gene transfer with lymphotactin (Ltn), which attracts CD4$^+$ T-lymphocytes in vitro. The delivery of Ltn alone by transfected fibroblasts into A20 myeloma in mice caused infiltration of CD4$^+$ T-lymphocytes in tumor tissue, but no tumor regression was achieved. The introduction of interleukin-2 (IL-2) into the tumor site also had little effect on tumor growth. However, coinjection of Ltn and IL-2-expressing fibroblasts greatly increased T-lymphocyte infiltration in myeloma, and the animals were protected from the growth of established tumor in a CD4$^+$ and CD8$^+$ T-cell-dependent manner *(25)*. Thus, T-cell migration and infiltration induced by Ltn alone is not associated with an increase in immunologic activity as measured by antitumor effect. The combination of Ltn with the T-cell-expanding and -activating cytokine IL-2 produces a synergistic antitumor response.

The consequences of angiogenic or angiostatic properties of some C-X-C chemokines on tumor growth have also been studied by gene transfer. When two closely related C-X-C chemokines, IP-10 and monokine induced by interferon-γ (which in addition possess angiostatic activity), were injected into nude mice bearing Burkitt lymphoma, tumor necrosis resulted in a proportion of the animals *(26,27)*. Burkitt lymphoma cells transfected to overexpress IP-10 had reduced ability to form sc tumors in nude mice. This effect of IP-10 was attributed to its ability to damage the tumor vasculature *(26)*. On the other hand, the C-X-C chemokine IL-8 has been reported as an essential growth factor for certain melanoma cell lines, and overexpression of IL-8 in the melanoma SB-2 line increased tumor cell invasiveness, tumorigenicity, and lung metastases *(28)*. Such tumor promoting activity of IL-8 is probably based on a direct mitogenic effect as well as an indirect angiogenic effect of IL-8 on melanoma cells.

2.3. Chemokines in Tumor Growth

C-X-C chemokines IL-8 and melanoma growth stimulating activity (MGSA)/ growth-related oncogene (GRO), in addition to their role as neutrophil chemoattractants and mediators of angiogenesis (as discussed in Section IV of this volume), have been implicated in the progression through various stages of melanocyte lesions toward malignant melanoma *(29,30)*. IL-8 is the prototype of C-X-C chemokines and was the first chemokine reported to induce melanoma cell chemotactic and haptotactic migration *(31)*. IL-8 was subsequently found to be an essential autocrine growth factor for some melanoma cell lines *(30)*. Six of the eight melanoma cell lines examined expressed detectable IL-8 by reverse transcriptase polymerase chain reaction (RT-PCR). Neutralizing anti-IL-8 antibodies as well as IL-8 antisense oligonucleotides inhibited the growth of two human malignant melanoma cell lines in soft agar *(30)*. Thus, some melanoma cells may rely on IL-8 as an endogenous growth-stimulating factor.

Another C-X-C chemokine, MGSA/GRO-α, was initially identified and purified from serum-free culture supernatants of malignant melanoma cell lines and characterized as an autocrine growth factor for melanoma cells *(30,32)*. The receptor type that mediates the action of MGSA/GRO-α on melanoma cells has been controversial. MGSA/GRO-α uses predominantly CXCR2 as a functional receptor and CXCR2 mRNA transcripts were found in Hs294T melanoma cell by RT-PCR *(33)*. In another study, CXCR1 but not CXCR2 transcripts were detected in a number of melanoma cell lines *(34)*. In binding competition experiments, Horuk et al. *(35)* reported that IL-8, which uses both CXCR1 and CXCR2, failed to compete with ^{125}I-MGSA/GRO-α for binding to melanoma cells. This led to the hypothesis that a unique receptor type MGSA/GRO-α might exist in these cells. However, by using RT-PCR, Norgauer and colleagues *(36)* detected the expression of CXCR2 in different melanoma cell lines and in normal human melanocytes. More important, antibodies raised against MGSA/GRO-α or the CXCR2 receptor were able to inhibit the growth of melanoma cells in vitro *(36)*.

Two highly related C-X-C chemokines, MGSA/GRO-β and MGSA/GRO-γ, which share receptor specificity with MGSA/GRO-α, have recently been studied for their role in melanocyte transformation and tumor growth *(37)*. As seen with MGSA/GRO-α gene transduction *(38)*, the mouse melanocyte cell line Melan-a transfected to overexpress MGSA/GRO-β, or MGSA/GRO-γ genes exhibited enhanced ability to form large colonies in soft agar and tumors in nude mice *(37)*. These cell clones formed highly pigmented tumors in nude mice within 2 mo after inoculation, and the tumors secreted immunoreactive MGSA/GRO-β or MGSA/GRO-γ. Although an autocrine growth-stimulatory effect of MGSA/GRO on melanocyte transformation and enhanced tumorigenicity was suggested, the angiogenic activity of MGSA/GRO may also contribute in sustaining and promoting tumor growth.

Owen and colleagues *(37)* examined the angiogenic potential of melanocyte clones engineered to overexpress MGSA/GRO-α, -β, and -γ using a rat cornea model. A marked angiogenesis was induced in response to the culture supernatants of GRO/MGSA-α-, -β-, or -γ-expressing cells, and this angiogenesis was specifically inhibited by antibodies to each of the GRO/MGSA chemokines. Histologic examination of the tumor tissues showed an extensive vascular system within and surrounding the tumor. The same investigators also used the SCID model to demonstrate that antibodies to MGSA/GRO-α or -γ retarded the tumor growth resulting from MGSA/GRO-α- or -γ-expressing melanocyte. This inhibition of tumor growth was attributed to a partial blockade of both melanocyte proliferation and angiogenesis.

Recently, Richards et al. *(39)* studied the expression of CXCR1 and CXCR2 in human head and neck squamous carcinoma specimens. By histochemistry, all of 38 stage I–IV tumor tissues were stained positive for CXCR1, whereas in only half of the specimens, CXCR1 staining was positive on microvascular endothelial cells. The CXCR2 staining pattern was similar to that of CXCR1. Since these tumors produce high levels of IL-8 ligand, the CXCR1 and CXCR2 expression by cancer cells and microvessel cells in head and neck squamous carcinoma may play an active role in tumor cell growth and angiogenesis. However, it is also intriguing that well-differentiated squamous carcinomas were more densely stained with both CXCR1 and CXCR2 than less differentiated tumors. Thus, the contribution of IL-8, and possibly other C-X-C chemokines, on squamous carcinoma growth requires further investigation.

2.4. Chemokines in the Metastatic Process

Tumor metastases develop most likely as a consequence of the interaction between selected tumor cells with a supportive environment. Malignant cells that exhibit the capacity to metastasize to a particular organ may have a variety of properties favoring their tissue invasion and growth *(40)*, including enhanced adherence to the microvascular endothelial cells of the organ, higher responsiveness to chemotactic signals released from the target organs, and increased response to local soluble or tissue-associated growth signals in the target organ. The target organs must possess suitable characteristics for the successful entry and growth of the metastatic tumor cells. These include an appropriate type of microvascular endothelium, organ stroma or matrix, and the presence of paracrine motility factors and growth factors *(40)*.

Relatively limited information is available as to the direct role of C-C chemokines on tumor metastasis. Young and colleagues *(41)* studied the directional migration of human breast adenocarcinoma cell lines in response to a variety of C-C and C-X-C chemokines. A well-differentiated breast carcinoma cell line, MCF-7, exhibited a significant chemotactic response to both C-C and C-X-C chemokines, with the C-C chemokines MIP-1α, MIP-1β, and RANTES being the most potent chemoattractants *(41)*. A lower order of response was also observed with the C-C chemokine MCP-1 as well as with the C-X-C chemokines IL-8 and GRO-α. Further experiments showed that the response of MCF-7 cells to C-C chemokines was sensitive to pertussis toxin and cholera toxin, suggesting the involvement of α-subunits of the chemokine receptor-associated G proteins. MCF-7 cells were also shown to specifically bind the radiolabeled C-C chemokines MIP-1α, MIP-1β, RANTES, and MCP-1 as well as the C-X-C chemokine IL-8, indicating that MCF-7 cells express multiple chemokine receptors. However, two other breast carcinoma cell lines showed weak or no responsiveness to some of the chemokines, suggesting that even carcinoma cells of similar origin may display distinct migratory responses to a given chemokine. This presumably depends on the level of receptor expression, as illustrated in the study with human head and neck squamous carcinomas in which well-differentiated tumors expressed a higher density of CXCR1 and CXCR2 receptors than poorly differentiated cells *(39)*.

Tumor cell motility is a pivotal step in the intricate process leading to the formation of metastases, and tumor cells that have increased metastatic potential are more motile than nonmetastatic tumor cells *(40)*. Morphologic studies of rat sarcoma cells have shown that the structure of the actin network relates to the degree of the malignancy and determines the cell motility *(41)*. In T-lymphoma cells such as the BW5147 cell line, the motility and F-actin content of noninvasive variants have been compared with invasive variants, and a higher level of actin polymerization is a prerequisite for pseudo-pod formation and a requirement for infiltration of the cells into tissue *(42)*. Young et al. *(41)* showed a significant increase in the level of F-actin in the MCF-7 breast carcinoma cell line after treatment with the C-C chemokines MIP-1α and MIP-1β. Confocal microscopy further indicated a redistribution of the cytoskeletal F-actin within 45 min after chemokine stimulation, with movement of F-actin toward the periphery of the cells in a polarized manner *(41)*.

The increased tumor cell motility may promote the random dissemination of the tumor cells. However, some malignant tumors preferentially metastasize to particular distant organs, suggesting a crucial role of the organ-microenvironment for the localization and proliferation of the metastatic tumor cells. Although several tissue-derived factors have been suggested *(40)*, the precise mechanism(s) determining such organ-specific metastasis has yet to be established. Chemokines not only chemoattract normal as well as malignant cells of the hematopoietic origin, but also endothelial cells, fibroblasts, melanoma cells, and epithelial tumor cells. Furthermore, chemokines are produced by virtually all types of tissues and organs constitutively and even more so if stimulated. Consequently, their attractive role in determining the organ-specific metastasis has been a subject of investigation. Wakabayashi et al. *(43)* reported that medium conditioned with mouse lung microvessel endothelial cells possessed chemotactic activity for a highly lung-metastasizing variant of the RAW117 murine large-cell lymphoma cell line, but not for the poorly metastatic parental cell or a liver-metastasizing variant. The chemotactic activity contained in the lung microvessel endothelial supernatants was purified to homogeneity and identified as murine JE, a counterpart of the human C-C chemokine MCP-1 *(1,17)*. The usage of recombinant JE and anti-JE antibody confirmed that JE indeed induced migration of the lung-metastasizing tumor variant but not of the nonmetastatic parental cell line.

Benke and Shirrmacher *(44)* studied the metastatic behavior of another murine tumor model. A highly metastatic variant tumor cell line, ESb, was derived from a chemically induced murine T-cell lymphoma. ESb-MP was isolated by plastic adherence from parental ESb cells. Although both cell lines form metastatic foci in the lung, liver, and brain when injected intravenously or intraperitoneally, ESb-MP cells metastasize into the kidney with high frequency, whereas the ESb cells only rarely infiltrate the kidney. ESb-MP cells exhibited greater cell mobility and an increased capacity to penetrate nitrocellulose filters than parental ESb cells. Moreover, ESb-MP cells migrated in response to kidney organ-conditioned media, to which the parental ESb cells did not respond. This raised the possibility that a kidney-derived chemotactic factor(s) may be involved in the attraction of ESb-MP cells in vitro, and may account for the kidney-specific localization of ESb-MP metastases in vivo. We purified and identified chemokines MCP-1/JE and RANTES from murine kidney-derived mesangial cell supernatant as inducers of in vitro migration of ESb-MP variant cells but not of the parental ESb cells *(45).* These two C-C chemokines accounted for a majority but not all of the chemotactic activity contained in the mesangial cell supernatant as well as in the conditioned media of normal kidney, as indicated by antibody neutralization experiments.

Further studies with radiolabeled chemokines revealed that although both the ESb-MP variant and parental ESb cells expressed similar levels of specific binding sites for several C-C chemokines including MCP-1, MCP-3, MIP-1α, MIP-1β, and RANTES, only ESb-MP cells migrated in response to C-C chemokines. These results suggest that cell-surface expression of chemokine receptors may not be sufficient for functional responsiveness to the specific ligands. To be responsive, the cells must possess the proper molecular array to transduce a receptor-triggered signaling cascade. For example, ESb-MP cells expressed a significantly higher level of CD11b, a β2 integrin crucial for ligand-activated cell adhesion and locomotion, than ESb parental cells.

Moreover, only ESb-MP cells were demonstrated to exhibit NF-κB activation by treatment with C-C chemokines. NF-κB participates in the regulation of many genes involved in immunologic and inflammatory responses, cell growth, and adhesion *(46).* NF-κB is an oxidative stress-responsive transcription factor, and the reactive oxygen intermediates, which are also induced by chemokines in leukocytes *(1,2),* are major mediators of NF-κB activation. The ceramide pathway has also been reported to be critical in initiating the intracellular events leading to NF-κB activation. Ceramide is generated by an acid sphingomyelinase through the production of diacylglycerol (DAG) by phosphatidylcholine-phospholipase C (PLC). The generation of DAG by PLC has been demonstrated to be initiated by many proinflammatory cytokines including IL-1, tumor necrosis factor-α (TNF-α) *(46),* and chemokines *(47).* Although the precise role of chemokines in NF-κB activation remains to be determined, selective effects of C-C chemokines on the kidney-metastasizing tumor variant suggest that NF-κB and consequent gene transcription may represent an important signaling event in chemokine-mediated cell activation.

Several of the murine kidney-derived cell lines tested, including endothelial, epithelial, and transitional cells, were able to produce chemotactic activity for the kidney-metastasizing tumor variant on stimulation by proinflammatory cytokines such as IL-1 and TNF-α. However, the mesangial cell line MES-13 constitutively produced the highest levels of chemotactic activity for ESb-MP cells. Mesangial cells are mesenchyme-derived, multipotential vascular pericytes that share some properties with smooth muscle cells and macrophages. These cells can produce a variety of proinflammatory cytokines and growth factors under pathologic conditions *(48).* Human mesangial cells have been shown to express the chemokines MCP-1 and IL-8 on stimulation in vitro *(48).* As a consequence of their ability to release inflammatory mediators, mesangial cells may play an important role not only in different glomerular diseases but also in attracting metastatic tumor cells that migrate in response to the C-C chemokine gradient. In fact, some tumors have been reported to metastasize preferentially to injured or inflamed tissue sites *(49),* where high levels of chemokines could be expected to be produced. It is somewhat unexpected to find that normal kidney produces low levels of chemokines. However, this is probably not an in vitro artifact since normal kidney tissue has been reported to express MCP-1/JE and RANTES genes *(50,51).* Concentrated normal human urine has also been reported to contain detectable MCP-1 protein *(52)*. While the role of chemokines in tumor metastasis must be further investigated in vivo, the foregoing observations suggest that some chemokines may promote the spread of certain tumors to "favored" sites.

3. CONCLUSION

Chemokines have been demonstrated to be key mediators in a number of infectious, inflammatory, and immunologic diseases. The use of in vitro and in vivo models provides a unique opportunity to exploit the beneficial as well as detrimental effects of known chemokines and their receptors in host defense. The beneficial and the deleterious effects of chemokines on tumor growth and metastasis also call for more rigorous investigation. Whereas many chemokines have been shown to have antitumor activity by activating immune cells or by inhibition of neovascularization of tumors, other chemokines may promote tumor growth and metastasis by direct growth stimulation, enhanced cell motility, or angiogenesis. Thus, in addition to expanding the research on the antitumor effects of chemokines, the development of chemokine or chemokine receptor antagonists may have promise in limiting the detrimental effects of chemokines in various disease states including malignant tumors.

ACKNOWLEDGMENTS

The authors thank Drs. O. M. Z. Howard and S. Su for reviewing the manuscript, and K. Bengali, W. Gong, and N. Dunlop for technical assistance. W. Shen is supported in part by a fellowship from the Office of the International Affairs, National Cancer Institute, National Institutes of Health.

REFERENCES

1. Rollins, B. J. 1997. Chemokines. *Blood* **90:** 909–928.
2. Murphy, P. M. 1996. Chemokine receptors: structure, function and role in microbial pathogenesis. *Cytokine Growth Factor Rev.* **7:** 47–64.
3. Svennevig, J. L., and H. Svaar. 1979. Content and distribution of macrophages and lymphocytes in solid malignant human tumors. *Int. J. Cancer* **24:** 754–758.
4. Mantovani, A. 1994. Biology of disease, tumor-associated macrophages in neoplastic progression: a paradigm for the in vivo function of chemokines. *Lab. Invest.* **71:** 5–16.
5. Bottazzi, B., N. Polentarutti, R. Acero, A. Balsari, D. Boraschi, P. Ghezzi, M. Salmona, and A. Mantovani. 1983. Regulation of the macrophage content of neoplasms by chemoattractants. *Science* **220:** 210–212.
6. Zachariae, C. O., A. O. Anderseon, H. L. Thompson, E. Appella, A. Mantovani, J. J. Oppenheim, and K. Matsushima. 1990. Properties of monocyte chemotactic and activating factor (MCAF) purified from a human fibrosarcoma cell line. *J. Exp. Med.* **171:** 2177–2182.
7. Yoshimura, T., E. A. Robinson, S. Tanaka, E. Appella, J. Kuratsu, and E. J. Leonard. 1989. Purification and amino acid analysis of two human glioma-derived monocyte chemoattractants. *J. Exp. Med.* **169:** 1449–1459.
8. Van Damme, J., P. Proost, J. P. Lenaerts, and G. Opdenakker. 1992. Structural and functional identification of two human, tumor-derived monocyte chemotactic proteins (MCP-2 and MCP-3) belonging to the chemokine family. *J. Exp. Med.* **176:** 59–65.
9. Negus, R. P. M., G. W. H. Stamp, J. Hadley, and F. R. Balkwill. 1997. Quantitative assessment of the leukocyte infiltrate in ovarian cancer and its relationship to the expression of C-C chemokines. *Am. J. Pathol.* **150:** 1723–1734.

10. Negus, R. P. M., G. W. H. Stamp, M. G. Relf, F. Burke, S. T. A. Malik, S. Bernasconi, P. Allavena, S. Sozzani, A. Mantovani, and F. R. Balkwill. 1995. The detection and localization of monocyte chemoattractant protein-1 (MCP-1) in human ovarian cancer. *J. Clin. Invest.* **95:** 2391–2396.

11. Mazzucchelli, L., P. Loetscher, A. Kappeler, M. Uguccioni, M. Baggiolini, J. A. Laissue, and C. Mueller. 1996. Monocyte chemoattractant protein-1 gene expression in prostatic hyperplasia and prostate adenocarcinoma. *Am. J. Pathol.* **149:** 501–509.

12. Huang, S., R. K. Singh, K. Xie, M. Gutman, K. K. Berry, C. D. Bucana, I. J. Fidler, and M. Bar-Eli. 1994. Expression of the JE/MCP-1 gene suppresses metastatic potential in murine colon carcinoma cells. *Cancer Immunol. Immunother.* **39:** 231–238.

13. Opdenakker, G., and J. Van Damme. 1992. Cytokines and proteases in invasive process: molecular similarities between inflammation and cancer. *Cytokine* **4:** 251–258.

14. Dranoff, G., E. Jaffee, A. Lazenby, P. Golumbek, H. Levisky, K. Brose, V. Jackson, H. Hamada, D. Pardoll, and R. C. Mulligan. 1993. Vaccination with irradiated tumor cells engineered to secrete murine granulocyte-macrophage colony-stimulating factors stimulates potent, specific, and long-lasting anti-tumor immunity. *Proc. Natl. Acad. Sci. USA* **90:** 3539–3543.

15. Tahara, H., H. J. Zeh, III, W. J. Storkus, I. Pappo, S. C. Watkins, U. Gubler, S. F. Wolf, P. D. Robbins, and M. T. Lotze. 1994. Fibroblasts genetically engineered to secrete interleukin 12 can suppress tumor growth and induce antitumor immunity to a murine melanoman in vivo. *Cancer Res.* **54:** 182–189.

16. Asher, A. L., J. J. Mule, A. Kasid, N. P. Restifo, J. C. Salo, C. M. Reichert, G. Jaffe, B. Fendly, M. Kriegler, and S. A. Rosenberg. 1991. Murine tumor cells transduced with the gene for tumor necrosis factor-alpha: evidence for paracrine immune effects of tumor necrosis factor against tumors. *J. Immunol.* **146:** 3227–3234.

17. Rollins, B. J., and M. E. Sunday. 1991. Suppression of tumor formation in vivo by expression of the JE gene in malignant cells. *Mol. Cell. Biol.* **11:** 3125–3131.

18. Bottazzi, B., W. Luini, D. Govoni, F. Colotta, and A. Mantovani. 1992. Monocyte chemotactic cytokine gene transfer modulates macrophage infiltration, growth, and susceptibility to IL-2 therapy of a murine melanoma. *J. Immunol.* **148:** 1280–1285.

19. Nakashima, E., N. Mukaida, Y. Kubota, K. Kuno, K. Yasumoto, F. Ichimura, I. Nakanishi, M. Miyasaka, and K. Matsushima. 1995. Human MCAF gene transfer enhances the metastatic capacity of a mouse cachectic adenocarcinoma cell line in vitro. *Pharm. Res.* **12:** 1598–1604.

20. Manome, Y., P. Y. Wen, A. Hershowitz, T. Tanaka, B. J. Rollins, D. W. Kufe, and H. A. Fine. 1995. Monocyte chemoattractant protein-1 (MCP-1) gene transduction: an effective tumor vaccine strategy for non-intracranial tumors. *Cancer Immunol. Immunother.* **41:** 227–235.

21. Luster, A. D., and P. Leder. 1993. IP-10, a -C-X-C- chemokine, elicits a potent thymus-dependent antitumor response in vivo. *J. Exp. Med.* **178:** 1057–1065.

22. Mule, J. J., M. Custer, B. Averbook, J. C. Yang, J. S. Weber, D. V. Goeddel, S. A. Rosenberg, and T. J. Schall. 1996. RANTES secretion by gene-modified tumor cells results in loss of tumorigenicity in vivo: role of immune cell subpopulations. *Hum. Gene Ther.* **7:** 1545–1553.

23. Laning, J., H. Kawasaki, E. Tanaka, Y. Luo, and M. E. Dorf. 1994. Inhibition of in vivo tumor growth by the β chemokine, TCA3. *J. Immunol.* **153:** 4625–4635.

24. Nakashima, E., A. Oya, Y. Kubota, N. Kanada, R. Matsushita, K. Takeda, F. Ichimura, K. Kuno, N. Mukaida, K. Hirose, I. Nakanishi, T. Ujiie, and K. Matsushima. 1996. A candidate for cancer gene therapy: MIP-1α gene transfer to an adenocarcinoma cell line reduced tumorigenicity and induced protective immunity in immunocompetent mice. *Pharm. Res.* **13:** 1896–1901.

25. Dilloo, D., K. Bacon, W. Holden, W. Zhong, S. Burdach, A. Zlotnik, and M. Brenner.

1996. Combined chemokine and cytokine gene transfer enhances antitumor immunity. *Nat. Med.* **2:** 1090–1095.

26. Sgadari, C., A. L. Angiolillo, B. W. Cherney, S. E. Pike, J. M. Farber, L. G. Koniaris, P. Vanguri, P. R. Burd, N. Sheikh, G. Gupta, J. Teruya-Feldstein, and G. Tosato. 1996. Interferon-inducible protein-10 identified as a mediator of tumor necrosis in vivo. *Proc. Natl. Acad. Sci. USA* **93:** 13,791–13,796.

27. Sgadari, C., J. M. Farber, A. L. Angiolillo, F. Liao, J. Teruya-Feldstein, P. R. Burd, L. Yao, G. Gupta, C. Kanegane, and G. Tosato. 1997. Mig, the monokine induced by interferon-gamma, promotes tumor necrosis in vivo. *Blood* **89:** 2635–2643.

28. Luca, M., S. Huang, J. E. Gershenwald, R. K. Singh, R. Reich, and M. Bar-Eli. 1997. Expression of interleukin-8 by human melanoma cells up-regulates MMP-2 activity and increases tumor growth and metastasis. *Am. J. Pathol.* **151:** 1105–1113.

29. Bordoni, R., R. Fine, D. Murray, and A. Richmond. 1990. Characterization of the role of melanoma growth stimulating activity (MGSA) in the growth of normal melanocytes, nevocytes, and malignant melanocytes. *J. Cell. Biochem.* **44:** 207–219.

30. Schadendorf, D., A. Moller, B. Algermissen, M. Worm, M. Sticherling, and B. M. Czarnetzki. 1993. IL-8 produced by human malignant melanoma cells in vitro is an essential autocrine growth factor. *J. Immunol.* **151:** 2267–2275.

31. Wang, J. M., G. Taraboletti, K. Matsushima, J. Van Damme, and A. Mantovani. 1990. Induction of haptotactic and chemotactic migration of melanoma cells by neutrophil activating protein/interleukin-8. *Biochem. Biophys. Res. Commun.* **169:** 165–170.

32. Richmond, A., and H. G. Thomas. 1986. Purification of melanoma growth stimulatory activity. *J. Cell. Physiol.* **129:** 375–384.

33. Mueller, S. G., W. P. Schraw, and A. Richmond. 1994. Melanoma growth stimulatory activity enhances the phosphorylation of the class II interleukin-8 receptor in nonhematopoietic cells. *J. Biol. Chem.* **269:** 1973–1980.

34. Moser, B., L. S. Barella, S. Mattei, C. Schumacher, F. Boulay, M. P. Colombo, and M. Baggiolini. 1993. Expression of transcripts for two interleukin-8 receptors in human phagocytes, lymphocytes, and melanoma cells. *Biochem. J.* **294:** 285–292.

35. Horuk, R., D. G. Yansura, D. Reilly, S. Spencer, J. Bourell, W. Henzel, G. Rice, and E. Unemori. 1993. Purification, receptor binding analysis, and biologic characterization of human melanoma growth-stimulating activity: evidence for a novel receptor. *J. Biol. Chem.* **268:** 541–546.

36. Norgauer, J., B. Metzner, and I. Schraufstatter. 1996. Expression and growth-promoting function of the IL-8 receptor β in human melanoma cells. *J. Immunol.* **156:** 1132–1137.

37. Owen, J. D., R. Strieter, M. Burdick, H. Haghnegahdar, L. Nanney, R. Shattuck-Brandt, and A. Richmond. 1997. Enhanced tumor-forming capacity for immortalized melanocytes expressing melanoma growth stimulatory activity/growth-regulated cytokine β and γ proteins. *Int. J. Cancer* **73:** 94–103.

38. Balentien, E., B. E. Mufson, R. L. Shattuck, R. Derynck, and A. Richmond. 1991. Effects of MGSA/GRO alpha on melanocyte transformation *Oncogene* **6:** 1115–1124.

39. Richards, B. L., R. J. Eisma, J. D. Spiro, R. L. Lindquist, and D. L. Kreutzer. 1997. Coexpression of interleukin-8 receptors in head and neck squamous cell carcinoma. *Am. J. Surg.* **174:** 507–512.

40. Nicolson, G. L. 1993. Paracrine and autocrine growth mechanisms in tumor metastasis to specific sites with particular emphasis on brain and lung metastasis. *Cancer Metastasis Rev.* **12:** 325–343.

41. Young, S. J., S. A. Ali, D. D. Taub, and R. C. Rees. 1997. Chemokines induce migrational responses in human breast carcinoma cells. *Int. J. Cancer* **71:** 257–266.

42. Verschueren, H., I. Van Der Taelen, J. Dewit, J. De Braekeleer, and P. De Baetselier. 1994. Metastatic competence of BW5147 T lymphoma cell lines is correlated with in vitro metastasis. *J. Leuk. Biol.* **55:** 552–556.

43. Wakabayashi, H., P. G. Cavanaugh, and G. L. Nicolson. 1995. Purification and identification of mouse microvessel endothelial cell-derived chemoattractant for lung-metastasizing murine RAW117 large-cell lymphoma cells: identification as mouse monocyte chemotactic protein. *Cancer Res.* **55:** 4458–4464.
44. Benke, R., and V. Schirrmacher. 1991. Change in organotropism of mouse lymphoma variants associated with selective chemotactic responsiveness to organ-derived chemoattractants. *Clin. Exp. Metastasis* **9:** 205–219.
45. Wang, J. M., O. Chertov, P. Proost, J.-J. Li, P. Menten, L. Xu, S. Sozzani, A. Mantovani, W. Gong, V. Schirrmacher, J. Van Damme, and J. J. Oppenheim. 1998. Purification and identification of chemokines potentially involved in kidney-specific metastasis by a murine lymphoma variant: induction of migration of NFκB activation. *Int. J. Cancer* **75:** 900–907.
46. Akira S., and T. Kishimoto. 1997. NF-IL6 and NF-κB in cytokine gene regulation. *Adv. Immunol.* **65:** 1–33.
47. Ben-Baruch, A., D. F. Michiel, and J. J. Oppenheim. 1995. Signals and receptors involved in recruitment of inflammatory cells. *J. Biol. Chem.* **270:** 11,703–11,706.
48. Zoja, C., J. M. Wang, S. Bettoni, M. Sironi, D. Renzi, F. Chiaffarino, H. E. Abboud, A. Mantovani, G. Remuzzi, and A. Rambaldi. 1991. Interleukin-1β and tumor necrosis factor-α induce gene expression and production of leukocyte chemotactic factors, colony stimulating factors and interleukin-6 in human mesangial cells. *Am. J. Pathol.* **138:** 991–1003.
49. Tang, W. W., S. Yin, A. J. Wittwer, and M. Qi. 1995. Chemokine gene expression in anti-glomerular basement membrane antibody glomerulonephritis. *Am. J. Physiol.* **269(3 Pt. 2):** F323–F330.
50. Murphy, P., P. Alexander, P. V. Senior, J. Fleming, N. Kirkham, and I. Taylor. 1988. Mechanisms of organ selective tumor growth by bloodborne cancer cells. *Br. J. Cancer* **57:** 19–31.
51. Wenzel, U. O., and H. E. Abboud. 1995. Chemokines and renal disease. *Am. J. Kidney Dis.* **26:** 982–994.
52. Noris, M., S. Bernasconi, F. Casiraghi, S. Sozzani, E. Gotti, G. Remuzzi, and A. Matovani. 1995. Monocyte chemoattractant protein-1 is excreted in excessive amounts in the urine of patients with Lupus nephritis. *Lab. Invest.* **73:** 804–809.
53. Hoshino, Y., K. Hatake, T. Kasahara, Y. Takahashi, M. Ikeda, H. Tomizuka, T. Ohtsuki, M. Uwai, N. Mukaida, K. Matsushima, and Y. Miura. 1995. Monocyte chemoattractant protein-1 stimulates tumor necrosis and recruitment of macrophages into tumors in tumor-bearing nude mice: increased granulocyte and macrophage progenitors in murine bone marrow. *Exp. Hematol.* **23:** 1035–1039.
54. Hirose, K., M. Hakozaki, Y. Nyunoya, Y. Kobayashi, K. Matsushita, T. Takenouchi, A. Mikata, N. Mukaida, and K. Matsushima. 1995. Chemokine gene transfection into tumor cells reduced tumorigenicity in nude mice in association with neutrophil infiltration. *Br. J. Cancer* **72:** 708–714.

9

C-X-C Chemokines and Lung Cancer Angiogenesis

Robert M. Strieter, Bruno DiGiovine, Peter J. Polverini,
Steven L. Kunkel, Armen Shanafelt, Joseph Hesselgesser,
Richard Horuk, and Douglas A. Arenberg

1. INTRODUCTION

Angiogenesis is an essential biologic event encountered in vertebrate animals *(6,35,36,38,39,60,92)*. Embryonic development, the formation of inflammatory granulation tissue during wound healing, chronic inflammation, and the growth of malignant solid tumors represent physiologic and pathologic processes that are strictly dependent on neovascularization. The rate of normal capillary endothelial cell turnover in adults is typically measured in months or years *(30,132)*. However, during wound repair and development of granulation tissue, resting endothelial cells become activated, leading to proteolytic degradation of their basement membrane and surrounding extracellular matrix, migration, proliferation, and establishment of newly functioning capillaries within a matter of days *(60)*. An important feature of wound-associated angiogenesis is that it is locally controlled and transient. As rapidly as neovascularization occurs, these new vessels virtually disappear, returning the tissue vasculature to a homeostatic environment. This abrupt termination of angiogenesis in the context of the resolution of wound repair supports the notion of two possible mechanisms of control. First, there is probably a marked reduction in the synthesis and/or elaboration of angiogenic mediators. Second, a simultaneous increase occurs in the levels of factors that inhibit neovascularization *(15)*. In contrast to the precise regulation of angiogenesis that accompanies wound repair, dysregulation of angiogenesis can lead to an imbalance in overexpression of angiogenic and underexpression of angiostatic factors that contributes to the pathogenesis of solid tumor growth. Thus, the complement of positive and negative regulators of angiogenesis may vary among different physiologic and pathologic settings. The recognition of this dual mechanism of control is critical in order to gain insight into this complex process and to understand its significance in regulating net angiogenesis.

2. THE PROCESS OF ANGIOGENESIS

The initiation of angiogenesis in the adult organism occurs in the postcapillary venule. Endothelial cells within these vessels are adjacent to basement membrane and surrounded by an interrupted layer of pericytes and smooth muscle cells invested by

From: *Chemokines and Cancer*
Edited by: B. J. Rollins © Humana Press Inc., Totowa, NJ

extracellular matrix. After injury, the initial angiogenic response is associated with a change in cellular adhesive interactions among adjacent endothelial cells, pericytes, and smooth muscle cells *(7–9,13,91,112).* Activated endothelial cells undergo reorganization of cytoskeletal elements and express cell surface adhesion molecules (e.g., integrins and selectins) followed by the generation of extracellular matrix components *(20,21,41,51,52,70,83).* These endothelial cells produce a variety of proteolytic enzymes, which lead to degradation of the basement membrane, allowing the cells to migrate into the surrounding extracellular matrix *(89,97).* This process initiates the formation of capillary buds, releases growth factors sequestered in the basal lamina and adjacent extracellular matrix, and induces endothelial cell and other mesenchymal cell–derived growth factor expression *(12,109).* This initial phase can proceed in the absence of endothelial proliferation *(109).* Subsequent phases of angiogenesis leading to the formation of microvessels requires continual exposure to angiogenic mediators *(12,42,61,101,138).* These molecules can function in an autocrine and a paracrine manner to control endothelial cell migration, proliferation, elongation, orientation, and differentiation, leading to reestablishment of the basement membrane, lumen formation, and anastomosis with other neovessels or preexisting vessels *(41,55,88).* The neovasculature may persist as capillaries, differentiate into mature venules or arterioles, or undergo regression. The signals responsible for this latter event are now being identified and may either function to initiate apoptosis or induce cell cycle arrest of endothelial cells *(21,63,95).*

2.1. Angiogenic and Angiostatic Factors Regulate Angiogenesis

Net angiogenesis is determined by a dual yet opposing system of angiogenic and angiostatic factors *(27,39,53,80,92,93)* (Table 1). The majority of angiogenic factors are polypeptides that induce endothelial cell migration, proliferation, and differentiation into tubular structures. These angiogenic molecules are produced by an array of cells and function as ligands in an autocrine and a paracrine manner to facilitate endothelial cell activation. These molecules can stimulate angiogenesis either by directly interacting with specific receptors on endothelial cells or by indirectly attracting and activating accessory cells, such as macrophages, that produce additional angiogenic factors *(92,93).* In addition, various molecules can function as cofactors for the promotion of angiogenesis. For example, proteases can lead to the release of an active angiogenic factor *(12,99).* Moreover, heparin, a glycosaminoglycan component of the extracellular matrix, can play a key role in stabilizing and/or enhancing the function of angiogenic molecules *(39,138).*

A role for inhibitors in the control of angiogenesis was first observed when hyaline cartilage was found to be resistant to vascular invasion *(28,116).* These studies demonstrated that a heat-labile guanidium chloride extract prepared from cartilage contained an inhibitor of neovascularization. Subsequently, other investigators showed that a similar or identical extract from either rodent neonatal or shark cartilage was able to block effectively neovascularization and the growth of tumors in vivo *(17,57).* Similar angiostatic factors have been reported for other cell and tissue extracts *(18,19,56,68),* and for a variety of natural and artificial agents including inhibitors of basement membrane biosynthesis *(51,52,70,75);* placental ribonuclease inhibitor *(105);* lymphotoxin *(102);* interferons *(110);* prostaglandin synthetase inhibitors *(90);* heparin-binding frag-

Table 1
Representative Examples of Angiogenic and Angiostatic Factors

Proangiogenic mediators of angiogenesis	*Endogenous inhibitors of angiogenesis*
Growth factors	*Proteins and peptides*
Acidic fibroblast growth factor	Angiostatin
bFGF	Eosinophilic major basic protein
Epidermal growth factor	Endostatin
IL-1	High molecular weight hyaluronan
IL-2	IFN-α
Scatter factor/hepatocyte growth factor	IFN-β
TGF-α	IFN-γ
TGF-β	Non-ELR–C-X-C chemokines
TNF-α	IL-1
VEGF	IL-4
Carbohydrates and lipids	IL-12
12(R)-hydroxyeicosatrienoic acid (compound D)	Laminin and fibronectin peptides
Hyaluronan fragments	Placental RNase (angiogenin) inhibitor
Lactic acid	Somatostatin
Monobutyrin	Substance P
Prostaglandins E_1 and E_2	Thrombospondin 1
Other proteins and peptides	Tissue inhibitor of metalloproteinases
Angiogenin	*Lipids*
Angiotensin II	Angiostatic steroids
Ceruloplasm	Retinoids
Fibrin	Vitamin A
Human angiogenic factor	*Others*
ELR–C-X-C chemokines	Nitric oxide
Plasminogen activator	Vitreous fluids
Polyamines	Prostaglandin synthetase inhibitor
Substance P	
Urokinase	
Others	
Adenosine	
Angiotropin	
Copper	
Heparin	
Nicatinamide	
ESAF	

ments of fibronectin *(49);* protamine *(135);* angiostatic steroids *(25,59);* several antineoplastic and antiinflammatory agents *(25,135);* platelet factor 4 (PF4) *(73);* interferon-γ-inducible protein-10 (IP-10) *(1,63,73,121,127–130);* monokine induced by interferon-γ (MIG) *(129);* thrombospondin-1 *(43,94,137);* angiostatin *(85);* endostatin *(84);* and antagonists to $\alpha v\beta 3$ integrins *(20,21).* Although most inhibitors can act directly on the endothelial cell to block migration and/or mitogenesis in vitro, their effects in vivo may be considerably more complex, involving additional cells and their products.

A significant feature of these opposing yet complementary systems is that, with rare exception, none of the angiogenic or angiostatic factors is endothelial-cell specific nor unique to the process of regulation of angiogenesis. Most of these factors have a wide range of functions and target cells. This concept is perhaps one of the most essential features of the angiogenic response, the ability of endothelial cells to respond to a variety of mediators. These features support the notion that angiogenesis has evolved as a highly conserved response with a redundant system of factors to ensure fruition of neovascularization. For example, during embryonic development, basic fibroblast growth factor (bFGF) and vascular endothelial growth factor (VEGF) have been shown to be principal mediators of vasculogenesis and angiogenesis *(22,34,98)*. By contrast, during wound repair, these angiogenic factors may have a more restricted role, whereas an entirely different complement of angiogenic mediators appears to play a role in mediating angiogenesis *(6,39,60,92,131)*. Although speculation may exist as to whether angiogenic or angiostatic factors are tissue or process specific, the sheer redundancy of positive and negative factors that regulate neovascularization affirms the fundamental nature of this process.

2.2. Dysregulation of Angiogenesis Can Lead to an Imbalance in Angiogenic and Angiostatic Factors That Contributes to the Pathogenesis of Solid Tumor Growth

Several lines of evidence suggest that an imbalance in the production of promoters and inhibitors of angiogenesis contributes to the pathogenesis of angiogenesis-dependent disorders. For solid tumor growth to succeed, a complex interplay must occur between transformed neoplastic cells and nontransformed resident and recruited immune and nonimmune cells. Although carcinogenesis or neoplastic transformation is dependent on multiple genetic and epigenetic events *(107)*, the salient feature of all solid tumor growth is the presence of neovascularization *(15,16,36,38)*. It appears that tumors are continually renewing and altering their vascular supply *(36)*. Interestingly, the normal vascular mass of tissue is approx 20%, whereas, during tumorigenesis, tumor vascular mass may be >50% of the total tumor *(36)*. In the absence of local capillary proliferation and delivery of oxygen and nutrients, neoplasms cannot grow beyond the size of 2 mm^3 *(15,16,36,38)*. In addition, the magnitude of tumor-derived angiogenesis has been directly correlated with metastasis of melanoma, prostate cancer, breast cancer, and non-small cell lung cancer (NSCLC) *(40,48,69,74,142–144)*. These findings support the notion that tumor-associated angiogenesis is dysregulated in such a manner that a biologic imbalance exists that favors either the overexpression of local angiogenic factors or the suppression of endogenous angiostatic factors *(28,36,40)*. Thus, the growth of solid tumors is associated with an enhanced angiogenic environment. Although the complement of positive and negative regulators of angiogenesis may vary among different physiologic and pathologic settings, the recognition of this dual mechanism of control is necessary to gain a more thorough understanding of this complex process and its significance in regulating net angiogenesis.

3. C-X-C CHEMOKINES

The human C-X-C chemokine family comprises cytokines that in their monomeric forms are <10 kDa, and are characteristically basic heparin-binding proteins (Table 2).

Table 2
The C-X-C Chemokines

Interleukin-8 (IL-8)
Epithelial cell–derived neutrophil-activating factor-78 (ENA-78)
Growth-related oncogene-α (GRO-α)
Growth-related oncogene-β (GRO-β)
Growth-related oncogene-γ (GRO-γ)
Granulocyte chemotactic protein-2 (GCP-2)
Platelet basic protein (PBP)
    Connective tissue activating protein-III (CTAP-III)
    β-thromboglobulin (β-TG)
    Neutrophil-activating peptide-2 (NAP-2)
Platelet factor 4 (PF4)
Interferon-γ-inducible protein (IP-10)
Monokine induced by interferon-γ (MIG)
Stromal cell–derived factor-1 (SDF-1)

This family displays four highly conserved cysteine amino acid residues, with the first two cysteines separated by one nonconserved amino acid residue *(10,11,77, 78,120,125,141)*. In general, these cytokines appear to have specific chemotactic activity for neutrophils. Because of their chemotactic properties and the presence of the C-X-C cysteine motif, these cytokines have been designated the C-X-C chemokine family. The genes encoding chemokines are all clustered on human chromosome 4 and exhibit between 20 and 50% homology at the amino acid level *(10,11,77,78,120, 125,141)*.

Since the late 1980s, several human C-X-C chemokines have been identified, and include PF4, NH_2-terminal truncated forms of platelet basic protein ([PBP]; connective tissue activating protein-III [CTAP-III], β-thromboglobulin [β-TG], and neutrophil-activating peptide-2 [NAP-2]), interleukin-8 (IL-8), growth-related oncogene-α (GRO-α), GRO-β, GRO-γ, IP-10, MIG, epithelial cell–derived neutrophil-activating factor-78 (ENA-78), granulocyte chemotactic protein-2 (GCP-2), and stromal cell–derived factor-1 (SDF-1) *(10,11,14,32,77,78,86,108,120,125,133,141)*. The NH_2-terminal truncated forms of PBP are generated when PBP is released from platelet α-granules and undergoes proteolytic cleavage by monocyte-derived proteases *(139)*. PF4, the first member of the C-X-C chemokine family to be described, was originally identified on the basis of its ability to bind to heparin, leading to inactivation of heparin's anticoagulant function *(26)*. Both IP-10 and MIG are interferon-inducible chemokines *(31–33,64–66)*. Although IP-10 appears to be induced by all three interferons (interferon-α [IFN-α], IFN-β, and IFN-γ), MIG is unique, in that it appears to be expressed only in the presence of IFN-γ *(31–33,64–66)*. Whereas IFN-γ induces the production of IP-10 and MIG, this cytokine attenuates the expression of IL-8, GRO-α, and ENA-78 *(44,103)*. These findings would suggest that members of the C-X-C chemokine family demonstrate disparate regulation in the presence of interferons (Table 3). GRO-α, GRO-β, and GRO-γ, are closely related C-X-C chemokines, with GRO-α originally described for its melanoma growth-

Table 3
Stimulus Specificity for the Expression and Production of C-X-C Chemokines

		Stimulus		
C-X-C chemokines	*Lipopolysaccharide*	*TNF*	*IL-1*	*IFN-γ*
IL-8	++++	++++	++++	----
ENA-78	+++	+++	+++	----
GRO-α	+++	+++	+++	----
IP-10	+	+	+	+++
MIG	–	–	–	+++

stimulatory activity *(2,3,96)*. IL-8, ENA-78, and GCP-2 were all initially identified on the basis of their ability to induce neutrophil activation and chemotaxis *(10,11,77,78,87,120,125,140,141)*. SDF-1 has been recently described for its ability to induce lymphocyte migration and prevent infection of T-cells by lymphotropic strains of human immunodeficiency virus-1 *(14,86,108,133)*. The C-X-C chemokines are produced by an array of cells *(10,11,29,76–78,87,100,117–120,123–126,136,140,141)*. Although numerous in vivo and in vitro investigations have shown the importance of C-X-C chemokines in acute inflammation as chemotactic/activating factors for neutrophils and mononuclear cells, only recently has it become apparent that these C-X-C chemokines may be important in the regulation of angiogenesis.

4. THE ROLE OF THE ELR MOTIF OF C-X-C CHEMOKINES IN THE REGULATION OF ANGIOGENESIS

Our laboratory and others have found that IL-8 can induce angiogenic activity, independent of inflammation *(50,54,122)*. The angiogenic activity of IL-8 is equivalent on a molar basis to other well-recognized promoters of angiogenesis, such as bFGF and VEGF, and was found to be a significant angiogenic factor present in extracts of freshly isolated human NSCLC, accounting for 42–80% of the overall angiogenic activity of these tumors *(50,54,115,122)*. Recombinant IL-8 mediates both in vitro endothelial cell chemotactic and proliferative activity *(54,122)*. In addition, IL-8 induces the full development of neovascularization, independent of inflammation in the cornea micropocket (CMP) assay *(54,122)*. Interestingly, another member of the C-X-C chemokine family, PF4, has been shown to have angiostatic properties *(71–73)*, as well as to attenuate angiogenesis during the growth of tumors *(106)*. These findings suggest that members of the C-X-C chemokine family can function as either angiogenic or angiostatic factors in regulating neovascularization.

Our laboratory has speculated that members of the C-X-C chemokine family may exert disparate effects in mediating angiogenesis as a function of the presence or absence of the ELR motif for four reasons. First, members of the C-X-C chemokine family that display binding to and activation of neutrophils share the highly conserved ELR motif that immediately precedes the first cysteine amino acid residue, whereas PF4, IP-10, MIG, and SDF-1 lack this motif and do not bind to neutrophils *(24,47)*. Second, IL-8 (contains ELR motif) is an angiogenic factor that mediates both endothelial cell chemotactic and proliferative activity in vitro and angiogenic activity in vivo *(50,54,122)*. By contrast, PF4 (lacking the ELR motif) is an angiostatic factor *(71–73)*, and attenuates growth of tumors in vivo *(106)*. Third, the interferons (IFN-α, IFN-β, and IFN-γ) are all known inhibitors of wound repair, especially angiogenesis *(36,37,39,53)*. These cytokines, however, upregulate IP-10 and MIG from a number of cells, including keratinocytes, fibroblasts, endothelial cells, and mononuclear phagocytes *(31–33,65,67,78)*. Fourth, we and others have found that IFN-α, IFN-β, and IFN-γ are potent inhibitors of the production of monocyte-derived IL-8, GRO-α, and ENA-78 *(44,103)*, supporting the notion that IFN-α, IFN-β, and IFN-γ may shift the biologic balance of ELR– and non-ELR–C-X-C chemokines toward a preponderance of angiostatic (non-ELR) C-X-C chemokines.

To evaluate whether C-X-C chemokines display disparate angiogenic activity, endothelial cell chemotaxis was performed in the presence or absence of IL-8, ENA-78, PF4, and IP-10 in varying concentrations. Both IL-8 and ENA-78 demonstrated a dose-dependent increase in endothelial migration that was significantly greater than that of the control *(129)*. By contrast, neither PF4 nor IP-10 induced significant endothelial cell chemotaxis *(129)*. Other C-X-C chemokines were tested for their ability to induce endothelial cell chemotaxis, including ELR–C-X-C chemokines IL-8, ENA-78, GCP-2, GRO-α, GRO-β, GRO-γ, PBP, CTAP-III, and NAP-2, or the non-ELR–C-X-C chemokines IP-10, PF4, and MIG. In a similar fashion to IL-8 or ENA-78, all the ELR–C-X-C chemokines tested demonstrated significant endothelial cell chemotactic activity over the background control, whereas the endothelial cell chemotactic activity induced by MIG was either similar to background control or to the endothelial cell chemotactic activity seen with either PF4 or IP-10 *(129)*. These findings demonstrated that C-X-C chemokines could be divided into two groups with defined biologic activities: one of which contains the ELR motif and is chemotactic for endothelial cells, and the other of which lacks the ELR motif and fails to induce endothelial chemotaxis.

4.1. ELR–C-X-C Chemokines Are Angiogenic and Non-ELR–C-X-C Chemokines Are Angiostatic Factors

The previously cited studies demonstrated that PF4, IP-10, and MIG were not significant chemotactic factors for endothelial cells, and suggested that these C-X-C chemokines may be potent inhibitors of angiogenesis *(129)*. To test this hypothesis, endothelial cell chemotaxis was performed (as previously) in the presence or absence of IL-8, ENA-78, or bFGF with or without combining varying concentrations of PF4, IP-10, or MIG. Endothelial cell migration in response to either IL-8, ENA-78, or bFGF was significantly inhibited by PF4, IP-10, or MIG in a dose-dependent manner *(129)*. PF4 and IP-10 inhibited either IL-8-, ENA-78-, or bFGF-induced endothelial chemotaxis. MIG, in a similar manner as PF4 and IP-10, inhibited endothelial cell chemotaxis in response to IL-8, ENA-78, and bFGF (Table 4). Interestingly, whereas IP-10 and MIG inhibited IL-8-induced endothelial cell chemotactic activity, neither IP-10 nor MIG were effective in attenuating IL-8-induced neutrophil chemotactic activity *(129)*.

To determine whether IP-10 or MIG could inhibit the angiogenic activity of either the ELR containing C-X-C chemokines, bFGF, or VEGF in vivo, the CMP assay of neovascularization was used *(129)*. Cytokines (IL-8, ENA-78, GRO-α, GCP-2, bFGF,

Table 4
The IC$_{50}$ of PF4, IP-10, and MIG for the Inhibition
of the Agonists IL-8, ENA-78, and bFGF

Agonist inhibitor (IC$_{50}$)	IL-8 (10 nM)	ENA-78 (10 nM)	bFGF (5 nM)
PF4	$5 \times 10^{-11}M$	$5 \times 10^{-11}M$	$1 \times 10^{-9}M$
IP-10	$5 \times 10^{-11}M$	$5 \times 10^{-11}M$	$1 \times 10^{-9}M$
MIG	$5 \times 10^{-10}M$	$5 \times 10^{-9}M$	$1 \times 10^{-9}M$

or VEGF, either alone or in combination with IP-10 or MIG) were implanted into the cornea *(129)*. The ELR–C-X-C chemokines (IL-8, ENA-78, GRO-α, or GCP-2), bFGF, or VEGF induced positive corneal angiogenic responses without evidence for significant leukocyte infiltration. By contrast, neither IP-10 nor MIG alone induced neovascular responses in the cornea. When combined with the ELR–C-X-C chemokines (IL-8, ENA-78, GRO-α, or GCP-2), bFGF, or VEGF, IP-10 significantly abrogated the ELR–C-X-C chemokine, bFGF, or VEGF-induced angiogenic activity. Furthermore, MIG and SDF-1, similar to IP-10, inhibited IL-8-, ENA-78-, bFGF-, and VEGF-induced corneal neovascularization (Fig. 1).

4.2. C-X-C Chemokines: The Role of the ELR Motif in the Regulation of Angiogenesis

To establish whether the ELR motif is the critical structural/functional domain that dictates angiogenic activity for members of the C-X-C chemokine family, muteins were constructed by site-directed mutagenesis of IL-8 that contained either TVR (from IP-10) or DLQ (from PF4) amino acid residue substitutions for the ELR motif, and a mutant of MIG was constructed that contained the ELR motif immediately adjacent to the first cysteine amino acid residue of the primary structure of MIG *(129)*. In endothelial cell chemotaxis assays, the TVR–IL-8 or DLQ–IL-8 muteins alone failed to induce endothelial cell chemotactic activity, yet these muteins inhibited the maximal endothelial chemotactic activity of wild-type IL-8 *(129)*. Neither TVR–IL-8 nor DLQ–IL-8 induced neutrophil chemotaxis, nor were they effective in attenuating neutrophil chemotaxis in response to IL-8. Using the in vivo CMP assay of neovascularization, neither the TVR–IL-8 nor the DLQ–IL-8 muteins alone induced a neovascular response. However, both TVR–IL-8 and DLQ–IL-8 muteins inhibited the angiogenic response of either wild-type IL-8 or ENA-78 *(129)*. Moreover, the angiostatic activity of the IL-8 muteins was not unique to the inhibition of ELR–C-X-C chemokine-induced angiogenic activity, as both TVR–IL-8 and DLQ–IL-8 mutants inhibited bFGF-induced endothelial cell chemotaxis and corneal neovascularization. In addition, when a mutant of MIG was produced containing the ELR motif (ELR-MIG), this molecule induced a significant angiogenic response, as compared to wild-type MIG *(129)*. Interestingly, wild-type MIG inhibited the angiogenic response of the ELR-MIG mutant in both endothelial migration and CMP neovascularization assays.

Although these studies support the contention that the ELR motif was important in dictating the angiogenic activity of ELR–C-X-C chemokines, a strategy of scanning mutagenesis was used to investigate the importance of each of the amino acid residues

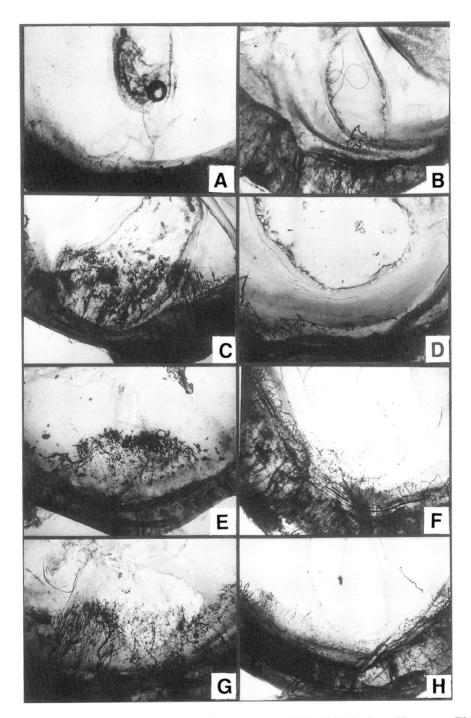

Fig. 1. Rat cornea neovascularization in response to ELR–C-X-C chemokines, non-ELR–C-X-C chemokines, bFGF, and VEGF, or combinations of these cytokines. **(A,B,C,E,G)** corneal neovascular response to a hydron pellet containing vehicle control, MIG (10 n*M*), ENA-78 (10 n*M*), bFGF (10 n*M*), or VEGF (10 n*M*), respectively; **(D,F,H)** corneal neovascular response to a hydron pellet containing ENA-78 + MIG, bFGF + MIG, VEGF + MIG, respectively. Magnification, X25.

Table 5
ELR- and non-ELR–C-X-C Chemokines Are Angiogenic and Angiostatic Factors

Angiogenic C-X-C chemokines containing the ELR motif
    Interleukin-8 (IL-8)
    Epithelial cell–derived neutrophil-activating factor-78 (ENA-78)
    Growth-related oncogene-α (GRO-α)
    Growth-related oncogene-β (GRO-β)
    Growth-related oncogene-γ (GRO-γ)
    Granulocyte chemotactic protein-2 (GCP-2)
    Platelet basic protein (PBP)
        Connective tissue activating protein-III (CTAP-III)
        β-thromboglobulin (β-TG)
        Neutrophil-activating peptide-2 (NAP-2)

Angiogenic C-X-C chemokines that lack the ELR motif
    Platelet factor 4 (PF4)
    Interferon-γ-inducible protein (IP-10)
    Monokine induced by interferon-γ (MIG)
    Stromal cell–derived factor-1 (SDF-1)

of the ELR motif. Muteins of wild-type GRO-α containing substitutions of the amino acid residues, E → A or L → A, demonstrated partial angiogenic activity, whereas the mutant containing the amino acid substitution of R → A failed to demonstrate any angiogenic activity in the CMP assay. Furthermore, the R → A mutant inhibited the angiogenic activity of wild-type GRO-α, as well as bFGF and VEGF in the CMP assay, suggesting that it behaves as an angiostatic factor. Although other structure domains (i.e., the hydrophobic pocket beyond the second cysteine amino acid residue) that may be important for alterations in angiogenic activity have not been studied, these results support the importance of the ELR motif, specifically the arginine amino acid residue, as a structural domain that is important in angiogenic activity of these C-X-C chemokines (Table 5).

5. POTENTIAL ENDOTHELIAL CELL C-X-C CHEMOKINE RECEPTORS THAT MAY BIND ANGIOGENIC AND ANGIOSTATIC C-X-C CHEMOKINES

Luster and colleagues *(34)* have found that IP-10 binds to a specific cell-surface site on endothelial cells that is shared by PF4, and appears to be a heparan sulfate proteoglycan receptor *(63)*. This binding site is specific for IP-10 and PF4, as neither ELR-containing C-X-C chemokines nor various C-C chemokines compete for binding on endothelial cells. Furthermore, these investigators demonstrated that the binding of IP-10 to endothelial cells resulted in an inhibition of proliferation that was independent of calcium flux and apoptosis and dependent on reversible cell cycle arrest. Although it is not clear that this receptor represents the recently identified receptors for IP-10/MIG (CXCR3) or SDF-1 (CXCR4) expressed on T-cells *(14,62,86)*, these findings suggest that IP-10, MIG, PF4, and potentially SDF-1 are unique members of the C-X-C chemokine family that share a heparan sulfate proteoglycan component of their receptor that accounts for their binding to endothelial cells and subsequent angiostatic activity.

In contrast to the recently described specific proteoglycan receptor for IP-10 and PF4 on endothelial cells, a specific endothelial receptor(s) has not been established for the activity of ELR–C-X-C chemokine–induced neovascularization. However, indirect evidence would suggest that the endothelial receptor for ELR–C-X-C chemokines is the C-X-C chemokine receptor, CXCR2. The following facts support this contention:

1. Although endothelial cells have been recently identified to express IL-8 receptor A (CXCR1) mRNA by reverse transcriptase-polymerase chain reaction. However the authors of this same study found that both IL-8 and NAP-2 could compete for binding on endothelial cells that was inhibited by heparin and heparan sulfate *(104)*. However, only IL-8, not NAP-2, can bind to CXCR1 *(58)*.
2. The expression of CXCR2 on neutrophils leads to binding of all ELR–C-X-C chemokines with high affinity *(58,134)*, and all ELR–C-X-C chemokines are angiogenic *(130)*.
3. Although the Duffy antigen receptor for chemokines has been identified on post-capillary venule endothelial cells *(45)*, this receptor binds not only ELR–C-X-C chemokines, but also C-C chemokines, monocyte chemoattractant protein-1 and regulates on activation normal T-cell expressed and secreted RANTES which are not angiogenic *(82)*.
4. Human burn tissue 2–12 d after injury has been demonstrated to express CXCR2 in association with capillary endothelial cells in areas of neovascularization *(81)*.

Nevertheless, further studies will be required to delineate the specific endothelial cell receptor(s) for the angiogenic activities of the ELR–C-X-C chemokines.

6. IL-8 IS AN ENDOGENOUS ANGIOGENIC FACTOR THAT PROMOTES NEOVASCULARIZATION DURING TUMOR GROWTH OF NSCLC

Our laboratory originally described the presence of elevated levels of IL-8 in NSCLC *(115)*. These studies demonstrated elevated levels of IL-8 in NSCLC, and determined that IL-8 significantly contributed to overall tumor-derived angiogenic activity. IL-8 accounted for 42–80% of the angiogenic activity contained in each of the tumor specimens, as determined by bioassays of angiogenesis *(115)*. While IL-8-dependent angiogenic activity represented a significant proportion of overall NSCLC-derived angiogenesis, the relative contribution of IL-8 was compared to other known angiogenic factors in NSCLC. Neutralizing antibodies to IL-8 resulted in a significant reduction of endothelial cell chemotactic activity in response to NSCLC tissue, with a decline to 75, 39, and 61% of the standard bioactivity, respectively, for adenocarcinoma, squamous cell carcinoma, and A549 (adenocarcinoma) samples *(115)*. By contrast, anti-bFGF antibodies had no significant effect on the endothelial cell chemotaxis in response to samples of A549 (adenocarcinoma) cells or squamous cell carcinoma tissue; however, neutralizing anti-bFGF antibodies reduced the endothelial cell chemotactic activity from adenocarcinoma tissue by 35% of the standard bioactivity *(115)*. Interestingly, the neutralization of transforming growth factor-α (TGF-α) had no significant effect on endothelial cell chemotaxis in response to adenocarcinoma or to the A549 cells; but, these antibodies resulted in a significant reduction in the endothelial cell chemotactic response to squamous cell carcinoma tissue *(115)*. Although bFGF and TGF-α have been previously described as potential angiogenic factors involved in tumor angiogen-

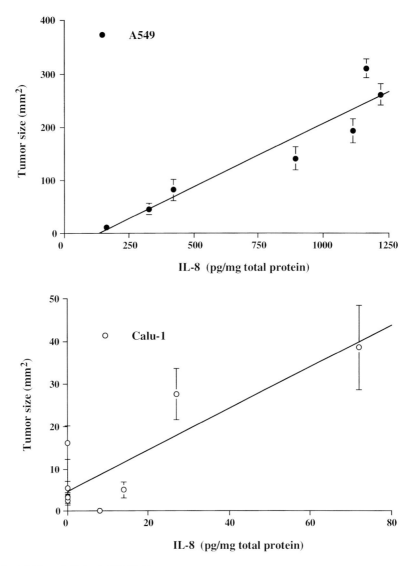

Fig. 2. A549 and Calu 1 NSCLC tumor growth and IL-8 production in SCID mice. **(Top)** time course of A549 (adenocarcinoma) tumor growth correlated ($r = 0.95$) with tumor-derived IL-8 normalized to total protein; **(bottom)** time course of Calu-1 (squamous cell carcinoma) tumor growth correlated ($r = 0.87$) with tumor-derived IL-8 normalized to total protein.

esis, our studies were the first to demonstrate that a primary angiogenic signal for NSCLC neovascularization was directly mediated by tumor-associated IL-8.

To extend the previously described studies to an in vivo model system of human tumorigenesis and to demonstrate proof of principle that C-X-C chemokines regulate tumor-derived angiogenesis, we utilized a human NSCLC/SCID mouse chimera by injecting either the human NSCLC cell lines A549 (adenocarcinoma) or Calu-1 (squamous cell carcinoma) into SCID mice *(4)*. There was a progressive increase in tumor size in A549-bearing animals beginning at wk 2 through wk 8. By contrast, animals bearing Calu-1 tumors demonstrated little growth until wk 8. The production of IL-8 from A549 tumors increased in direct correlation with tumor size and mass. By contrast, the production of IL-8 by Calu-1 tumors was delayed, yet correlated with tumor size *(4)* (Fig. 2). A549 (adenocarcinoma) tumors produced markedly greater levels of IL-8 and were 50-fold larger in size than Calu-1 (squamous cell carcinoma) tumors by 8 wk. Plasma levels of IL-8 from both A549 and Calu-1 tumor-bearing animals paralleled the production of IL-8 from the primary tumors.

Histology of A549 tumors demonstrated a paucity of infiltrating neutrophils. This apparent lack of neutrophil infiltration within the tumors, despite an appropriate chemotactic signal and the ability of murine neutrophils to respond to human IL-8 *(111)*, remains perplexing. This lack of neutrophil infiltration in these tumors is similar to our previous observations of freshly isolated human NSCLC tumors *(115)*. The relative absence of neutrophil infiltration in NSCLC may reflect the attenuation of inflammatory cell chemotactic signal by other tumor-derived factors. Our description of the production of IL-1 receptor antagonist and IL-10 by human NSCLC lends support to this concept *(113,114)*. Alternatively, the presence of IL-8 in circulation (plasma) of SCID mice, which parallels the tumor production of IL-8, may simulate a phenomenon recently described in the IL-8 transgenic mouse *(111)*. In this model, human IL-8 overexpression has been associated with increased circulating levels of IL-8, similar to what we have observed in the human NSCLC/SCID mice during tumorigenesis. These levels correlated with a proportional decrease in L-selectin expression *(111)*. The IL-8 transgenic mice demonstrated a defect in neutrophil recruitment to the peritoneal cavity after ip injection of either exogenous IL-8 or thioglycollate *(111)*. Although the IL-8 transgenic mouse model exemplifies the importance of localized production of IL-8 in order to establish a chemotactic gradient and target leukocytes to sites of inflammation, our study establishes a potential mechanism whereby the tumor may evade an innate host response by releasing sufficient IL-8 into the circulation and attenuating neutrophil extravasation at the site of the tumor.

To delineate whether IL-8 contributed to the tumorigenesis of A549 cells in SCID mice, animals were subjected to a strategy of IL-8 depletion. A549 (adenocarcinoma) tumor–bearing animals were treated in one of the following ways: passive immunization with neutralizing IL-8 antibodies, with control antibodies, or untreated. A549 tumor–bearing animals treated with neutralizing antibodies to IL-8 demonstrated a >40% reduction in tumor growth, as compared with animals bearing A549 tumors that were either untreated or treated with control antibodies *(4)*. There was no significant difference in the neutrophil infiltration of the tumors treated with anti-IL-8 or control antibody. SCID mice bearing A549 tumors treated with neutralizing antibodies to IL-8 demonstrated a reduction in the number of metastases to the lung, as compared with SCID mice treated with control antibodies *(4)*.

To further determine the mechanism of tumor growth inhibition, ex vivo angiogenic activity was evaluated from A549 tumors of animals that had been treated in vivo with either control or neutralizing anti-IL-8 antibodies. Five of the six A549 tumor samples from control antibody-treated animals induced positive corneal angiogenic responses. By contrast, four of six A549 tumor samples from anti-IL-8-treated animals induced no corneal neovascular response, with the remaining two inducing only weak angiogenic activity. More important, there was no infiltration of the corneal tissue by inflammatory cells in any of the test samples, suggesting that the angiogenic responses were mediated entirely by factors present in tumor tissue, rather than by products of infiltrating inflammatory cells. To further confirm that decreased angiogenic activity correlated with a reduction in tumor vascularity, vessel density was quantified from A549 tumors of SCID mice treated with either control or neutralizing IL-8 antibodies. Tumor vessel density in animals passively immunized with neutralizing IL-8 antibodies was significantly lower than in tumors of control antibody-treated animals. These studies demonstrated that a primary angiogenic signal for A549 (adenocarcinoma) tumor neovascularization in vivo was directly mediated by tumor-associated IL-8.

7. IP-10 IS AN ENDOGENOUS ANGIOSTATIC FACTOR THAT INHIBITS NEOVASCULARIZATION DURING TUMOR GROWTH OF NSCLC

To determine whether IP-10 protein was present in human NSCLC in a similar manner as IL-8 in the previously described study, freshly isolated specimens of bronchogenic tumors were assessed by specific IP-10 enzyme-linked immunosorbent assay *(5)*. The levels of IP-10 from tumor specimens were significantly higher than in normal lung tissue. To ascertain whether the presence of IP-10 protein varied by histologic cell type, results were further subdivided by cell type (squamous cell carcinoma vs adenocarcinoma). The increase in IP-10 from NSCLC tissue was entirely attributable to the higher levels of IP-10 present in squamous cell carcinoma, as compared to adenocarcinoma. The observation of a marked difference in the levels of IP-10 associated with squamous cell carcinoma, as compared to adenocarcinoma, in freshly isolated NSCLC tumor specimens is pathophysiologically relevant and represents a possible mechanism for the biologic differences of these two cell types of NSCLC. Patient survival and metastatic potential for NSCLC are significantly different for these two cell types. For example, patient survival is lower and metastatic potential is higher for adenocarcinoma, as compared to squamous cell carcinoma of the lung *(23,79)*. This difference may be due, in part, to the greater IP-10-dependent angiostatic activity found in freshly isolated squamous cell carcinoma tumor specimens. This is supported by the recent findings that squamous cell carcinoma specimens displayed less tumor-derived vasculature than adenocarcinomas of the lung *(145)*. The finding of higher levels of IP-10 in freshly isolated specimens of squamous cell carcinoma, as compared to adenocarcinoma, demonstrates a potential inverse relationship between IP-10 and tumor vasculature, which may explain the behavioral differences of squamous cell carcinoma vs adenocarcinoma NSCLC.

Although these experiments demonstrated that IP-10 protein was significantly elevated in specimens of freshly isolated squamous cell carcinoma, we postulated that IP-10 may be acting in vivo to regulate tumor-derived angiogenesis *(5)*. To test this hypothesis, we preincubated specimens of human squamous cell carcinoma in the presence of either control or neutralizing antibodies to IP-10 and assessed their angiogenic activity using either in vitro endothelial cell chemotaxis or CMP assays. Squamous cell carcinoma samples preincubated with neutralizing IP-10 antibodies, as compared to control antibodies, demonstrated a significant increase in their endothelial cell chemotactic activity. These findings were further confirmed using CMP assay, as squamous cell carcinoma specimens preincubated in the presence of neutralizing antibodies to IP-10, as compared to control antibodies, demonstrated an augmented neovascular response in the cornea suggesting that IP-10 is an endogenous angiostatic factor in squamous cell carcinoma.

The foregoing findings suggested that IP-10 represented an important endogenous angiostatic factor in squamous cell carcinoma of the lung. However, to determine whether this angiostatic activity was physiologically relevant during the course of in vivo tumor growth, a human NSCLC/SCID mouse model of human NSCLC tumorigenesis was utilized. SCID mice were inoculated with either A549 (adenocarcinoma) or Calu-1 (squamous cell carcinoma) cells in a similar manner as the experiments previously outlined for assessing IL-8 *(4,5)*. The production of IP-10 from A549 and Calu-1 tumors was inversely correlated with tumor growth. In addition, IP-10 levels were significantly higher in the Calu 1 (squamous cell carcinoma) tumors, as compared to A549 tumors. Plasma IP-10 levels from tumor-bearing SCID mice paralleled the findings from the primary tumors. Furthermore, the appearance of spontaneous lung metastases in SCID mice bearing A549 tumors occurred after IP-10 levels from either the primary tumor or plasma reached a nadir. To determine whether IP-10 in vitro was an autocrine growth factor for these cell lines, A549 and Calu-1 cells were cultured in the presence or absence of recombinant IP-10 for 24 and 48 h. The presence of exogenous IP-10 did not alter proliferation, as compared to appropriate controls. These findings suggested that IP-10 neither functions as an autocrine growth factor nor as an inhibitor of cellular proliferation of human NSCLC cell lines.

Since IP-10 was found to be a potent endogenous angiostatic molecule in squamous cell carcinoma, the reduced expression of IP-10 in A549 (adenocarcinoma) tumors, as compared to Calu 1 (squamous cell carcinoma) tumors, may contribute to their more aggressive behavior. We hypothesized that the restoration of tumor-associated IP-10 in A549 tumors could lead to the inhibition of tumorigenesis via an IP-10-dependent decrease in tumor-associated angiogenic activity and neovascularization. SCID mice bearing A549 tumors were injected (intratumor) with recombinant human IP-10, as compared to an equimolar concentration of an irrelevant human protein, every 48 h for 8 wk beginning at the time of tumor cell inoculation. The intratumor administration of IP-10 resulted in a 40 and 42% reduction in tumor size and mass, respectively. To exclude that IP-10 inhibited tumor growth by recruiting tumoricidal leukocytes, quantitation of tumor-infiltrating leukocytes was performed. A549 tumors from SCID mice treated with IP-10 revealed no evidence for alterations in intratumor leukocyte populations.

Lung sections from each lung of SCID mice treated with either intratumor IP-10 or control protein were examined for evidence of spontaneous metastases *(5)*. The number of metastases was significantly reduced in mice treated with IP-10, as compared with controls. In addition, the size (area) of the lung metastases per section was also dramatically reduced in the IP-10-treated group. To further demonstrate the importance of endogenous IP-10 in the regulation of human NSCLC (squamous cell carcinoma) tumor growth, we passively immunized SCID mice bearing Calu 1 tumors with either neutralizing rabbit antihuman IP-10 or control antibodies. Calu-1 tumors from animals that were passively immunized with neutralizing antibodies to IP-10 demonstrated a 1.8- to 2.9-fold increase in tumor size, as compared with tumors from animals that had received control antibodies.

To further determine the mechanism of growth inhibition by intratumor administration of IP-10, we directly evaluated angiogenic activity in the CMP assay from A549 tumors of animals that had been treated in vivo with IP-10. Nine of 12 A549 tumor

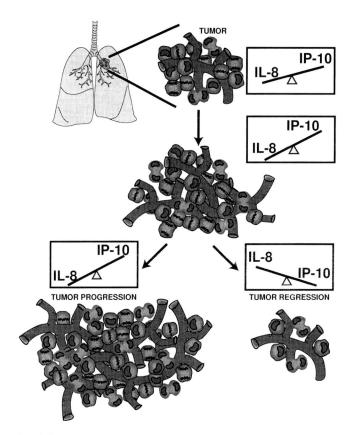

Fig. 3. The role of C-X-C chemokines in mediating angiogenesis in the context of tumorigenesis. The over- and underexpression of the angiogenic and angiostatic C-X-C chemokines IL-8 and IP-10, respectively, leads to tumor progression via the promotion of tumor-associated neovascularization. By contrast, attenuation of the angiogenic and reconstitution of the angiostatic C-X-C chemokines IL-8 and IP-10, respectively, leads to tumor regression via the inhibition of tumor-associated neovascularization.

samples from IP-10-treated tumors induced no significant neovascular response, with the remaining 3 inducing only weak angiogenic activity. By contrast, 11 of 12 A549 tumor samples from control-treated tumors induced positive angiogenic responses. To further confirm that the decreased angiogenic activity correlated with a reduction in tumor vasculature, vessel density by flourescence-activated cell sorting (FACS) analysis of factor VIII–related antigen-expressing endothelial cells from the primary tumors was quantified from A549 tumors of SCID mice treated with intratumor IP-10 or control protein. Tumor-derived factor VIII–related antigen-expressing endothelial cells were markedly reduced in primary tumors treated with IP-10, supporting the notion that IP-10 is a potent angiostatic factor for the attenuation of tumor-derived neovascularization, leading to reduced tumorigenicity and spontaneous metastases. These studies confirm our hypothesis that an imbalance in the over- and underexpression of angiogenic and angiostatic C-X-C chemokines, respectively, exist during tumorigenesis of NSCLC, and that the attenuation and reconstitution of angiogenic and angiostatic C-X-C chemokines, respectively, leads to reduced tumor-derived angiogenesis and growth (Fig. 3).

8. C-X-C CHEMOKINE COMPOSITION OF STAGE I ADENOCARCINOMA OF THE LUNG CORRELATES WITH CLINICAL OUTCOME

Recent studies have shown that the degree of angiogenesis is a predictor of metastases in stage I NSCLC *(46)*. However, these studies used morphometric analysis of vessel density. The studies outlined above support the contention that an imbalance in the overexpression of angiogenic and the underexpression of angiostatic C-X-C chemokines, in part, dictate NSCLC-derived angiogenic activity. Our laboratory has investigated whether the presence of angiogenic, as opposed to angiostatic, C-X-C chemokines in tumor specimens obtained from individuals with surgical stage I adenocarcinoma of the lung were correlated with clinical outcome. Levels of IL-8, GRO-α, and ENA-78 (angiogenic C-X-C chemokines), and IP-10 and MIG (angiostatic C-X-C chemokines) were measured from the tumor specimens. The patients were followed for a range of 6–48 mo and divided according to whether they developed metastases. Our study group consisted of 28 patients, 4 of whom developed metastases during the study period. In comparing the two groups, patients that developed metastases had significantly higher and lower levels of ENA-78 and MIG in their tumors, respectively. When the combined levels of the angiostatic C-X-C chemokines were subtracted from the combined levels of the angiogenic C-X-C chemokines, an "angiogenic index" was generated for each individual tumor specimen. The angiogenic C-X-C chemokine index was significantly higher in patients who developed metastases. Furthermore, if the patients were divided into either "high" or "low" risk for metastases based on their angiogenic index, patients in the high-risk group were >32 times more likely to develop metastases than those in the low-risk group. These results support the notion that the C-X-C chemokines are important determinants of angiogenesis in stage I adenocarcinoma. If further prospective studies show that these levels are in fact predictive of outcome, then they would be an easily obtainable and hence clinically useful measure of metastatic potential of stage I adenocarcinoma of the lung.

9. CONCLUSION

Angiogenesis is regulated by a dual, yet opposing, balance of angiogenic and angiostatic factors. For example, the magnitude of the expression of angiogenic and angiostatic factors in a primary tumor correlates with both tumor growth and the potential of spontaneous metastases. The previously discussed studies using both in vitro and in vivo systems have demonstrated that as a family, the C-X-C chemokines behave as either angiogenic or angiostatic factors, depending on the presence of the ELR motif that immediately precedes the first cysteine amino acid residue of the primary structure of these cytokines. In addition, in the context of NSCLC and perhaps other solid tumors, C-X-C chemokines are important endogenous factors that regulate tumor growth, tumor-derived angiogenic activity and neovascularization, and the potential for spontaneous metastases. Furthermore, the imbalance in the expression of angiogenic and angiostatic C-X-C chemokines may have a predictive value for determining which patients are at increased risk for potential metastases. These findings support the notion that therapy directed at either attenuating angiogenic or augmenting angiostatic C-X-C chemokines may be a novel intervention for the treatment of NSCLC.

ACKNOWLEDGMENTS

This work was supported, in part, by NIH grants CA72543 (D.A.A.), CA66180, P50 HL56402, and P50 CA69568 (R.M.S.), HL39926 (P.J.P.), and HL31693 and HL35276 (S.L.K.).

REFERENCES

1. Angiolillo, A. L., C. Sgadari, D. T. Taub, F. Liao, J. M. Farber, S. Maheshwari, H. K. Kleinman, G. H. Reaman, and G. Tosato. 1995. Human Interferon-inducible protein 10 is a potent inhibitor of angiogenesis in vivo. *J. Exp. Med.* **158:** 155–162.
2. Ansiowicz, A., L. Bardwell, and R. Sager. 1987. Constitutive overexpression of a growth-regulated gene in transformed Chinese hamster and human cells. *Proc. Natl. Acad. Sci. USA* **84:** 7188–7192.
3. Ansiowicz, A., D. Zajchowski, G. Stenman, and R. Sager. 1988. Functional diversity of gro gene expression in human fibroblasts and mammary epithelial cells. *Proc. Natl. Acad. Sci. USA* **85:** 9645–9649.
4. Arenberg, D. A., S. L. Kunkel, P. J. Polverini, M. Glass, M. D. Burdick, and R. M. Strieter. 1996. Inhibition of interleukin-8 reduces tumorigenesis of human non-small cell lung cancer in SCID mice. *J. Clin. Invest.* **97(12):** 2792–2802.
5. Arenberg, D. A., S. L. Kunkel, P. J. Polverini, S. B. Morris, M. D. Burdick, M. Glass, D. T. Taub, M. D. Iannetoni, R. I. Whyte, and R. M. Strieter. 1996. Interferon-γ-inducible protein 10 (IP-10) is an angiostatic factor that inhibits human non-small cell lung cancer (NSCLC) tumorigenesis and spontaneous metastases. *J. Exp. Med.* **184(3):** 981–992.
6. Auerbach, R. 1981. *Angiogenesis-Inducing Factors: A Review,* vol. 69. Academic, New York.
7. Ausprunk, D. H., and J. Folkman. 1977. Migration and proliferation of endothelial cells in preformed and newly formed blood vessels during tumor angiogenesis. *Microvas. Res.* **14:** 53–65.
8. Ausprunk, D. H., and J. Folkman. 1978. The sequence of events in the regression of corneal capillaries. *Lab. Invest.* **38:** 284–296.
9. Ausprunk, D. H., D. R. Knighton, and J. Folkman. 1974. Differentiation of vascular endothelium in the chick chorioallantois: a structure and autoradiographic study. *Dev. Biol.* **38:** 237–248.
10. Baggiolini, M., B. Dewald, and A. Walz. 1992. Interleukin-8 and related chemotactic cytokines, in *Inflammation: Basic Principles and Clinical Correlates.* (Gallin, J. I., I. M. Goldstein, and R. Snyderman, eds.), Raven, New York.
11. Baggiolini, M., A. Walz, and S. L. Kunkel. 1989. Neutrophil-activating peptide-1/interleukin 8, a novel cytokine that activates neutrophils. *J. Clin. Invest.* **84:** 1045–1049.
12. Baird, A., and N. Ling. 1985. Fibroblast growth factors are present in the extracellular matrix produced by endothelial cells in vitro: implications for a role for heparinase-like enzymes in the neovascular response. *Biochem. Biophys. Res. Commun.* **126:** 358–364.
13. Bar, T. H., and J. R. Wolff. 1972. The formation of capillary basement membrane during vascularization of the rat's cerebral cortex. *Z. Zellforsch.* **133:** 231–248.
14. Bleul, C. C., M. Farzan, H. Choe, C. Parolin, I. Clark-Lewis, J. Sodroski, and T. A. Springer. 1996. The lymphocyte chemoattractant SDF-1 is a ligand for LESTR/fusin and blocks HIV-1 entry. Nature **382:** 829–833.
15. Bouck, N. 1992. Angiogenesis: a mechanism by which oncogenes and tumor suppressor genes regulate tumorigenesis. *Cancer Treat. Res.* **63:** 359–371.
16. Bouck, N. 1990. Tumor angiogenesis: the role of oncogenes and tumor suppressor genes. *Cancer Cells* **2:** 179–185.
17. Brem, H., and J. Folkman. 1975. Inhibition of tumor angiogenesis mediated by cartilage. *J. Exp. Med.* **141:** 427–439.

18. Brem, H., I. Gresser, J. Grosfeld, and J. Folkman. 1993. The combination of antiangiogenic agents to inhibit primary tumor growth and metastasis. *J. Pediatr. Surg.* **28(10):** 1253–1257.

19. Brem, S., I. Preis, R. Langer, H. Brem, J. Folkman, and A. Patz. 1977. Inhibition of neovascularization by an extract derived from vitreous. *Am. J. Ophthalmol.* **84:** 323–328.

20. Brooks, P. C., R. A. Clark, and D. A. Cheresh. 1994. Requirement of vascular integrin alpha v beta 3 for angiogenesis. *Science* **264(5158):** 569–571.

21. Brooks, P. C., A. M. Montgomery, M. Rosenfeld, R. A. Reisfeld, T. Hu, G. Klier, and D. A. Cheresh. 1994. Integrin alpha v beta 3 antagonists promote tumor regression by inducing apoptosis of angiogenic blood vessels. *Cell* **79(7):** 1157–1164.

22. Carmeliet, P., V. Ferreira, G. Breier, S. Pollefeyt, L. Kieckens, M. Gertsenstein, M. Fahrig, A. Vandenhoeck, K. Harpal, C. Eberhardt, C. Declercq, J. Pawling, L. Moons, D. Collen, W. Risau, and A. Nagy. 1996. Abnormal blood vessel development and lethality in embryos lacking a single VEGF allele. *Nature* **380:** 435–439.

23. Carney, D. N. 1988. Cancers of the lungs. In *Pulmonary Diseases and Disorders,* 2nd ed. (Fishman, A. P., ed.), McGraw-Hill, New York, pp. 1885–2068.

24. Clark-Lewis, I., B. Dewald, T. Geiser, B. Moser, and M. Baggiolini. 1993. Platelet factor 4 binds to interleukin 8 receptors and activates neutrophils when its N terminus is modified with Glu-Leu-Arg. *Proc. Natl. Acad. Sci. USA* **90:** 3574–3577.

25. Crum, R., S. Szabo, and J. Folkman. 1985. A new class of steroids inhibits angiogenesis in the presence of heparin or a heparin fragment. *Science* **230:** 1375–1378.

26. Deutsch, E., and W. Kain. 1961. Studies on platelet factor 4, in *Blood Platelets.* (Jonson, S. A., R. W. Monto, J. W. Rebuck, and R. C. Horn eds.) Little-Brown, Boston.

27. DiPietro, L. A., and P. J. Polverini. 1993. Angiogenic macrophages produce the angiogenic inhibitor thrombospondin 1. *Am. J. Pathol.* **143:** 678–684.

28. Eisenstein, R., K. E. Kuettner, C. Neopolitan, L. W. Sobel, and N. Sorgente. 1975. The resistance of certain tissues to invasion III: cartilage extracts inhibit the growth of fibroblasts and endothelial cells in culture. *Am. J. Pathol.* **81:** 337–347.

29. Elner, V. M., R. M. Strieter, S. G. Elner, M. Baggiolini, I. Lindley, and S. L. Kunkel. 1990. Neutrophil chemotactic factor (IL-8) gene expression by cytokine-treated retinal pigment epithelial cells. *Am. J. Pathol.* **136:** 745–750.

30. Engerman, R. L., D. Pfaffenbach, and M. D. Davis. 1967. Cell turnover of capillaries. *Lab. Invest.* **17:** 738–743.

31. Farber, J. M. 1992. A collection of mRNA species that are inducible in the RAW 264.7 mouse macrophage cell line by gamma interferon and other agents. *Mol. Cell Biol.* **12(4):** 1535–1545.

32. Farber, J. M. 1993. HuMIG: a new member of the chemokine family of cytokines. *Biochem. Biophys. Res. Commun.* **192:** 223–230.

33. Farber, J. M. 1990. A macrophage mRNA selectively induced by gamma-interferon encodes a member of the platelet factor 4 family of cytokines. *Proc. Natl. Acad. Sci. USA* **87(14):** 5238–5242.

34. Ferrara, N., K. Carver-Moore, H. Chen, M. Dowd, L. Lu, K. S. O'Shea, L. Powell-Braxton, K. J. Hillan, and M. W. Moore. 1996. Heterozygous embryonic lethality induced by targeted inactivation of the VEGF gene. *Nature* **380(6573):** 439–442.

35. Folkman, J. 1995. Angiogenesis in cancer, vascular, rheumatoid and other disease. *Nat. Med.* **1(1):** 27–31.

36. Folkman, J. 1993. Tumor angiogenesis. In *Cancer Medicine,* 3rd ed. (vol. 1., Holland, J. F., E. Frye III, R. C. Bast Jr., D. W. Kufe, D. L. Morton, and R. R. Weischelbaum eds.), Lea & Febiger, Philadelphia, pp. 153–170.

37. Folkman, J., and H. Brem. 1992. Angiogenesis and inflammation, in *Inflammation: Basic Principles and Clinical Correlates,* 2nd ed. (Gallin, J. J., I. M. Goldstein, and R. Snyderman eds.), Raven, New York, pp. 821–839.

38. Folkman, J., and R. Cotran. 1976. Relation of vascular proliferation to tumor growth. *Int. Rev. Exp. Pathol.* **16:** 207–248.

39. Folkman, J., and M. Klagsbrun. 1987. Angiogenic factors. *Science* **235:** 442–447.

40. Folkman, J., K. Watson, D. Ingber, and D. Hanahan. 1989. Induction of angiogenesis during the transition from hyperplasia to neoplasia. *Nature* **339:** 58–61.

41. Gamble, J. R., U. Matthias, and G. Meyer. 1993. Regulation of in vitro capillary tube formation by anti-integrin antibodies. *J. Cell Biol.* **121:** 921–943.

42. Gerritsen, M. E., and C. M. Bloor. 1993. Endothelial cell gene expression in response to injury. *FASEB J.* **7:** 523–532.

43. Good, D. J., P. J. Polverini, F. Rastinejad, M. M. Le Beau, R. S. Lemons, W. A. Frazier, and N. P. Bouck. 1990. A tumor suppressor-dependent inhibitor of angiogenesis is immunologically and functionally indistinguishable from a fragment of thrombospondin. *Proc. Natl. Acad. Sci. USA* **87(17):** 6624–6628.

44. Gusella, G. L., T. Musso, M. C. Bosco, I. Espinoza-Delgado, K. Matsushima, and L. Varesio. 1993. IL-2 up-regulates but IFN-g suppresses IL-8 expression in human monocytes. *J. Immunol.* **151:** 2725–2732.

45. Hadley, T. J., Z. Lu, K. Wasniowska, S. C. Peiper, J. Hesselgesser, and R. Horuk. 1994. Postcapillary venule endothelial cells in kidney express a multispecific chemokine receptor that is structurally and functionally identical to the erythroid isoform, which is the Duffy blood group antigen. *J. Clin. Invest.* **94:** 985–991.

46. Harpole, D. H., Jr., W. G. Richards, J. E. N. Herndon, and D. J. Sugarbaker. 1996. Angiogenesis and molecular biologic substaging in patients with stage I non-small cell lung cancer. *Ann. Thorac. Surg.* **61(5):** 1470–1476.

47. Hebert, C. A., R. V. Vitangcol, and J. B. Baker. 1991. Scanning mutagenesis of interleukin-8 identifies a cluster of residues required for receptor binding. *J. Biol. Chem.* **266:** 18,989–18,994.

48. Herlyn, M., W. H. Clark, U. Rodeck, M. L. Manciati, J. Jambrosic, and H. Koprowski. 1987. Biology of tumor progression in human melanocytes. *Lab. Invest.* **56:** 461–474.

49. Homandberg, G. A., J. Kramer-Bjerke, D. Grant, G. Christianson, and R. Eisenstein. 1986. Heparin-binding fragments of fibronectin are potent inhibitors of endothelial cell growth: structure-function correlations. *Biochim. Biophys. Acta* **874(1):** 61–71.

50. Hu, D. E., Y. Hori, and T. P. D. Fan. 1993. Interleukin-8 stimulates angiogenesis in rats. *Inflammation* **17:** 135–143.

51. Ingber, D. E. 1991. Extracellular matrix and cell shape: potential control points for the inhibition of angiogenesis. *J. Cell. Biochem.* **47:** 236–241.

52. Ingber, D. E., and J. Folkman. 1989. Mechanochemical switching between growth and differentiation during fibroblast growth factor-stimulated angiogenesis in vitro: role of extracellular matrix. *J. Cell Biol.* **109(1):** 317–330.

53. Klagsbrun, M., and P. A. D'Amore. 1991. Regulators of angiogenesis. *Annu. Rev. Physiol.* **53:** 217–239.

54. Koch, A. E., P. J. Polverini, S. L. Kunkel, L. A. Harlow, L. A. DiPietro, V. M. Elner, S. G. Elner, and R. M. Strieter. 1992. Interleukin-8 (IL-8) as a macrophage-derived mediator of angiogenesis. *Science* **258:** 1798–1801.

55. Konerding, M. A., C. VanAckern, F. Steinberg, and C. Streffer. 1992. Combined morphological approaches in the study of network formation in tumor angiogenesis, in *Angiogenesis: Key Principles*. Birkhauser Verlag, Basel, Switzerland, pp. 40–58.

56. Langer, R., H. Conn, J. Vacanti, C. C. Haudenschild, and J. Folkman. 1980. Control of tumor growth in animals by infusion of an antiangiogenesis inhibitor. *Proc. Natl. Acad. Sci. USA* **77:** 4331–4335.

57. Lee, A., and R. Langer. 1983. Shark cartilage contains inhibitors of tumor angiogenesis. *Science* **221:** 1185–1187.

58. Lee, J., R. Horuk, G. C. Rice, G. L. Bennett, T. Camerato, and W. I. Wood. 1992. Characterization of two high affinity human interleukin-8 receptors. *J. Biol. Chem.* **267**: 16,283–16,287.

59. Lee, K., E. Erturk, R. R. Mayer, and A. T. K. Cockett. 1987. Efficacy of antitumor chemotherapy in C3H mice enhanced by the antiangiogenesis steroid, cortisone acetate. *Cancer Res.* **47**: 5021.

60. Leibovich, S. J., and D. M. Weisman. 1988. Macrophages, wound repair and angiogenesis. *Prog. Clin. Biol. Res.* **266**: 131–145.

61. Liaw, L., and S. M. Schwartz. 1993. Comparison of gene expression in bovine aortic endothelium in vivo versus in vitro. *Arterioscl. Thromb.* **13**: 985–993.

62. Loetscher, M., B. Gerber, P. Loetscher, S. A. Jones, L. Piali, I. Clark-Lewis, M. Baggiolini, and B. Moser. 1996. Chemokine receptor specific for IP-10 and Mig: structure, function, and expression in activated T-lymphocytes. *J. Exp. Med.* **184**: 963–969.

63. Luster, A. D., S. M. Greenberg, and P. Leder. 1995. The IP-10 chemokine binds to a specific cell surface heparan sulfate shared with platelet factor 4 and inhibits endothelial cell proliferation. *J. Exp. Med.* **182**: 219–232.

64. Luster, A. D., S. C. Jhanwar, R. S. Chaganti, J. H. Kersey, and J. V. Ravetch. 1987. Interferon-inducible gene maps to a chromosomal band associated with a (4;11) translocation in acute leukemia cells. *Proc. Natl. Acad. Sci. USA.* **84(9)**: 2868–2871.

65. Luster, A. D., and J. V. Ravetch. 1987. Biochemical characterization of a gamma interferon-inducible cytokine (IP-10). *J. Exp. Med.* **166(4)**: 1084–1097.

66. Luster, A. D., J. C. Unkeless, and J. V. Ravetch. 1985. Gamma-interferon transcriptionally regulates an early-response gene containing homology to platelet proteins. *Nature* **315(6021)**: 672–676.

67. Luster, A. D., R. L. Weinshank, R. Feinman, and J. V. Ravetch. 1988. Molecular and biochemical characterization of a novel gamma-interferon-inducible protein. *J. Biol. Chem.* **263(24)**: 12,036–12,043.

68. Lutty, G. A., D. C. Thompson, J. Y. Gallup, R. J. Mello, and A. Fenselau. 1983. Vitreous: an inhibitor of retinal extract-induced neovascularization. *Inv. Opthalmol. Vis. Sci.* **24**: 52–56.

69. Macchiarini, P., G. Fontanini, M. J. Hardin, F. Squartini, and C. A. Angeletti. 1992. Relation of neovascularization to metastasis of non-small cell lung cancer. *Lancet* **340**: 145–146.

70. Madri, J. A., B. M. Pratt, and A. M. Tucker. 1988. Phenotypic modulation of endothelial cells by transforming growth factor-beta depends upon the composition and organization of the extracellular matrix. *J. Cell Biol.* **106**: 1375–1384.

71. Maione, T. E., G. S. Gray, A. J. Hunt, and R. J. Sharpe. 1991. Inhibition of tumor growth in mice by an analogue of platelet factor 4 that lacks affinity for heparin and retains potent angiostatic activity. *Cancer Res.* **51(8)**: 2077–2083.

72. Maione, T. E., G. S. Gray, J. Petro, A. J. Hunt, A. L. Donner, S. I. Bauer, H. F. Carson, and R. J. Sharpe. 1990. Inhibition of angiogenesis by recombinant human platelet factor-4. *Science* **247**: 77–79.

73. Maione, T. E., G. S. Gray, J. Petro, A. J. Hunt, A. L. Donner, S. I. Bauer, H. F. Carson, and R. J. Sharpe. 1990. Inhibition of angiogenesis by recombinant human platelet factor-4 and related peptides. *Science* **247(4938)**: 77–79.

74. Maiorana, A., and P. M. Gullino. 1978. Acquisition of angiogenic capacity and neoplastic transformation in the rat mammary gland. *Cancer Res.* **38**: 4409–4414.

75. Maragoudakis, M. E., M. Sarmonika, and N. Panoutscaopoulou. 1988. Inhibition of basement membrane biosynthesis prevents angiogenesis. *J. Pharmacol. Exp. Ther.* **244**: 729–733.

76. Matsushima, K., K. Morishita, T. Yoshimura, S. Lavu, Y. Kobayashi, W. Lew, E. Appella,

H. F. Kung, E. J. Leonard, and J. J. Oppenheim. 1988. Molecular cloning of a human monocyte-derived neutrophil chemotactic factor (MDNCF) and the induction of MDNCF mRNA by interleukin-1 and tumor necrosis factor. *J. Exp. Med.* **167:** 1883–1893.

77. Matsushima, K., and J. J. Oppenheim. 1989. Interleukin 8 and MCAF: novel inflammatory cytokines inducible by IL-1 and TNF. *Cytokine* **1:** 2–13.

78. Miller, M. D., and M. S. Krangel. 1992. Biology and biochemistry of the chemokines: a family of chemotactic and inflammatory cytokines. *Crit. Rev. Immunol.* **12:** 17–46.

79. Minna, J. D. 1991. Neoplasms of the lung, in *Principles of Internal Medicine,* 12th ed. (Isselbacher, K. J., ed.), McGraw-Hill, New York, pp. 1102–1110.

80. Moses, M. A., and R. Langer. 1991. Inhibitors of angiogenesis. *Biotechnology* **9:** 630–634.

81. Nanney, L. B., S. G. Mueller, R. Bueno, S. C. Peiper, and A. Richmond. 1995. Distributions of melanoma growth stimulatory activity or growth-related gene and the interleukin-8 receptor type B in human wound repair. *Am. J. Pathol.* **147(5):** 1248–1260.

82. Neote, K., W. Darbonne, J. Ogez, R. Horuk, and T. Schall. 1993. Identification of a promiscuous inflammatory peptide receptor on the surface of red blood cells. *J. Biol. Chem.* **268:** 985–991.

83. Nguyen, M., N. A. Strubel, and J. Bischoff. 1993. A role for Lewis-X/A glycoconjugates in capillary morphogenesis. *Nature* **365:** 267–269.

84. O'Reilly, M., T. Boehm, Y. Shing, N. Fukai, G. Vasios, W. Lane, E. Flynn, J. Birkhead, B. Olsen, and J. Folkman. 1997. Endostatin: an endogenous inhibitor of angiogenesis and tumor growth. *Cell* **88:** 277–285.

85. O'Reilly, M. S., L. Holmgren, C. Chen, and J. Folkman. 1996. Angiostatin induces and sustains dormancy of human primary tumors in mice. *Nat. Med.* **2(6):** 689–692.

86. Oberlin, E., A. Amara, F. Bachelerie, C. Bessia, J.-L. Virelizier, F. Arenzana-Seisdedos, O. Schwartz, J.-M. Heard, I. Clark-Lewis, D. F. Legler, M. Loetscher, M. Baggiolini, and B. Moser. 1996. The CXC chemokine SDF-1 is the ligand for LESTR/fusin and prevents infection by T-cell-line-adapted HIV-1. *Nature* **382:** 833–835.

87. Oppenheim, J. J., O. C. Zachariae, N. Mukaida, and K. Matsushima. 1991. Properties of the novel proinflammatory supergene "intercrine" cytokine family. *Annu. Rev. Immunol.* **9:** 617–648.

88. Paweletz, N., and M. Knierim. 1989. Tumor-related angiogenesis. *Crit. Rev. Oncol. Hematol.* **9:** 197–242.

89. Pepper, M. S., J. D. Vassaui, L. Orci, and R. Montesano. 1992. Proteolytic balance and capillary morphogenesis in vitro, in *Angiogenesis: Key Principles.* (Steiner, R., P. B. Weisz, and R. Langer eds.), Birkhauser Verlag, Basel, pp. 137–145.

90. Peterson, H.-I. 1986. Tumor angiogenesis inhibition by prostaglandin synthetase inhibitors. *Anticancer Res.* **6:** 251–254.

91. Phillips, G. D., R. A. Whitehead, and D. R. Knighton. 1991. Initiation and pattern of angiogenesis in wound healing in the rat. *Am. J. Anat.* **192:** 257–262.

92. Polverini, P. J., P. S. Cotran, M. A. Gimbrone, and E. R. Unanue. 1977. Activated macrophages induce vascular proliferation. *Nature* (Lond.) **269(5631):** 804–806.

93. Polverini, P. J., and S. J. Leibovich. 1984. Induction of neovascularization in vivo and endothelial cell proliferation in vitro by tumor-associated macrophages. *Lab. Invest.* **51:** 635–642.

94. Rastinejad, F., P. J. Polverini, and N. P. Bouck. 1989. Regulation of the activity of a new inhibitor of angiogenesis by a cancer suppressor gene. *Cell* **56(3):** 345–355.

95. Re, F., A. Zanetti, M. Sironi, N. Polentarutti, L. Lanfrancone, E. Dejana, and F. Colotta. 1994. Inhibition of anchorage-dependent cell spreading triggers apoptosis in cultured human endothelial cells. *J. Cell Biol.* **127:** 537–546.

96. Richmond, A., and H. G. Thomas. 1988. Melanoma growth stimulatory activity: isolation from human melanoma tumors and characterization of tissue distribution. *J. Cell Biochem.* **36:** 185–198.

97. Rifkin, D. B., J. L. Gross, D. Moscatelli, and E. Jaffe. 1982. Proteases and angiogenesis: production of plasminogen activator and collagenase by endothelial cells, in *Pathobiology of the Endothelial Cell* (Nossel, H., and H. J. Vogel eds.), Academic, New York, pp. 191–197.

98. Risau, W. 1991. Vasculogenesis, angiogenesis and endothelial cell differentiation during embryonic development, in *The Development of the Vascular System* (Feinberg, R. N., G. K. Sherer, and R. Auerbach eds.), K. Karger, Basel, Switzerland, pp. 58–68.

99. Roberts, R. B., and M. B. Spom. 1989. Regulation of endothelial cell growth, architecture, and matrix synthesis by TGF-Beta. *Am. Rev. Respir. Dis.* **140:** 1126–1128.

100. Rolfe, M. W., S. L. Kunkel, T. J. Standiford, S. W. Chensue, R. M. Allen, H. L. Evanoff, S. H. Phan, and R. M. Strieter. 1991. Pulmonary fibroblast expression of interleukin-8: a model for alveolar macrophage-derived cytokine networking. *Am. J. Respir. Cell. Mol. Biol.* **5:** 493–501.

101. Sarma, V., F. W. Wolf, R. M. Marks, T. B. Shows, and V. M. Dixit. 1992. Cloning of a novel tumor necrosis factor-alpha-inducible primary response gene that is differentially expressed in development and capillary-tube-like formation in vitro. *J. Immunol.* **148:** 3302–3312.

102. Sato, N., K. Fukuda, H. Nariuchi, and N. Sagara. 1987. Tumor necrosis factor inhibits angiogenesis in vitro. *JNCI* **79:** 1383.

103. Schnyder-Candrian, S., R. M. Strieter, S. L. Kunkel, and A. W. A. 1995. Interferon-a and interferon-g downregulate the production of interleukin-8 and ENA-78 in human monocytes. *J. Leuk. Biol.* **57(6):** 929–935.

104. Schönbeck, U., E. Brandt, F. Petersen, H. Flad, and H. Loppnow. 1995. IL-8 specifically binds to endothelial but not to smooth muscle cells. *J. Immunol.* **154:** 2375–2383.

105. Shapiro, R., and B. L. Vallee. 1987. Human placental ribonuclease inhibitor abolishes both angiogenic and ribonucleolytic activities of angiogenin. *Proc. Natl. Acad. Sci. USA* **84:** 2238.

106. Sharpe, R. J., H. R. Byers, C. F. Scott, S. I. Bauer, and T. E. Maione. 1990. Growth inhibition of murine melanoma and human colon carcinoma by recombinant human platelet factor 4. *J. Natl. Cancer Inst.* **82(10):** 848–853.

107. Shields, P. G., and C. C. Harris. 1993. Genetic predisposition to cancer, in *Lung Cancer* (Roth, J. A., J. D. Cox, and W. K. Hong, eds.), Blackwell, Boston, pp. 3–19.

108. Shirozu, M., T. Nakano, J. Inazawa, K. Tashiro, H. Tada, T. Shinohara, and T. Honjo. 1995. Structure and chromosomal localization of the human stromal cell-derived factor 1 (SDF-1) gene. *Genomics* **28:** 495–500.

109. Sholly, M. M., G. P. Fergusen, H. R. Seibel, J. L. Montour, and J. D. Wilson. 1984. Mechanisms of neovascularization: vascular sprouting can occur without proliferation of endothelial cells. *Lab. Invest.* **51:** 624–634.

110. Sidky, Y. A., and E. C. Borden. 1987. Inhibition of angiogenesis by interferons: effects on tumor- and lymphocyte-induced vascular responses. *Cancer Res.* **47:** 5155–5161.

111. Simonet, W. S., T. M. Hughes, H. Q. Nguyen, L. D. Trebasky, D. M. Danilenko, and E. S. Medlock. 1994. Long term impaired neutrophil migration in mice overexpressing human interleukin-8. *J. Clin. Invest.* **94:** 1310–1319.

112. Sims, D. E. 1986. The pericyte: a review. *Tissue Cell* **18:** 153–174.

113. Smith, D. R., S. L. Kunkel, M. D. Burdick, C. M. Wilke, M. B. Orringer, R. I. Whyte, and R. M. Strieter. 1994. Production of Interleukin-10 by human bronchogenic carcinoma. *Am. J. Pathol.* **145:** 18–25.

114. Smith, D. R., S. L. Kunkel, T. J. Standiford, S. W. Chensue, M. W. Rolfe, M. B. Orringer, R. I. Whyte, M. D. Burdick, J. M. Danforth, A. R. Gilbert, and R. M. Strieter. 1993. The production of Interleukin-1 receptor antagonist by human bronchogenic carcinoma. *Am. J. Pathol.* **143:** 794–803.

115. Smith, D. R., P. J. Polverini, S. L. Kunkel, M. B. Orringer, R. I. Whyte, M. D. Burdick,

C. A. Wilke, and R. M. Strieter. 1994. IL-8 mediated angiogenesis in human bronchogenic carcinoma. *J. Exp. Med.* **179:** 1409–1415.

116. Sorgente, N., K. E. Kuettner, L. W. Soble, and R. Eisenstein. 1975. The resistance of certain tissues to invasion. II. Evidence for extractable factors in cartilage which inhibit invasion by vascularized mesenchyme. *Lab. Invest.* **32:** 217–222.

117. Standiford, T. J., S. L. Kunkel, M. A. Basha, S. W. Chensue, J. P. Lynch III, G. B. Toews, J. Westwick, and R. M. Strieter. 1990. Interleukin-8 gene expression by a pulmonary epithelial cell line: a model for cytokine networks in the lung. *J. Clin. Invest.* **86:** 1945–1953.

118. Strieter, R. M., K. Kasahara, R. Allen, H. J. Showell, T. J. Standiford, and S. L. Kunkel. 1990. Human neutrophils exhibit disparate chemotactic factor gene expression. *Biochem. Biophys. Res. Commun.* **173(2):** 725–730.

119. Strieter, R. M., K. Kasahara, R. M. Allen, T. J. Standiford, M. W. Rolfe, F. S. Becker, S. W. Chensue, and S. L. Kunkel. 1992. Cytokine-induced neutrophil-derived interleukin-8. *Am. J. Pathol.* **141:** 397–407.

120. Strieter, R. M., and S. L. Kunkel. 1997. Chemokines and the lung, in *Lung: Scientific Foundations,* 2nd ed. (Crystal, R., J. West, E. Weibel, and P. Barnes eds.), Raven, New York, pp. 155–186.

121. Strieter, R. M., S. L. Kunkel, D. A. Arenberg, M. D. Burdick, and P. J. Polverini. 1995. Interferon gamma-inducible protein 10 (IP-10), a member of the C-X-C chemokine family, is an inhibitor of angiogenesis. *Biochem. Biophys. Res. Commun.* **210(1):** 51–57.

122. Strieter, R. M., S. L. Kunkel, V. M. Elner, C. L. Martonyl, A. E. Koch, P. J. Polverini, and S. G. Elner. 1992. Interleukin-8: a corneal factor that induces neovascularization. *Am. J. Pathol.* **141:** 1279–1284.

123. Strieter, R. M., S. L. Kunkel, H. Showell, D. G. R. H. Phan, P. A. Ward, and R. M. Marks. 1989. Endothelial cell gene expression of a neutrophil chemotactic factoor by TNF-a, LPS, and IL-1b. *Science* **243:** 1467–1469.

124. Strieter, R. M., S. L. Kunkel, H. J. Showell, and R. M. Marks. 1988. Monokine-induced gene expression of human endothelial cell-derived neutrophil chemotactic factor. *Biochem. Biophys. Res. Commun.* **156:** 1340–1345.

125. Strieter, R. M., N. W. Lukacs, T. J. Standiford, and S. L. Kunkel. 1993. Cytokines and lung inflammation. *Thorax* **48:** 765–769.

126. Strieter, R. M., S. H. Phan, H. J. Showell, D. G. Remick, J. P. Lynch, M. Genord, C. Raiford, M. Eskandari, R. M. Marks, and S. L. Kunkel. 1989. Monokine-induced neutrophil chemotactic factor gene expression in human fibroblasts. *J. Biol. Chem.* **264:** 10,621–10,626.

127. Strieter, R. M., P. J. Polverini, D. A. Arenberg, and S. L. Kunkel. 1995. The role of CXC chemokines as regulators of angiogenesis. *Shock* **4(3):** 155–160.

128. Strieter, R. M., P. J. Polverini, D. A. Arenberg, A. Walz, G. Opdenakker, J. Van Damme, and S. L. Kunkel. 1995. Role of C-X-C chemokines as regulators of angiogenesis in lung cancer. *J. Leukoc. Biol.* **57(5):** 752–762.

129. Strieter, R. M., P. J. Polverini, S. L. Kunkel, D. A. Arenberg, M. D. Burdick, J. Kasper, J. Dzuiba, J. V. Damme, A. Walz, D. Marriott, S. Y. Chan, S. Roczniak, and A. B. Shanafelt. 1995. The functional role of the 'ELR' motif in CXC chemokine-mediated angiogenesis. *J. Biol. Chem.* **270(45):** 27,348–27,357.

130. Strieter, R. M., P. J. Polverini, S. L. Kunkel, D. A. Arenberg, M. D. Burdick, J. Kasper, J. Dzuiba, J. Van Damme, A. Walz, D. Marriott, S. Chan, S. Roczniak, and A. Shanafelt. 1995. The functional role of the ELR motif in CXC chemokine-mediated angiogenesis. *J. Biol. Chem.* **270(45):** 27,348–27,357.

131. Sunderkotter, C., M. Goebeler, K. Schulze-Osthoff, R. Bhardwaj, and C. Sorg. 1991. Macrophage-derived angiogenesis factors. *Pharmacol. Ther.* **51(2):** 195–216.

132. Tannock, I. F., and H. S. Hayashi. 1972. The proliferation of capillary and endothelial cells. *Cancer Res.* **32:** 77–82.

133. Tashiro, K., H. Tada, R. Heilker, M. Shirozu, T. Nakano, and T. Honjo. 1993. Signal sequence trap: a cloning strategy for secreted proteins and type I membrane proteins. *Science* **261:** 600–603.

134. Taub, D. D., and J. J. Oppenheim. 1994. Chemokines, inflammation and immune system. *Ther. Immunol.* **1:** 229–246.

135. Taylor, S., and J. Folkman. 1982. Protamine is an inhibitor of angiogenesis. *Nature* **297:** 307–312.

136. Thornton, A. J., R. M. Strieter, I. Lindley, M. Baggiolini, and S. L. Kunkel. 1990. Cytokine-induced gene expression of a neutrophil chemotactic factor/interleukin-8 by human hepatocytes. *J. Immunol.* **144:** 2609–2613.

137. Tolsma, S. S., O. V. Volpert, D. J. Good, W. A. Frazier, P. J. Polverini, and N. Bouck. 1993. Peptides derived from two separate domains of the matrix protein thrombospondin-1 have anti-angiogenic activity. *J. Cell Biol.* **122(2):** 497–511.

138. Vlodavsky, I., J. Folkman, R. Sullivan, R. Fridman, R. Ishai-Michaeli, J. Sasse, and M. Klagsbrun. 1987. Endothelial cell-derived basic fibroblast growth factor: synthesis and deposition into subendothelial extracellular matrix. *Proc. Natl. Acad. Sci. USA* **84:** 2292–2296.

139. Walz, A., and M. Baggiolini. 1990. Generation of the neutrophil-activating peptide NAP-2 from platelet basic protein or connective tissue-activating peptide III through monocyte proteases. *J. Exp. Med.* **171:** 449–454.

140. Walz, A., R. Burgener, B. Car, M. Baggiolini, S. L. Kunkel, and R. M. Strieter. 1991. Structure and neutrophil-activating properties of a novel inflammatory peptide (ENA-78) with homology to interleukin-8. *J. Exp. Med.* **174:** 1355–1362.

141. Walz, A., S. L. Kunkel, and R. M. Strieter. 1996. CXC chemokines—an overview, in *Chemokines in Disease* (Koch, A. E., and R. M. Strieter eds.), R. G. Landes, Austin, pp. 1–26.

142. Weidner, N. 1995. Intratumor microvessel density as a prognostic factor in cancer. *Am. J. Pathol.* **147(1):** 9–19.

143. Weidner, N., P. R. Carroll, J. Flax, W. Blumenfeld, and J. Folkman. 1993. Tumor angiogenesis correlates with metastasis in invasive prostate carcinoma. *Am. J. Pathol.* **143:** 401–409.

144. Weidner, N., J. P. Semple, W. R. Welch, and J. Folkman. 1991. Tumor angiogenesis and metastasis—correlation in invasive breast carcinoma. *N. Engl. J. Med.* **324:** 1–8.

145. Yuan, A., Y. Pan-Chyr, Y. Chong-Jen, Y. Lee, Y. Yu-Tuang, C. Chi-Long, L. Lee, K. Sow-Hsong, and L. Kwen-Tay. 1995. Tumor angiogenesis correlates with histologic type and metastasis in non-small cell lung cancer. *Am. J. Respir. Crit. Care Med.* **152:** 2157–2162.

10

The Role of Melanoma Growth-Stimulatory Activity in Melanoma Tumorigenesis and Angiogenesis

**Ann Richmond, Hamid Haghnegahdar,
Rebecca Shattuck-Brandt, Lauren D. Wood,
Chaitanya S. Nirodi, James D. Owen,
Robert Strieter, Marie Burdick, and Jing Luan**

1. INTRODUCTION

1.1. Melanoma Growth Stimulatory Activity/Growth-Regulated Gene

Melanoma growth-stimulatory activity/growth-regulated genes (MGSA/GROs) encode proteins that are important mediators of the wound healing and immune response. MGSA/GRO-α is a secreted 7894-Dalton protein that is derived from a 11,391-Dalton precursor protein *(2,4,42)*. At physiologic concentrations (0.1–100 n*M*), the monomer structure of MGSA/GRO-α is favored. The monomer–dimer equilibrium exhibits a K_d of ~5 μ*M,* and solution pH has an effect on the stabilization of the dimer structure *(41)*. Dimerization is not required for biologic activity *(41)*. In humans, three different genes have been identified that encode highly related forms of MGSA/GRO, and these have been named MGSA/GRO-α, -β, and -γ*(3,13,17,44,58)*. In mice two MGSA/GRO homologs have been identified, KC and macrophage inflammatory protein-2 (MIP-2) *(39,44,58)*. Numerous other homologs have since been identified in rats, rabbits, chickens, pigs, and sheep *(3,44* for review). These proteins are members of the rapidly growing family of chemokines and, based on their structural properties, are in the C-X-C chemokine subfamily along with interleukin-8 (IL-8), neutrophil-activating peptide-2, epithelial cell–derived neutrophil-activating factor-78 (ENA-78), granulocyte chemotactic protein-2, stromal cell–derived factor-1, monokine induced by interferon-γ (MIG), and interferon-γ-inducible protein-10 (IP-10) *(3,* for a review). The C-X-C chemokines are chemotactic for a number of cells expressing receptors for these chemokines *(3)*. In addition, they are growth regulatory for a variety of cell types including melanocytes, keratinocytes, and endothelial cells *(44,* for a review). These biologic activities of chemokines are mediated through seven-transmembrane G protein–coupled chemokine receptors. MGSA/GRO molecules have been shown to bind to the C-X-C chemokine receptor identified as CXCR2, the Duffy antigen receptor for chemokines (DARC), and two virally encoded chemokine receptors, HSV-ECRF3 and the KSHV-encoded G protein–coupled receptor *(1,3,14,16,34,35,57)*. The presence of the ELR motif in MGSA/GRO proteins is required for receptor activation *(44,56)*.

From: *Chemokines and Cancer*
Edited by: B. J. Rollins © Humana Press Inc., Totowa, NJ

2. DEREGULATION OF EXPRESSION OF MGSA/GRO GENES IN MELANOMA

2.1. Regulation of Expression of MGSA/GRO Genes in Melanocytic Cells

The expression of chemokines is normally tightly regulated and is only transiently induced in response to mediators of the inflammatory response such as IL-1, tumor necrosis factor-α (TNF-α), and a variety of other agents *(3)*. Interestingly, during tumor progression and chronic inflammation, this tight regulation of chemokine expression is disturbed such that numerous tumor lesions and chronically inflamed tissues have been reported to express chemokines continuously *(2,6,44,46,50,63,66)*. For example, in the absence of cytokine stimulation, the expression of MGSA/GRO is very low in normal melanocytes and normal retinal pigment epithelial cells, but is quite high in malignant melanoma *(7,10,47,63,64)*. In normal skin keratinocytes, MGSA/GRO expression appears to coincide with differentiation, as noted by the presence of immunoreactive MGSA/GRO in suprabasal keratinocytes and in the hair follicles, sebaceous glands, and sweat ducts. By contrast, lesional tissue from 7/7 squamous cell carcinoma tumors was moderately positive, whereas basal cell carcinoma tissue was negative for immunoreactive MGSA/GRO in four of six tumor samples *(59)*.

2.2. MGSA/GRO as an Effector of Melanocyte Tumorigenesis

Although normal melanocytes express little MGSA/GRO, when there is dysplasia or a congenital proliferation of melanocytes, the incidence of MGSA/GRO expression is increased *(59)*. Immunoreactive MGSA/GRO-α protein is expressed in >70% of the melanoma tumors we have studied, although there is considerable heterogeneity within the tumors regarding MGSA/GRO-α expression *(27,37,40,43,44a,45)*. Melanoma tumors often contain infiltrating lymphocytes and inflammatory infiltrates *(8,62)*, suggesting that secreted MGSA/GRO-α is biologically active in these tumors. MGSA/GRO-α predominates in melanoma lesions, with only very low levels of expression of MGSA/GRO-β or -γ based on reverse transcriptase-polymerase chain reaction (RT-PCR), *in situ* hybridization, and immunohistochemistry *(66)*. This is consistent with our purification of the MGSA/GRO-α protein from melanoma tumors and melanoma conditioned medium. It is also consistent with the prior reports that a screen of melanoma tumors by PCR consistently detects MGSA/GRO-α mRNA expression *(10,27)*.

It will be important to determine the ratio of MIG and IP-10 to other C-X-C chemokines in developing melanoma lesions. Work from Strieter's laboratory suggests that during tumor progression, the balance of chemokines becomes altered, so that non-ELR-containing C-X-C chemokines, which negatively affect tumor growth through their antiangiogenic activity (MIG and IP-10), are decreased and so that the ELR-containing C-X-C chemokines, which positively affect cell growth through stimulation of angiogenesis (MGSA/GRO, IL-8, and ENA-78), are increased *(55)*. Thus, it has been suggested that the shift in the balance of ELR- and non-ELR-containing chemokines can enhance tumor progression.

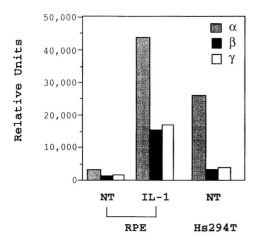
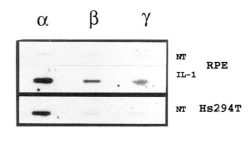

Fig. 1. Nuclear run-on analysis of MGSA/GRO transcription in Hs294T and RPE cells. Confluent RPE cells (45×10^6 cells/assay) were either not treated (NT) or treated with 5 U of IL-1/mL for 1 h. Untreated Hs294T cells (45×10^6) were similarly taken for each assay. Transcribed RNA was labeled and purified. Equal counts of purified, labeled RNA were hybridized to MGSA/GRO-α, -β, and -γ genomic fragments and to Bluescript (SK+) (not shown). The signal was quantitated and the resulting values are shown in the bar graphs. (Reprinted from *Mol. Cell. Biol.* **14:** 791–802, 1994, with permission).

2.3. In Vitro Models Exploring Mechanisms of Regulation of MGSA/GRO Expression in Tumorigenesis

MGSA/GRO-α, -β, and -γ mRNA expression has been examined in normal human epidermal melanocytes (NHEMs), retinal pigment epithelial (RPE) cells, and melanoma cells by PCR and Northern analysis using oligonucleotide probes specific for each of the three mRNAs *(50)*. This highly sensitive PCR shows that MGSA/GRO-α, -β, and -γ mRNAs can be detected in both normal melanocytes and Hs294T melanoma cells. IL-1 treatment substantially amplifies the PCR product for the α, β, and γ cDNAs *(27,50)*. Hs294T melanoma cells, but not NHEM or RPE cells, constitutively express sufficient MGSA/GRO-α for detection by Northern blot analysis. This enhanced expression of MGSA/GRO-α mRNA in Hs294T melanoma is, in part, owing to constitutive transcriptional activation of this gene. Nuclear run-on analyses verified that there is an 8- to 30-fold enhanced endogenous transcription of the MGSA/GRO genes in Hs294T cells as compared to RPE cells. IL-1 markedly enhanced transcription of MGSA/GRO in RPE cells (10- to 20-fold), but did not increase the already elevated constitutive transcription of the MGSA/GRO in melanoma cells *(50)* (Fig. 1). Transformed fibroblasts from hamster and chicken have also been shown to exhibit transcriptional deregulation of the MGSA/GRO homologs. Transformed Chinese hamster embryo fibroblasts (CHEF) show a 50-fold enhanced transcription of hamster GRO as compared to nontransformed CHEF cells *(2)*, and RSV-transformed fibroblasts express 10-fold higher levels of pCEF4, the chicken homolog of MGSA/GRO *(6)*. Moreover, MIP-2, one of the murine homologs of MGSA, is also transcriptionally deregulated in B-16 melanoma *(63)*.

2.4. Mechanism for Constitutive Transcription of the MGSA/GRO in Hs294T Melanoma Cells

Three experimental approaches have been used to show that differences in MGSA/GRO-α expression in RPE vs Hs294T cells were not owing to differences in the DNA copy number, position, or sequence of the promoter/enhancer:

1. Southern blot analysis of genomic DNA isolated from RPE and Hs294T melanoma cells demonstrated that there are no gross differences in the restriction pattern of the MGSA/GRO-α gene in these two cell lines, suggesting that the MGSA/GRO-α gene has not been amplified or rearranged in the melanoma cells.
2. Sequence analysis of 350 bp of the immediate MGSA/GRO-α promoter from Hs294T cells amplified by PCR demonstrated that there were no mutations or deletions that would affect MGSA/GRO-α gene transcription, although this does not rule out alterations at more distant 5′ loci.
3. DNase hypersensitivity demonstrated that there were no differences in chromatin structure affecting MGSA/GRO-α transcription in Hs294T as compared to RPE cells (R. Shattuck-Brandt, unpublished data).

Altogether, these data demonstrated that the differences in MGSA/GRO expression in Hs294T cells as compared to RPE cells were not owing to differences in the DNA sequence of the promoter/enhancer. Rather, the differences in expression may result from alterations in the interaction of the *trans*-acting factors with the DNA.

To further characterize the role of *trans*-acting factors in the enhanced MGSA/GRO-α transcription in Hs294T cells, we constructed a series of MGSA/GRO promoter/chloramphenicol-acetyltransferase (CAT) reporter genes. In transient transfection assays in which CAT expression was placed under the transcriptional control of the initial 1000 bp of the MGSA/GRO-α, -β, or -γ promoter/enhancer, IL-1 only minimally increased CAT activity in Hs294T cells, but strongly stimulated CAT activity in RPE cells. These results corroborate the results obtained by nuclear run-on assay in which Hs294T melanoma cells exhibited constitutive transcription of MGSA/GRO-α, but in which the transcription was not further increased by IL-1, whereas, by contrast, RPE cells did not constitutively express MGSA/GRO-α, -β, or -γ but exhibited marked enhancement of MGSA/GRO transcription in response to IL-1 *(50)*. A series of deletions in the MGSA/GRO-α promoter were introduced into the CAT-reporter gene to characterize further the region within the 1000 bp of 5′ regulatory sequence responsible for induction by IL-1 and TNF-α in RPE cells. Five regulatory regions appear to be essential for basal- as well as cytokine-induced transcription of the gene:

1. A TATA box (–23 to –29 nt)
2. An NF-κB binding element (–62 to –77 nt)
3. An AT-rich HMGI(Y) binding element, nestled within the NF-κB sequence
4. An apparently novel *cis* element upstream to the NF-κB site, the immediate upstream region (IUR) (–77 to –97 nt)
5. A GC-rich sequence containing Sp1 binding element (–115 to –132 nt).

A dramatic decrease in basal CAT activity and a loss of cytokine induction was noted when the NF-κB element located between MGSA/GRO-α 145 and MGSA/GRO-α89/CAT was deleted or mutated. From gel shift analyses we know that IL-1 and TNF-α induce NF-κB binding activity in both RPE and Hs294T cells. However, in Hs294T cells IL-1/TNF-α-induced transactivation does not occur, probably because the NF-κB complex is already involved in the high constitutive expression of MGSA/GRO-α *(50)*.

2.5. MGSA/GRO-α CAT Activity Is Increased
by Nuclear Import of an Activated NF-κB Complex

When a Rel-A expression vector was cotransfected with MGSA/GRO-α 350/CAT in RPE or Hs294T cells, an increase in CAT activity above that found with the reporter plasmid alone was observed in both cell types. However, the RPE cells demonstrated a much larger increase in CAT activity compared with the four-fold increase demonstrated by the Hs294T cells. In both cell types, cotransfection of NF-κB p65 with either reporter gene plasmids containing two copies of the MGSA/GRO-NF-κB or the HIV-NF-κB element also resulted in a strong increase in CAT activity *(65)*. These data demonstrate that altering the ratios of Rel A (NF-κB p65) within the chosen cell types can differentially affect MGSA/GRO transcription.

2.6. NF-κB Is Constitutively Activated
in Hs294T Melanoma Cells but Not in RPE Cells

Based on studies demonstrating a role for NF-κB in tumorigenesis and the importance of IκB in regulating NF-κB activity, we characterized the regulation of IκBα expression in response to the cytokine IL-1 in Hs294T melanoma and RPE cells. IκBα mRNA is constitutively expressed in the Hs294T cells at levels 9-fold higher than those detected in RPE cells. IL-1 increases IκBα expression in Hs294T cells no greater than 2-fold, whereas in RPE cells the increase is 53-fold. Electromobility shift assay (EMSA) demonstrated that despite the high constitutive levels of IκBα mRNA in Hs294T cells, a constitutive NF-κB complex was present in Hs294T nuclei (Fig. 2). These results are similar to those seen in mature B-cells in which NF-κB is constitutively activated and IκBα mRNA and protein expression are high *(60)*. However, in contrast to the study in B-cells, we observed that IκB protein levels are lower in the cytoplasm of Hs294T melanoma cells as compared to the retinal pigment epithelial cell line (ARPE) (Fig. 3). IκBα is more rapidly degraded in Hs294T cells than in ARPE cells, in which no constitutive nuclear NF-κB complex is seen (Fig. 4). Interestingly, in the Hs294T cells, EMSA and Western analysis indicate that IL-1 does not induce further NF-κB binding in Hs294T cells (Fig. 2).

2.7. An IUR in Addition to the NF-κB Site Is Required
for MGSA/GRO-α CAT Activity in RPE Cells

Mukaida et al. *(36,37)* have shown that both the NF-κB and the C/EBP binding sites are required for the IL-1 and TNF-α activation of IL-8 *(32,33)*. Previous work in other systems has demonstrated a physical association *(25)* and cross-coupling of NF-κB and C/EBP family members *(22,53,54)*. In particular, regulation of IL-8 gene expression depends on the ratio of NF-κB and C/EBP complexes. C/EBP has an inhibitory effect through the adjacent NF/κB element whereas NF-κB p65 enhances transactivation through the C/EBP element *(23)*. Unlike IL-8, the sequence immediately upstream to the NF-κB site in the MGSA/GRO-α promoter, IUR, does not bind C/EBP members nor is MGSA/GRO-α transactivation affected by C/EBP overexpression. However, Rel-A expression resulted in a substantial increase in activ-

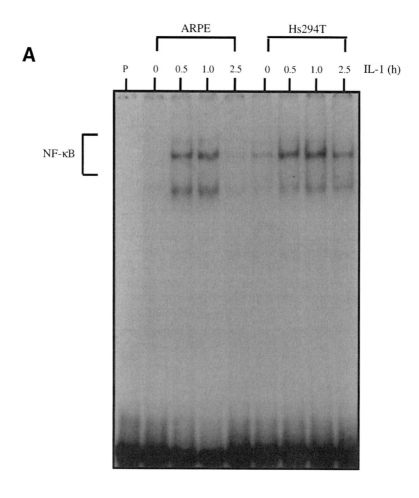

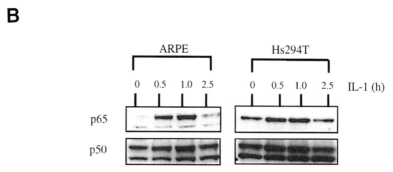

Fig. 2. In Hs294T cells a constitutive NF-κB complex is detected and the time course for NF-κB deactivation is delayed. ARPE and Hs294T cells were stimulated with IL-1 (5 U/mL) for 0.5, 1, and 2.5 h. Following stimulation, nuclei were isolated by sucrose gradient purification and nuclear extracts were obtained. **(A)** NF-κB activity was determined by EMSA using the 36-bp NF-κB element from the MGSA/GRO-α gene. **(B)** Nuclear extracts were analyzed by Western analysis for p65 and p50. Nuclear extracts were separated on a 7.5% sodium dodecyl sulfate-polyacrylamide gel. Following transfer of the proteins to polyvinylidene difluoride (PVDF)-Immobilon, p65 and p50 were detected by enhanced chemiluminescence (ECL) using antibodies to these proteins. (Reprinted with permission from *Cancer Res.* **57**: 3032–3039, 1997.)

A

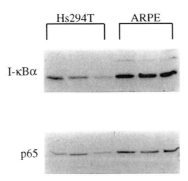

B

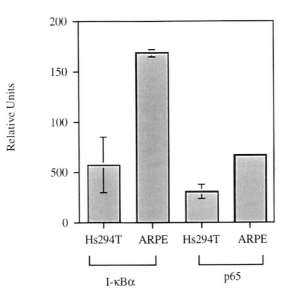

Fig. 3. Hs294T cells contain low levels of IκBα. **(A)** Total cellular protein was solubilized from unstimulated Hs294T and ARPE cells in radioimmuno-protein assay (RIPA) buffer. Whole-cell extracts (30 μg) were analyzed by Western analysis for p65 and IκBα immunoreactivity. **(B)** Autoradiograms obtained from ECL were quantitated by densitometric scanning. Whole-cell extracts from three independent experiments were analyzed, and the results are presented as the average of the relative units. (Reprinted with permission from *Cancer Res.* **57:** 3032–3039, 1997.)

ity from wild-type as well as with mutant IUR or mutant NF-κB MGSA/GRO-α350/ CAT. The data indicate that Rel A transactivates through both the NF-κB and upstream IUR in MGSA/GRO-α *(65)*.

Sequence analysis of IL-8 and MGSA/GRO-α promoter regions indicates a conserved NF-κB element with an IUR resembling a C/EBP site, but C/EBP proteins do

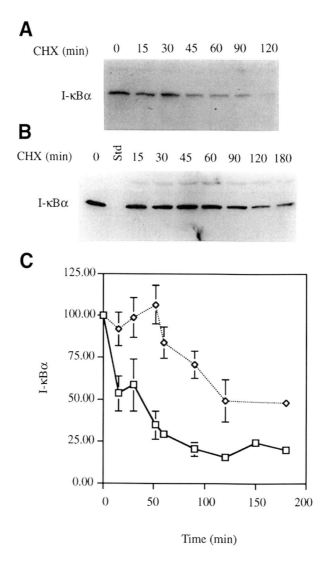

Fig. 4. IκBα is rapidly degraded in Hs294T cells. Hs294T (**A, □**) and ARPE (**B, ◇**) cells were treated with 10 µg/mL of cycloheximide for the indicated period of time. Total cellular protein was solubilized from both cell types. Whole-cell extracts were analyzed for IκBα immunoreactivity by Western analysis. Different amounts of protein and exposure times were utilized in order to equalize the signal from Hs294T and ARPE cells. For the data shown from ARPE cells, 30 µg of whole-cell extract were analyzed and the exposure time after ECL was 30 min. For the data from Hs294T cells, 50 µg of whole-cell extract were analyzed and the exposure time was 1 h. Autoradiographs were quantitated by densitometric scanning. Representative experiments are shown and the plotted data are the averages of three separate determinations with the standard error of the mean. (Reprinted with permission from *Cancer Res.* **57:** 3032–3039, 1997.)

not bind to the IUR element *(65)*. Mutation of either the NF-κB element or the IUR within the context of the MGSA/GRO-α 350-bp CAT promoter/enhancer markedly reduces the constitutive CAT activity in the Hs294T and RPE cells, and also eliminates the cytokine-induced CAT activity in the RPE cells *(65)*. Based on the observation that

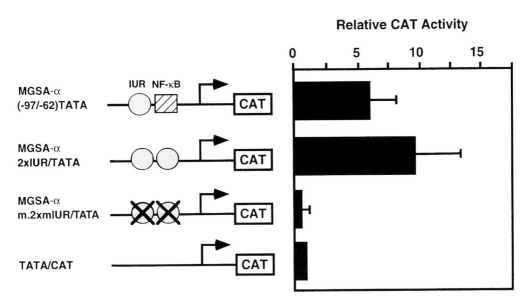

Fig. 5. Basal promoter activity through MGSA/GRO-α IUR. RPE cells were transfected with 10 μg of the indicated TATA/CAT construct. Transfection efficiencies were normalized by immunodetection of secreted growth hormone. At 48 h after transfection, whole-cell extracts were collected. Results are relative to CAT activity for parental TATA/CAT, to which a value of 1.0 was assigned. Values with standard deviation of error from duplicates of three separate experiments were TATA/CAT (1.0), MGSA-α –97/–62/TATA (6.25 ± 2.30), MGSA-α 2×IUR/TATA (9.40 ± 3.50), and mutant IUR MGSA-α 2xmIUR/TATA (0.50 ± 0.42). (Reprinted with permission from *J. Biol. Chem.* **270:** 10439–10448, 1995.)

the IUR contributes to MGSA/GRO-α basal promoter activity and that Rel A transactivates, we went on to characterize the IUR binding factor. Gel-shift analyses revealed the binding of protein(s) to an oligo composed of two copies of the sequence (2xIUR). Using a series of mutated 2xIUR oligonucleotides as competitors for the binding of the nuclear proteins to the IUR probe, we were able to determine that the nucleotides *TCGAT* formulate the binding region. Minimal promoter constructs containing a single copy of the IUR plus the NF-κB element MGSA/GRO-α(–97/–62) or two copies of the IUR, demonstrated that both constructs had a higher level of basal promoter activity as compared with the parental vector. Furthermore, point mutations in the IUR, which resulted in loss of the constitutively bound IUR complexes, effectively eliminated all basal promoter activity (Fig. 5). These data indicated that the IUR-bound complexes significantly contributed to MGSA/GRO-α basal promoter activity *(65)*.

When NF-κB p65 was overexpressed in cells cotransfected with this 2xIUR minimal promoter construct, basal CAT activity was much stronger, suggesting that NF-κB proteins interact with a protein binding to this site and enhance basal transcription. Ultraviolet (UV)-crosslinking experiments demonstrated that two proteins bound to this element but not to the mutant IUR *(65)*. We have recently demonstrated by Southwestern blot and gel-shift analysis of partially purified preparations of the IUR binding protein (IUR-F) that the major protein that binds the *TCGAT* sequence is approx 115 kDa (Fig. 6). The IUR sequence motif is also present in the 5′ regulatory region of

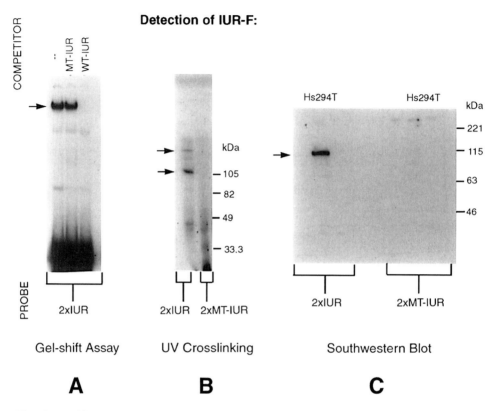

Fig. 6. Specificity and size of the IUR binding proteins. **(A)** Gel-shift assays: Hs294T nuclear extracts were analyzed by gel-shift assay using ^{32}P labeled 2xIUR as a probe. Competitions with mutant IUR (MT-IUR) oligonucleotides (which do not bind the factor) or wild-type IUR (WT-IUR) (which do bind the factor) reveal an IUR-specific activity in these extracts. **(B)** UV-crosslinking: Hs294T nuclear extracts were probed with 2xIUR or 2xMT-IUR and DNA-protein complexes were crosslinked by UV, digested with DNaseI and resolved by sodium dodecyl sulfate-polyacrylamide gel electrophoresis (SDS-PAGE). Note that ~100 kDa of protein crosslinked with 2xIUR but not the 2xMT-IUR. The fainter complexes >100 and ~57 kDa probably represent poorly digested protein-DNA complexes. The DNA has a mobility of ~20 kDa. **(C)** Southwestern blot analysis: Hs294T nuclear extracts and prestained molecular size markers were resolved by SDS-PAGE, transblotted under renaturing conditions to nitrocellulose filters, and probed with either 2xIUR or 2xMT-IUR. An ~100-kDa protein is detected by the 2xIUR but not the 2xMT-IUR probe. (Reprinted with permission from *J. Leuk. Biol.* **62:** 588–597, 1997.)

CXCR2 and a number of cytokine genes, suggesting that this motif may participate in the coordinate regulation of cytokines during the inflammatory response.

2.8. Sequence Analysis of the MGSA/GRO-α Promoter Revealed Binding/Transactivating Capacity of Sp1 and HMGI(Y) Proteins to the MGSA/GRO-α Promoter

Two other regulatory regions within the MGSA/GRO-α350/CAT are the Sp1 and HMGI(Y) elements. MGSA/GRO-α, -β, and -γ have Sp1 elements within 1000 bp; MGSA/GRO-α has an additional Sp1 element. Mutation of this Sp1 element reduces basal- but not cytokine-induced transactivation of MGSA/GRO in both Hs294T and RPE cells *(64)*. Recent gel-shift data demonstrate clearly that Sp1 and Sp3 proteins are present in the nuclear extracts of both RPE and Hs294T cells. We have been able to demonstrate that for the RPE cells, phosphoserine antibodies will also eliminate the shift, suggesting that the Sp1/Sp3 proteins in the extract are indeed phosphorylated on serine, a requirement for the transactivating capacity of Sp1 *(18–20)*.

There is a perfect HMGI(Y) consensus within the NF-κB element for the MGSA/GRO-α, -β, and -γ genes. By gel-shift assay we demonstrate the binding of a poorly retarded complex that is competed with the wild-type oligonucleotide but not by oligonucleotide mutated in the AT-rich region nested within the GC-rich region of the NF-κB element. Antibody to HMGI(Y) eliminates this retarded complex, suggesting that this protein may bind the NF-κB element and stabilize any TATA binding protein complexes that form, thus facilitating transactivation. Mutation of the AT-rich region of the NF-κB element within the context of the MGSA/GRO-α350/CAT reporter gene results in a marked reduction of basal transcription along with a reduction in cytokine-enhanced transactivation. Thus, loss of either NF-κB or HMGI(Y) complex binding by selected point mutations in the NF-κB element results in decreased basal- and cytokine-induced MGSA/GRO-α promoter activity. Therefore, these results indicate that transcriptional regulation of this chemokine requires at least three transcription factors—Sp1, NF-κB, and HMG(I)Y—*(50,64,65)* in addition to the IUR-F *(66)* and thus might constitute an enhanceosome similar to that described for the regulation of interferon-β *(11,60)*. Since the major difference in these promoters/enhancers were noted in the NF-κB activity between Hs294T and RPE cells by gel-shift assay and CAT assay, this element in combination with the IUR is hypothesized to be regulating the high constitutive expression in Hs294T melanoma cells.

3. HOW DOES DEREGULATION OF C-X-C CHEMOKINES INFLUENCE MELANOMA TUMOR PROGRESSION?

In addition to the effects of C-X-C chemokines on leukocyte chemotaxis, the C-X-C chemokines MGSA/GRO-α and IL-8 are reported to enhance the growth of normal melanocytes, nevocytes, and melanoma cells *(4,5,7,15,44a)*. The expression of MGSA/GRO or IL-8 in immortalized melanocytes is also associated with an enhanced ability to form colonies in soft agar and tumors in nude mice *(5,16,47,48)*. IL-8 expression has also been correlated with an enhanced metastatic capacity for melanoma tumors *(52)*. Antibodies to MGSA/GRO-α, IL-8, or CXCR2 can block this autocrine loop, slow the growth of the cells in vitro, and reduce formation of colonies in soft agar *(24,37,48)*. Thus, the deregulation of expression of these chemokines can have important effects on melanocyte tumor progression.

An essential component of the autocrine loop for C-X-C chemokines in melanoma is the expression of receptors for MGSA/GRO proteins in melanocytes and malignant melanoma cells. Moser et al. *(54)* examined the expression of C-X-C chemokine receptors in melanoma cells and demonstrated that melanoma cells express CXCR1 and CXCR2 mRNA in 2 melanocyte and 19 melanoma cell lines tested *(29)*. We have shown that the mRNAs for the CXCR1 and CXCR2, as well as variant forms of CXCR2, are present in cultured Hs294T melanoma cells *(30)* and (Richmond, unpublished). Metzner et al. *(56)* have shown that MGSA/GRO-α mobilizes calcium in

Hs294T cells and, thus, confirmed the expression of biologically active MGSA/GRO receptors in these melanoma cells *(28)*. We have demonstrated that antibodies to MGSA/GRO-α *(24)* and its receptor (Richmond, unpublished) block >50% of the growth of the Hs294T cells. Using Fab fragments of a blocking CXCR2 antibody, Norgauer et al. *(37)* recently demonstrated that this receptor is expressed on five malignant melanoma cell lines at levels 1.3- to 7-fold greater than the Hs294T cells, indicating that the majority of melanomas have elevated MGSA receptor expression. The level of expression for normal melanocytes was only 50% of Hs294T and 15-fold less than for the A2058 melanoma line. Antibodies to this receptor blocked ~50% of the binding of iodinated MGSA/GRO-α to these cell lines. The secretion of MGSA/GRO-α over 24 h ranged from 784 to 2060 pg, as compared to 126 pg for melanocytes. Antibody (Fab fragment) to CXCR2 blocked the proliferative response of these cell lines to exogenous MGSA/GRO-α. The failure of the receptor antibody to block 100% of the binding of ligand is expected, based on the prior observation that melanoma cells also express a novel receptor for MGSA/GRO *(15,45)*.

Horuk et al. *(50)* as well as Roby and Page *(31)* have suggested that melanoma cells might make a novel receptor for MGSA/GRO proteins *(15,45)*. Such a novel receptor may be responsible for the growth response of melanoma cells to MGSA/GRO-α or IL-8, which is not inhibited by antibody to CXCR2. Although antibodies to both the MGSA/GRO-α ligand and receptor have been shown to block the growth of six different melanoma cell lines, owing to the redundancy of MGSA/GRO-α, -β, and -γ and the stability of the MGSA/GRO proteins, antisense experiments are not informative and do not reduce the levels of protein sufficiently to inhibit growth (Richmond, unpublished). Recently, Olbina et al. *(57)* have demonstrated that antisense oligonucleotides to CXCR2 will inhibit the growth of tumors from nonsmall-cell lung cancer *(38)*. An important experiment will involve the expression of antisense CXCR2 constructs in melanoma cells to determine whether this alters the growth and transformation properties of these cells.

C-X-C chemokines are haptotactic for melanoma cells in vitro, possibly contributing to the secondary localization of tumors at sites of inflammation *(61,62)*. Singh et al. *(52)* have recently shown that highly metastatic melanoma cell lines produce higher levels of IL-8 than melanoma cell lines with low metastatic potential, and that the addition of IL-8 to those melanoma cell lines with low metastatic potential stimulated the proliferation of those cells. UV irradiation of a culture established from a primary melanoma that did not express IL-8 and was neither tumorigenic nor metastatic in nude mice led to elevations in IL-8 mRNA. This coincided with the onset of tumor-forming capacity and metastasis in Balb/c nude mice *(52)*. It was postulated that IL-8 might act through autocrine and paracrine mechanisms to affect tumor growth and metastatic potential *(49,* for a review). However, unlike Singh et al. *(52)*, Schadendorf et al. *(24,51)* found no correlation between IL-8 expression and metastasis of melanoma tumors *(47,48)*.

4. EFFECTS OF C-X-C CHEMOKINES ON ENDOTHELIAL CELLS AND ANGIOGENESIS

MGSA/GRO proteins, like IL-8, are angiogenic both in the in vitro endothelial chemotaxis assay and in the in vitro corneal neovascularization assay *(55)*. MGSA/GRO-α is equivalent to IL-8, whereas MGSA/GRO-β is less angiogenic *(55,56)*. This angiogenic activity requires the presence of a conserved amino-terminal ELR motif *(56).* IP-10 and antibodies to MGSA/GRO-α will block a large percentage of the angiogenic response from squamous cell carcinoma *(55,56).* Shono et al. *(59)* have verified that IL-8 enhances tubular morphogenesis in microvascular endothelial cells and that antibody to IL-8 will block that response *(51).* By contrast, a recent study by Cas et al. *(60)* suggests that the MGSA/GRO-β protein inhibits angiogenesis when introduced at microgram concentrations *(9).* However, continuous exposure to microgram concentrations of chemokine might be expected to cause downregulation and desensitization of receptors for the chemokine *(31).* Culturing endothelial cells on the appropriate collagen matrix is required to preserve the expression of the MGSA/GRO receptor on these endothelial cells normally observed in vivo at sites of neovascularization *(26).* Postcapillary venule endothelial cells also express DARC *(12).* We have documented the expression of the MGSA/GRO receptor, CXCR2, on endothelial cells undergoing neovascularization in human burn wounds *(36).* We have also demonstrated that MGSA/GRO proteins produced by melanocytes expressing the MGSA/GRO-α, -β, and -γ transgenes are angiogenic and that antibodies specific for these MGSA/GRO proteins will block that angiogenic response *(40).* Thus, activation of the CXCR2 receptor by either MGSA/GRO, IL-8, or other C-X-C chemokines binding to this receptor is a major mode of tumor-induced angiogenesis to provide nutrients for the growing tumor body.

5. CONTINUOUS MGSA/GRO EXPRESSION CONTRIBUTES TO TUMOR FORMATION IN MELANOCYTES

5.1. Overexpression of MGSA/GRO Proteins in Immortalized Melanocytes Contributes to Transformation

Reports from a number of laboratories have shown that MGSA/GRO-α, -β, and -γ have similar neutrophil chemotactic activities, though there are differences in potencies. We demonstrated that overexpression of MGSA/GRO-α in the immortalized mouse melanocyte cell line, melan-a, enabled these cells to form an increased number of large colonies in soft agar and to form tumors in nude mice *(5).* The melanoma tumors from the mice injected with mel-a-6 clone of melan-a cells overexpressing the human MGSA/GRO-α transgene were poorly differentiated based on the loss of melanin production, reduced S-100 protein, and increased levels of the melanoma-specific antigen HMB-45 *(5).* To determine whether other forms of MGSA/GRO have similar properties, we expressed MGSA/GRO-β and -γ in immortalized melan-a cells and evaluated the in vitro growth and tumor-forming capacity of these cells. Stable melan-a clones expressing MGSA/GRO-β and stable melan-a clones expressing MGSA/GRO-γ exhibited enhanced ability to form large colonies in soft agar and tumors in nude mice (Tables 1 and 2). These tumors were highly pigmented and expressed immunoreactive MGSA/GRO-β and -γ protein. The histology resembled that of a melanoma. When culture medium concentrates from clonal melan-a cell lines expressing MGSA/GRO-α, -β, or -γ were examined for the potential to induce angiogenesis in the rat cornea, strong angiogenic responses were observed (Fig. 7). The angiogenic response was blocked by antibodies to the chemokine produced by the stably transfected melan-a cells, but not by normal rabbit serum (NRS). By contrast, angiogenic

Table 1
Colony Formation in Soft Agar[a]

Melan-a clone	Mean number of colonies (80–100 μM)	Mean total colonies
Parental melan-a	3	15
V_6	6	37
β2-13	17	55
β2-5	32	139
β2-19	1655	5369
γ1-37	3	35
γ3-12	67	235
γ3-14	68	342

[a] 1×10^5 cells from each clone were plated into 35-mm dishes in melanocyte growth medium supplemented with 20% fetal boviric serum, G-418 (except for parental melan-a cells), and TPA; made 0.4% in Noble agar; and overlaid over the same medium containing 0.5% agar. Cells were fed weekly with 1 mL of growth medium made 0.4% in agar. After 3 wk of growth, colonies were read on an automated colony counter. The data shown here are from one experiment representative of a series of four separate experiments. The mean of three separate cultures is reported for each experiment. (Reprinted with permission from *Int. J. Cancer* **73:** 94–103, 1997.)

responses were observed in only 2 of 12 implants (16%) from the culture medium of melan-a clones expressing the cytomegalovirus (CMV)-driven neomycin-resistance marker alone. These data demonstrate that tumor formation resulting from overexpression of the MGSA/GRO chemokine occurs through autocrine mechanisms by altering the capacity of the cells to exhibit anchorage-independent growth, and through paracrine mechanisms by enhancing the angiogenic response to the growing tumor (Haghnegahdar et al., submitted).

5.2. SCID Mouse Model for MGSA/GRO in Melanoma Tumorigenesis

The nude mouse model cannot be used for testing the effectiveness of rabbit antibodies to MGSA/GRO in blocking the growth of melan-a tumors since the mouse would develop antibodies to the rabbit antibody. Therefore, for these experiments, we turned to the SCID mouse, which is deficient in both T- and B-lymphocytes. We injected the melan-a cells expressing human MGSA/GRO-α, -β, and -γ into young female SCID mice. Mice from each group (expressing MGSA/GRO-α or MGSA/GRO-γ) were injected every other day with complement-inactivated blocking antibodies to these respective chemokines, or with complement-inactivated NRS. We compared the tumor appearance and growth rate in the group injected with antibodies to MGSA/GRO-α or -γ to that of the group injected with NRS. At the end of the experiment, the tumors that formed were subjected to CD-31 immunostaining to quantitate the number of vascular endothelial cells in the tumors to monitor the effects of blocking the chemokine on angiogenesis. Mice treated with the antibody to the MGSA/GRO-γ slowly developed very small tumors (2.5 mo) in only three of six mice, whereas those treated with NRS quickly developed very large tumors (1.6 mo) (10 times the tumor volume for the group receiving MIP-2 antibodies) in all six mice by 8 wk after the initial injection of melan-a cells expressing MGSA/GRO-γ. Only one tumor in the antibody-treated group was large enough for analysis of CD-31–positive cells. That tumor did not differ from the control in the percentage of CD-31–positive cells.

Table 2
Summary of Tumor-Forming Ability of Melan-a Clones

	Cell lines Tested	Number of tumors formed/ number of mice injected	Weeks after injection of tumor onset
MGSA/GRO-β-expressing melan-a clones	β2-19	9/9	3–4
	β2-5	9/9	3–4
	β2-13	9/9	3–4
MGSA/GRO-γ-expressing melan-a clones	γ3-14	7/9	3–4
	γ1-37	9/9	3–4
	γ3-12	9/9	3–4
MGSA/GRO-α-expressing melan-a clones	mel-a-6	6/6	3–4
	B16 Melanoma	6/6	1
	Hs294T	5/5	3–4
CMV/neovector alone expressing melan-a clones	Vector 1	0/15	0
	Vector 4	0/6	0
	Vector 6	2/6	>12

[a] Melan-a clones expressing MGSA-α, -β, -γ were subcutaneously injected into 6- to 8-wk-old female athymic *nu/nu* Harlan Sprague-Dawley mice and monitored for tumor formation over a period of 9 mo. The number of mice injected and those that developed tumors are shown. (Reprinted with permission from *Int. J. Cancer* **73:** 94–103, 1997.)

The mel-a-6 cells expressing the human MGSA/GRO-α transgene made tumors in five of six mice injected with antibody to MGSA/GRO-α, whereas tumors arose in all six of the mice injected with the same cells and treated with NRS. Although the tumors appeared in the mice injected with antibody to MGSA/GRO-α first, the tumors that arose in the group injected with NRS grew faster and to a twofold larger volume than those injected with the blocking antibody to MGSA/GRO-α. It is not yet clear why the antibody to MGSA/GRO-α was not as effective at slowing tumor formation/growth as the antibody to MGSA/GRO-γ. Both antibodies were able to block the angiogenic response to these chemokines in the rat cornea micropocket assay. These differences could be due to clonal differences in the melan-a cells expressing MGSA/GRO-α as compared to MGSA/GRO-γ. Malignant melanoma cells produce and are regulated by a variety of factors, some of which could be differentially expressed in the melan-a clones studied here *(21)*. By contrast, melan-a cells expressing the neomycin resistance vector alone (V-6) did not form tumors in the SCID mice (no tumors in 12 mice injected).

6. CONCLUSION

In conclusion, continuous MGSA/GRO expression in immortalized melanocytes results in tumor formation both through autocrine effects on the melanocytes and

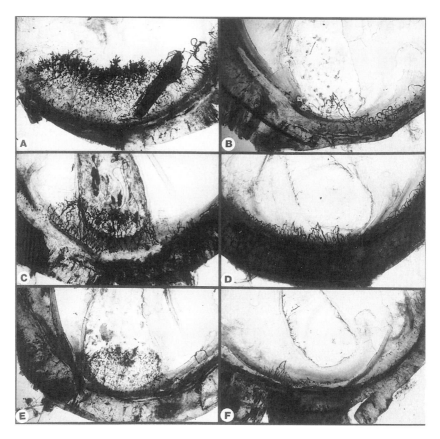

Fig. 7. Angiogenesis in response to culture medium concentrates from MGSA/GRO-α, -β, -γ transgene-expressing clones. The conditioned medium from confluent cultures of transgene-expressing melan-a cultures were collected, concentrated, and processed. Equal amounts of protein were combined with sterile Hydron casting solution, implanted into rat cornea, and harvested 6 d later. **(A)** Angiogenic response to Hydron pellet implants containing concentrated conditioned medium from melan-a cultures β2-19, γ3-14, mel-a-6, and V-1. **(B)** Angiogenic response to Hydron implants in the presence of blocking antibodies to MGSA/GRO-α, -β, -γ. A and B represent angiogenic responses to Hydron pellets prepared from conditioned medium from Mel-a-6 cells expressing MGSA/GRO-α and NRS (A) or anti-MGSA/GRO-α (B). **(C, D)** Angiogenic responses to Hydron pellets containing conditioned medium from β2-19 cells expressing MGSA/GRO-β and NRS (C) or anti-MGSA/GRO-β. **(E,F)** Angiogenic responses to Hydron pellets containing conditioned medium from γ3-14 cells expressing MGSA/GRO-γ and NRS (E) or anti-GRO-γ (F). (Reprinted with permission from *Int. J. Cancer* **73:** 94–103, 1997.)

through paracrine interactions with endothelial cells to stimulate angiogenesis in response to the growing tumor. Thus, the deregulation of expression of C-X-C chemokines such as MGSA/GRO has very important biologic consequences for the melanocyte that can lead to tumor progression and enhanced growth of tumors. The development of CXCR2 antagonists, which are readily soluble and have a half-life sufficiently long to block appropriately MGSA/GRO or IL-8 stimulation of melanocyte tumor progression, could provide a very effective mechanism for therapeutic intervention of these deadly tumors.

ACKNOWLEDGMENTS

This work was funded by a Merit Review Award and Associate Career Scientist Award from the Department of Veteran's Affairs (AR), and grants from the NCI-CA34560 and CA56704 (AR). The authors are indebted to Repligen Corporation for providing recombinant MGSA, to Stephen Haskill for antibodies to MGSA/GRO-γ, to Angelika Bodenteich and Joerg Berg of Topcro Pharma Research GmbH for antibody to MGSA/GRO-β, and to Lillian Nanney and the Skin Disease Research Center (AR41943) for assistance in the immunohistology.

REFERENCES

1. Aarvanitakis, L., E. Geras-Raaka, A. Varma, M. D. Gershengorn, and E. Cesarman. 1997. Human herpesvirus KSHV encodes a constitutively active G-protein-coupled receptor linked to cell proliferation. *Nature* **385**: 347–350.
2. Anisowicz, A., L. Bardwell, and R. Sager. 1987. Constitutive overexpression of a growth-regulated gene in transformed Chinese hamster and human cells. *Proc. Natl. Acad. Sci. USA* **84**: 7188–7192.
3. Baggiolini, M., B. Dewald, and B. Moser. 1994. Interleukin-8 and related chemotactic cytokines—CXC and CC chemokines. *Adv. Immunol.* **55**: 97–179.
4. Balentien, E., J. H. Han, H. G. Thomas, D. Wen, A. K. Samantha, C. O. Zachariae, P. R. Griffin, R. Brachmann, W. L. Wong, K. Matsushima, et al. 1990. Recombinant expression, biochemical characterization, and biological activities of the human MGSA/gro protein. *Biochemistry* **29**: 10,225–10,233.
5. Balentien, E., B. E. Mufson, R. L. Shattuck, R. Derynck, and A. Richmond. 1991. Effects of MGSA/GRO alpha on melanocyte transformation. Oncogene **6**: 1115–1124.
6. Bedard, P., D. Alcorta, D. L. Simmons, K. Luk, and R. L. Erikson. 1987. Constitutive expression of a gene encoding a polypeptide homologous to biologically active human platelet protein in Rous sarcoma virus-transformed fibroblasts. *Proc. Natl. Acad. Sci. USA* **84**: 6715–6719.
7. Bordoni, R., R. Fine, D. Murray, and A. Richmond. 1990. Characterization of the role of melanoma growth stimulatory activity (MGSA) in the growth of normal melanocytes, nevocytes, and malignant melanocytes. *J. Cell. Biochem.* **44**: 207–219.
8. Bröcker, E. B., G. Zwadlo, B. Holzman, E. Macher, and C. Sorg. 1988. Inflammatory cell infiltrates in human melanoma at different stages of tumor progression. *Int. J. Cancer* **41**: 562–567.
9. Cao, Y. H., C. Chen, J. A. Weatherbee, M. Tsang, and J. Folkman. 1995. gro-Beta, Alpha-C-X-C- chemokine, is an angiogenesis inhibitor that suppresses the growth of Lewis lung carcinoma in mice. *J. Exp. Med.* **182**: 2069–2077.
10. Chenevix-Trench, G., N. G. Martin, and K. A. O. Ellem. 1990. Gene expression in melanoma cell lines and cultured melanocytes: correlation between levels of c-*src*-1, c-*myc* and p53. *Oncogene* **5**: 1187–1193.
11. Du, W., and T. Maniatis. 1994. The high mobility group protein HMG I(Y) can stimulate or inhibit DNA binding of distinct transcription factor ATF-2 isoforms. *Proc. Natl. Acad. Sci. USA* **91**: 11,318–11322.
12. Hadley, T. J., Z. H. Lu, K. Wasneowska, A. W. Martin, S. C. Peiper, J. Hesselgesser, and R. Horuk. 1994. Post capillary venule endothelial cells in kidney express a multispecific chemokine receptor that is structurally and functionally identical to the erythroid isoform, which is the Duffy blood group antigen. *J. Clin. Invest.* **94**: 985–991.
13. Haskill, S., A. Peace, J. Morris, S. A. Sporn, A. Anisowicz, S. W. Lee, T. Smith, G. Martin, P. Ralph, and R. Sager. 1990. Identification of three related human GRO genes encoding cytokine functions. *Proc. Natl. Acad. Sci. USA* **87**: 7732–7736.

14. Holmes, W. E., J. Lee, W. J. Kuang, G. Rice, and W. I. Wood. 1991. Structure and functional expression of a human interleukin-8 receptor. *Science* **253:** 1278–1280.

15. Horuk, R., D. G. Yansura, D. Reilly, S. Spencer, J. Bourell, W. Henzel, G. Rice, and E. Unemori. 1993. Purification, receptor binding analysis, and biological characterization of human melanoma growth stimulating activity (MGSA): evidence for a novel MGSA receptor. *J. Biol. Chem.* **268:** 541–546.

16. Horuk, R., T. J. Colby, W. C. Darbonne, T. J. Schall, and K. Neote. 1993. The human erythrocyte inflammatory peptide (chemokine) receptor: biochemical characterization, solubilization, and development of a binding assay for the soluble receptor. *Biochemistry* **32:** 5733–5738.

17. Iida, N., and G. R. Grotendorst. 1990. Cloning and sequencing of a new gro transcript from activated human monocytes: expression in leukocytes and wound tissue, *Mol. Cell Biol.* **10:** 5596–5599 (published erratum appears in *Mol. Cell. Biol.* 1990; **10(12):** 6821).

18. Jackson, S., T. Gottlieb, and K. Hartley. 1993. Phosphorylation of transcription factor Sp1 by the DNA-dependent protein kinase. *Adv. Sec. Mes. Phosphop. Res.* **28:** 279–286 (review).

19. Jackson, S. P. 1992. Regulating transcriptioon factor activity by phosphorylation. *Trends Cell Biol.* **2:** 104–108.

20. Jackson, S. P., J. J. MacDonald, S. Lees-Miller, and R. Tjian. 1993. GC box binding induces phosphorylation of Sp1 by DNA-dependent protein kinase. *Cell* **63:** 155–165.

21. Kerbel, R. S. 1993. Growth factors are mediators of malignant tumor progression. *Cancer Metastasis Rev.* **12:** 215–217.

22. Kunsch, C., R. K. Lang, C. A. Rosen, and M. F. Shannon. 1994. Synergistic transcriptional activation of the IL-8 gene by NF-kappaB p65 (RelA) and NF-IL-6. *J. Immunol.* **153:** 153–164.

23. Kunsch, C., and C. A. Rosen. 1993. NF-kappaB subunit-specific regulation of the interleukin-8 promoter. *Mol. Cell. Biol.* **13:** 6137–6146.

24. Lawson, D. H., H. G. Thomas, R. G. Roy, D. S. Gordon, R. K. Chawla, D. W. Nixon, and A. Richmond. 1987. Preparation of a monoclonal antibody to a melanoma growth-stimulatory activity released into serum-free culture medium by Hs0294 malignant melanoma cells. *J. Cell. Biochem.* **34:** 169–185.

25. LeClair, K. P., M. A. Blanar, and P. A. Sharp. 1992. The p50 subunit of NF-kappaB associates with the NF-IL6 transcription factor. *Proc. Natl. Acad. Sci. USA* **89:** 8145–8149.

26. Lusti-Narasimhan, M., A. Chollet, C. A. Power, B. Allet, A. E. I. Proudfoot, and T. N. C. Wells. 1996. A molecular switch of chemokine receptor selectivity. *J. Biol. Chem.* **271:** 3148–3153.

27. Mattei, S., M. P. Colombo, C. Melani, A. Silvani, G. Parmiani, and M. Herlyn. 1994. Expression of cytokine/growth factors and their receptors in human melanoma and melanocytes. *Int. J. Cancer* **56:** 853–857.

28. Metzner, B., F. Parlow, R. Kownatzki, O. Spleiss, F. McConnel, I. Schraufstatter, and J. Norgauer. 1994. Identification of the GRO-alpha involved signal pathway components in Hs294T melanoma cells. *J. Invest. Dermatol.* **102:** 553–A177.

29. Moser, B., L. Barella, S. Mattei, C. Schumacher, F. Boulay, M. P. Colombo, and M. Baggiolini. 1993. Expression of transcripts for two interleukin 8 receptors in human phagocytes, lymphocytes and melanoma cells. *Biochem. J.* **294:** 285–292.

30. Mueller, S. G., W. P. Schraw, and A. Richmond. 1994. Melanoma growth stimulatory activity enhances the phosphorylation of the class II interleukin-8 receptor in non-hematopoietic cells. *J. Biol. Chem.* **269:** 1973–1980.

31. Mueller, S. G., J. R. White, W. P. Schraw, V. Lam, and A. Richmond. 1997. Ligand induced desensitization of CXCR2 requires multiple serine residues. *J. Biol. Chem.* **272:** 8207–8214.

32. Mukaida, N., Y. Mahe, and K. Matsushima. 1990. Cooperative interaction of nuclear factor-kb- and cis-regulatory enhancer binding protein-like factor binding elements in activating the interleukin-8 gene by pro-inflammatory cytokines. *J. Biol. Chem.* **265:** 21,128–21,133.

33. Mukaida, N., M. Morita, Y. Ishikawa, N. Rice, S. Okamoto, T. Kasahara, and K. Matsushima. 1994. Novel mechanism of glucocorticoid-mediated gene repression: nuclear factor-kappa B is target for glucocorticoid-mediated interleukin 8 gene repression. *J. Biol. Chem.* **269:** 13,289–13,295.

34. Murphy, P. M. 1997. Pirated genes in Kaposi's sarcoma. *Nature* **385:** 296, 297.

35. Murphy, P. M., and H. L. Tiffany. 1991. Cloning of complementary DNA encoding a functional human interleukin-8 receptor. *Science* **253:** 1280–1283.

36. Nanney, L. B., S. G. Muller, R. Bueno, S. C. Peiper, and A. Richmond. 1995. Distributions of melanoma growth stimulatory activity or growth-regulated gene and the interleukin-8 receptor B in human wound repair. *Am. J. Pathol.* **147:** 1248–1260.

37. Norgauer, J., B. Metzner, and I. Schraufstatter. 1996. Expression and growth-promoting function of the IL-8 receptor beta in human melanoma cells. *J. Immunol.* **156:** 1132–1137.

38. Olbina, G., D. Cieslak, S. Ruzdijic, C. Esler, Z. An, X. Wang, R. Hoffman, W. Seifert, and Z. Pietrzkowski. 1996. Reversible inhibition of IL-8 receptor B mRNA expression and proliferation in non-small cell lung cancer by antisense oligonucleotides. *Anticancer Res.* **16:** 3525–3530.

39. Oquendo, P., J. Alberta, D. Z. Wen, J. L. Graycar, R. Derynck, and C. D. Stiles. 1989. The platelet-derived growth factor-inducible KC gene encodes a secretory protein related to platelet alpha-granule proteins. *J. Biol. Chem.* **264:** 4133–4137.

40. Owen, J. D., R. Strieter, M. Burdick, H. Haghnegahdar, L. Nanney, R. Shattuck-Brandt, and A. Richmond. 1997. Enhanced tumor-forming capacity for immortalized melanocytes expressing melanoma growth stimulatory activity/growth-regulated cytokine β and γ proteins. *Int. J. Cancer* **73:** 94–103.

40. Priest, J. H., C. N. Phillips, Y. Wang, and A. Richmond. 1988. Chromosome and growth factor abnormalities in melanoma. *Cancer Genet. Cytogenet.* **35:** 253–262.

41. Rajarathnam, K., C. M. Kay, B. Dewald, M. Wolf, M. Baggiolini, I. Clark-Lewis, and B. D. Sykes. 1997. Neutrophil-activating peptide-2 and melanoma growth-stimulatory activity are functional as monomers for neutrophil activation. *J. Biol. Chem.* **272:** 1725–1729.

42. Richmond, A., E. Balentien, H. G. Thomas, G. Flaggs, D. E. Barton, J. Spiess, R. Bordoni, U. Francke, and R. Derynck. 1988. Molecular characterization of melanoma growth stimulatory activity, a growth factor structurally related to β-thromboglobulin. *EMBO J.* **7:** 2025–2033.

43. Richmond, A., R. Fine, D. Murray, D. H. Lawson, and J. Priest. 1986. Growth factor and cytogenetic abnormalities in nevus and malignant melanoma cells. *J. Invest. Dermatol.* **86:** 295–302.

44. Richmond, A., and R. L. Shattuck. 1996, in Melanoma growth stimulatory activity: physiology, biology, structure/function, and role in disease, *Chemoattractant Ligands and Their Receptors*. CRC Press, Boca Raton, FL. pp. 87–124.

44a. Richmond, A., and H. G. Thomas. 1988. Melanoma growth stimulatory activity: isolation from human melanoma tumors and characterization of tissue distribution. *J. Cell. Biochem.* **36:** 185–198.

45. Roby, P., and M. Page. 1995. Cell-binding and growth-stimulating activities of the C-terminal part of human MGSA/Gro alpha. *Biochem. Biophys. Res. Commun.* **206:** 792–798.

46. Rodeck, U., K. Melber, R. Kath, H.-D. Menssen, M. Varello, B. Atkinson, and M. Herlyn. 1991. Constitutive expression of multiple growth factor genes by melanoma cells but not normal melanocytes. *J. Invest. Dermatol.* **97:** 20–26.

47. Schadendorf, D., I. Fichtner, A. Makki, S. Alijagic, M. Kupper, U. Mrowietz, and B. M. Henz. 1996. Metastatic potential of human melanoma cells in nude mice—characterization of phenotype, cytokine secretion and tumor-associated antigens. *Br. J. Cancer* **74:** 194–199.

48. Schadendorf, D., A. Moller, B. Algermissen, M. Worm, M. Sticherling, and B. M. Czarnetzki. 1993. IL-8 produced by human malignant melanoma cells in vitro is an essential autocrine growth factor. *J. Immunol.* **151:** 2667–2675 (published erratum appears in *J. Immunol.* 1994; **153(7):** 3360).

49. Shattuck, R., and A. Richmond. 1997. Melanoma growth stimulatory activity (MGSA/GRO). Human Cytokines III, in press.

50. Shattuck, R. L., L. D. Wood, G. J. Jaffe, and A. Richmond. 1994. MGSA/GRO transcription is differentially regulated in normal retinal pigment epithelial and melanoma cells. *Mol. Cell. Biol.* **14:** 791–802 (publ. erratum in *Mol. Cell. Biol.* **15:** 1136, 1995).

51. Shono, T., M. Ono, H. Izumi, S.-I. Jimi, K. Matsushima, T. Okamoto, K. Kohno, and M. Kuwano. 1996. M. Involvement of the transcription factor NF-kappaB in tubular morphogenesis of human microvascular endothelial cells by oxidative stress. *Mol. Cell. Biol.* **16:** 4231–4239.

52. Singh, R. K., M. Gutman, R. Radinsky, C. D. Bucana, and L. J. Fidler. 1994. Expression of interleukin 8 correlates with the metastatic potential of human melanoma cells in nude mice. *Cancer Res.* **54:** 3242–3247.

53. Stein, B., and A. S. Baldwin, Jr. 1993. Distinct mechanisms for regulation of the interleukin-8 gene involve synergism and cooperativity between C/EBP and NF-kappaB. *Mol. Cell. Biol.* **13:** 7191–7198.

54. Stein, B., P. C. Cogswell, and A. S. Baldwin, Jr. 1993. Functional and physical associations between NF-kappa B and C/EBP family members: a Rel domain-bZIP interaction. *Mol. Cell. Biol.* **13:** 3964–3974.

55. Strieter, R. M., P. J. Polverini, D. A. Arenberg, A. Walz, G. Opdenakker, J. Van Damme, and S. L. Kunkel. 1995. Role of C-X-C chemokines as regulators of angiogenesis in lung cancer. *J. Leuk. Biol.* **57:** 752–762.

56. Strieter, R. M., P. J. Polverini, S. L. Kunkel, D. A. Arenberg, M. D. Burdick, J. Kasper, J. Dzuiba, J. Van Damme, J. Walz A, Marriott D, et al. 1995. The functional role of the ELR motif in CXC chemokine-mediated angiogenesis. *J. Biol. Chem.* **270:** 27,348–27,357.

57. Szabo, M. C., K. S. Soo, A. Zlotnik, and T. J. Schall. 1995. Chemokine class differences in binding to the Duffy antigen-erythrocyte chemokine receptor. *J. Biol. Chem.* **270:** 25348–25351.

58. Tekamp-Olson, P., C. Gallegos, D. Bauer, J. McClain, B. Sherry, M. Fabre, S. van Deventer, and A. Cerami. 1990. Cloning and characterization of cDNAs for murine macrophage inflammatory protein 2 and its human homologues. *J. Exp. Med.* **172:** 911–919.

59. Tettlebach, W., L. Nanney, D. Ellis, L. E. King, and A. Richmond. 1993. Localization of MGSA/GRO protein in cutaneous lesions. *J. Cutan. Pathol.* **20:** 259–266.

60. Thanos, D., and T. Maniatis. 1995. Identification of the rel family members required for virus induction of the human beta interferon gene. *Mol. Cell. Biol.* **15:** 152–164.

61. Tschen, J. A., D. Bhasin Fordice, M. Reddick, and J. Stehlin. 1992. Amelanotic melanoma presenting as inflammatory plaques. *J. Am. Acad. Dermatol.* **27:** 464–465.

62. Wang, J. M., G. Taraboletti, K. Matsushima, J. Van Damme, and A. Mantovani. 1990. Induction of haptotactic migration of melanoma cells by neutrophil activating protein/Interleukin-8. *Biochem. Biophys. Res. Commun.* **169:** 165–170.

63. Widmer, U., K. R. Manogue, A. Cerami, and B. Sherry. 1993. Genomic cloning and promoter analysis of macrophage inflammatory protein (MIP)-2, MIP-1α, and MIP-1β, members of the chemokine superfamily of proinflammatory cytokines. *J. Immunol.* **150:** 4996–5012.

64. Wood, L. D., A. A. Farmer, and A. Richmond. 1995. HMGI(Y) and Sp1 in addition to NF-kappa B regulate transcription of the MGSA/GRO alpha gene. *Nucleic Acids Res.* **23:** 4210–4219.
65. Wood, L. D., and A. Richmond. 1995. Constitutive and cytokine-induced expression of the melanoma growth stimulatory activity/GROalpha gene requires both NF-κB and novel constitutive factors. *J. Biol. Chem.* **270:** 30619–30626.
66. Luan, J., R. L. Shattuck-Brandt, H. Haghnegahdar, J. D. Owen, R. Strieter, M. Burdick, C. S. Nirod, D. Beauchamp, K. N. Johnson, and A. Richmond. 1997. Mechanism and biological significance of constitutive expression of the MGSA/GRO chemokines in malignant melanoma tumor progression. *J. Leuk. Biol.* **62:** 588–597.

V
Chemokines and Specific Malignancies

11

Chemokines and Gynecologic Malignancies

Rupert P. M. Negus and Frances R. Balkwill

1. INTRODUCTION

Gynecologic malignancies consist of tumors of the ovary, cervix, and uterus. Little is known of the role of chemokines in carcinoma of the cervix or endometrium, although they are expressed in conditions such as endometriosis *(1)*. This chapter reviews the expression of chemokines in carcinoma of the ovary in the context of the leukocyte infiltrate associated with this tumor. Most work to date concerns monocyte chemoattractant protein-1 (MCP-1). The expression of this chemokine is considered in more detail, and some of the mechanisms by which its production may be regulated in vivo are discussed.

2. OVARIAN CANCER

The incidence of ovarian cancer is approx 5000 cases annually in the United Kingdom and 26,600 annually in the United States *(2)*. Of these patients, more than 60% will be expected to die of their disease within 5 yr. The highest incidence of cancers of the ovary occurs in the white population in western and northern Europe and North America *(3,4)*. Compared with other malignancies, ovarian cancers account for a disproportionate number of deaths. This is owing to the fact that these tumors tend to spread silently throughout the peritoneal cavity often presenting as stage III or IV disease, although, matched stage for stage, the 5-yr survival rate from all ovarian tumors is comparable to that for breast, colorectal, and cervical carcinomas. At present, stage I ovarian cancers are diagnosed only in about 20% of cases as compared with more than 50% of breast cancers *(5)*. It is this skew toward late presentation, rather than marked differences in mortality at any given stage, that results in the high death rate associated with ovarian cancer.

Ninety percent of ovarian cancers are of epithelial origin. The malignant cells probably have a clonal origin *(6)*, and are thought to arise either directly from the surface epithelium of the ovary or from inclusion cysts *(7)*. Ovulation appears to be a major risk factor for ovarian cancer, since pregnancy *(8)*, the contraceptive pill *(9)*, and breast feeding *(10)* are all associated with a decreased relative risk of developing the disease, although there is evidence that ovarian hyperstimulation may increase the risk *(11)*. A great deal needs to be learned about the natural history of the various forms of this

From: *Chemokines and Cancer*
Edited by: B. J. Rollins © Humana Press Inc., Totowa, NJ

disease. Our work has focused on epithelial ovarian malignancies and the potential role played by a variety of chemokines in promoting the infiltration of leukocytes.

3. THE NATURE OF THE LEUKOCYTE INFILTRATE IN HUMAN OVARIAN CANCER

3.1. Introduction

The presence of lymphocytes and "round" cells in human tumors has long been recognized (reviewed in ref. *12*). In the late 1970s, several carcinomas were noted to contain mainly lymphocytes and macrophages *(13,14)*, often with a predominance of macrophages. Alpha-napthyl esterase–positive macrophages localized to necrotic areas in addition to being found within and around the tumor parenchyma. Other cell types, particularly granulocytes, have not been found so consistently. More recent studies have used immunohistochemistry with specific monoclonal antibodies to deduce the phenotype of infiltrating cells. CD3[+], CD45RO[+], and CD68[+] populations were all found in a series of 75 formalin-fixed, paraffin-embedded thyroid carcinomas *(15)*, with CD3[+] T-cells and macrophages occurring in comparable numbers. In colonic carcinomas, the infiltrate consisted of macrophages and CD4[+] α:β T-cells. CD8[+] T-cells were also abundant, particularly in close association with tumor cells *(16)*. In carcinoma of the breast, high numbers of CD45RO[+] T-cells, CD68[+] macrophages, and B-cells have been found *(17)*. Lwin et al. *(18)* obtained similar results for carcinomas of the breast. In the tumor stroma, there were roughly equal numbers of suppressor/cytotoxic T-cells, macrophages, and plasma cells, but within the tumor epithelium, the infiltrating population consisted largely of suppressor/cytotoxic T-lymphocytes with a smaller number of macrophages. CD8[+] cells also predominated in hepatocellular carcinomas *(19)*.

3.2. Infiltrating Cells in Ovarian Cancer

Several studies have specifically addressed the nature of the leukocyte infiltrate in ovarian cancer. Haskill et al. *(20)* used sedimentation-velocity to separate the components of the inflammatory infiltrate in 38 ovarian carcinomas. They concluded that T-cells and macrophages were the dominant components and that very few B-cells and natural killer (NK) cells were present. However, Kabawat et al. *(21)*, in an immunohistochemical analysis of cryostat sections from 70 tumors, concluded that the majority of the infiltrate consisted of CD4[+] T-cells with very few macrophages. Again they found few B-cells and NK cells. In frozen sections, CD4[+] cells again made up the majority of the T-cell infiltrate *(22)*. However, CD4[+] T-cells are difficult to assess owing to the expression of CD4 by other mononuclear cells *(23)*. In a study of dysgerminoma of the ovary using paraffin-embedded sections, Dietl et al. *(24)* concluded that infiltrating lymphocytes were predominantly CD8[+]. Fluorescence-activated-cell-sorter (FACS) analysis has been utilized to assess the infiltrate in disaggregated whole tumors and ascites *(25,26)*. It is reasonable to conclude that T-cells form the majority of the infiltrate whereas B-cells and NK cells account for <5% of the infiltrating cell population.

We used an immunohistochemical approach to examine the phenotypes of infiltrating cells in sections from 20 paraffin-embedded ovarian carcinomas *(27)*. The infiltrate was primarily composed of CD68[+] macrophages and CD3[+] T-cells (median values 3700 cells/mm^3 and 2200 cells/mm^3, respectively) (Fig. 1). There was a significant correlation between the CD3[+] counts and counts performed on sections stained with markers

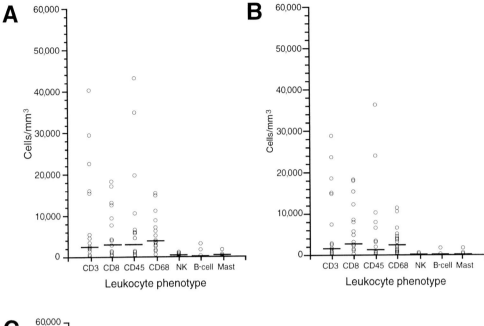

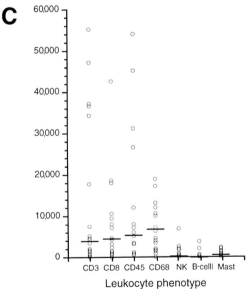

Fig. 1. Scatter plots of the calculated numbers of infiltrating leukocytes. Graphs of results in whole tumor (**A**), tumor parenchyma (**B**), and stroma (**C**). Cell numbers are expressed as (cells/mm^3) for each of the seven phenotypic markers. Horizontal bars represent median values. For each tumor compartment, there was a significant difference ($p < 0.0005$, Wilcoxon's matched pairs signed rank test) between the number of cells positive for CD3, CD8, CD45RO, and CD68 and those positive for NK cell, B-cell, and mast cell markers.

for CD8 and CD45RO ($r_s > 0.7$ and $p < 0.005$, Spearman's rank correlation), suggesting that the majority of infiltrating T-cells have a cytotoxic memory phenotype. NK cells, B-cells, and mast cells occurred in lower numbers (median values 0–200 cells/mm^3). Eosinophils were rarely seen and neutrophils were mainly confined to the

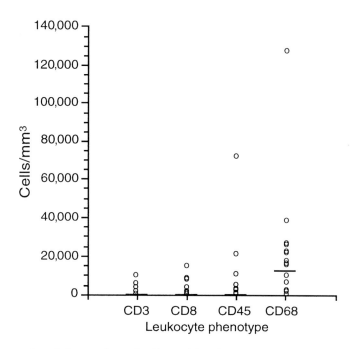

Fig. 2. Scatter plot of the number of cells positive for the T-cell phenotypic markers CD3, CD8, and CD45RO and the number positive for CD68, in regions of necrosis. Macrophages in these areas occurred at significantly higher density than any other cell type ($p < 0.0005$, Wilcoxon's matched pairs signed rank test). The horizontal bars represent median values.

lumina of blood vessels. In general, the infiltrating cell density was significantly higher in the stroma than the tumor parenchyma. For instance, the median value for the number of $CD3^+$ T-cells found within the stroma was 3800 cells/mm^3 compared with 1600 cells/mm^3 in the tumor parenchyma ($p < 0.005$, Wilcoxon's matched pairs signed rank test). Median values for $CD68^+$ macrophages were 6700 cells/mm^3 and 2100 cells/mm^3 in stroma and parenchyma, respectively ($p < 0.05$). The most striking differences in cell density were seen in regions of necrosis. Here, a significantly greater number of macrophages were observed than any other cell type (median 12,700 cells/mm^3, range 0–128,000 cells/mm^3; $p < 0.0005$, for all comparisons) (Fig. 2). The composition of the cellular infiltrate strongly favored a role for C-C chemokines.

3.3. The Role of the Host Infiltrate in Ovarian Cancer

Whether the infiltrating cell population represents a specific antitumor immune response or is simply the result of aberrant activation of innate response mechanisms remains disputed. The existence of a lymphocyte infiltrate has attracted attention because of the potential of these cells to destroy tumor cells. T-cells activated in vitro will kill autologous tumor cells, particularly when stimulated with cytokines such as interleukin-2 (IL-2) and interferon-γ. This approach has been used in clinical trials of therapy for advanced ovarian cancers with modest success. For instance, therapy with autologous T-cells activated with IL-2 resulted in complete surgical and histologic responses in 3 of 19 patients with stage III and IV disease, which lasted up to 26 mo *(28)*. Cytotoxic T-cells from ovarian tumors can recognize the mucin (Muc-1) core peptide of polymorphic epithelial mucins that is expressed by a variety of epithelial cancers *(29)*. On the other hand, defective expression of the TCR ζ-chain has been found in T-cells and NK cells from patients with ovarian cancer *(30)*. This may, in part, explain the observation that isolated T-cells do not display tumoricidal activity when unstimulated *(13,31)*.

Other reasons for the observed lack of cytotoxic T-cells in solid tumors have been proposed. In breast carcinomas, expression of the mucin antigen DF3/MUC1 by tumor cells can induce apoptosis in activated T-cells *(32)*, and HepG2 hepatoblastoma cells expressing CD95L (FasL) mRNA were capable of killing CD95$^+$ Jurkat lymphocytes *(33)*. Another factor that may be important is the lack of costimulatory molecules that characterizes some tumors *(34)*. Finally, chemokines may inhibit the activation of T-cells *(35)*.

Like T-cells, macrophages freshly isolated from ovarian tumors are poor at killing tumor cell targets *(36,37)*. Similarly, this activity can be stimulated in vitro with cytokines such as IL-1 and tumor necrosis factor-α (TNF-α), or with lipopolysaccharide *(38)*. The function of tumor-associated macrophages (TAMs) remains disputed. Mantovani *(39)* tested the affect on tumor cell proliferation of TAMs isolated from a chemically induced murine sarcoma. He found that at low macrophage-to-tumor cell ratios (≤2:1), proliferation of tumor cells was consistently observed, although at high ratios (≤20:1), nonspecific cytotoxicity occurred. Neither of these ratios is inconsistent with the local concentrations of macrophages that we observed within the different tumor compartments. Macrophages are a rich source of cytokines and other growth factors. They are associated with TNF-α production in ovarian tumors *(40)*, and macrophages isolated from ovarian tumors can secrete IL-1 and IL-6 *(41)*. Furthermore, TNF-α can act as a growth factor for ovarian cancer cells *(42)* and may promote angiogenesis *(43)*, although this is likely to be an indirect effect *(44)*.

These findings indicate that although in the natural course of the disease, infiltrating host leukocytes may be irrelevant, or may actually help promote tumor growth and development, there is the potential to harness this population to destroy tumor cells.

4. CHEMOKINE EXPRESSION IN OVARIAN CANCER

4.1. Introduction

The presence of a predominantly mononuclear infiltrate in human ovarian cancers, together with the relative absence of granulocytes, suggested that C-C chemokines may play an important role in determining the leukocyte infiltrate. Furthermore, the presence of large numbers of macrophages and the earlier work by Mantovani *(39)* in establishing the presence of a tumor-derived chemotactic factor (TDCF) for monocytes in ovarian cancers indicated that MCP-1 was produced by these tumors. In the early 1980s, Bottazzi et al. *(45)* used chemotaxis assays to determine the chemotactic activity for monocytes of culture supernatants from both murine sarcomas and freshly disaggregated human ovarian carcinomas *(46)*. A significant correlation was found between the activity of the supernatants from cultured murine tumor cells and the percentage of TAMs within the tumors. In both human and murine tumors, the activity appeared to be a protein, since the ability to chemoattract macrophages was lost after treatment with heat or proteases. Fractionation of the chemotactic activity suggested a mol wt of approx 12 kDa. Other tumor cells derived from a melanoma, osteosarcoma, glioblastoma, fibrosarcoma, and rhabdomyosarcoma were also able to produce monocyte chemotactic activity *(47)*. In 1989, MCP-1 was purified from the glioma cell line U-105MG *(48),* which constitutively expresses high levels, and cloned from both this cell line *(49)* and stimulated myelomonocytic cell lines *(50)*. Shortly afterward, TDCF derived from experimental sarcomas was found to be the same as MCP-1 *(51)*.

4.2. C-C Chemokine Expression

Using *in situ* hybridization to mRNA, we examined expression of the chemokines MCP-1, macrophage inflammatory protein-1α (MIP-1α), MIP-1β, and RANTES in frozen sections of human ovarian carcinomas. The total number of cells expressing MCP-1 or MIP-1α was significantly greater than the number expressing MIP-1β or RANTES ($p < 0.005$, Wilcoxon's matched pairs signed rank test) (Fig. 3A). MCP-1 was expressed by more cells within tumor islands than any other chemokine ($p < 0.0005$, median value 72.5 cells/mm^2) (Fig. 3B), but there was no significant difference between the number of MCP-1-expressing cells in tumor and stroma ($p < 0.03$). No correlation was found between the number of MCP-1-expressing cells and tumor grade. Within the stroma the number of cells expressing MCP-1 and MIP-1α was similar (median values 21 cells/mm^2 and 26 cells/mm^2, respectively) (Fig. 3C). MIP-1α was also expressed by more stromal cells than MIP-1β or RANTES ($p < 0.0005$). MCP-1-expressing cells within the tumor islands frequently occurred in clusters, but within the stroma tended to occur alone. The mean percentage of tumor cells expressing MCP-1 within a cluster was 8.2% (±5.8%) *(52)*. In the stroma the median number of cells expressing MIP-1β and RANTES was 2/mm^2 and 7/mm^2, respectively. Cells positive for MCP-1 signal were also occasionally seen within gland spaces, associated with nuclei possessing morphology typical of that for macrophages. In 9 of 20 frozen sections processed for *in situ* hybridization for MCP-1, it was possible to distinguish regions of necrosis. However, none of these was associated with the expression of MCP-1. A significant correlation was found between the total number of CD8$^+$ T-cells and the number of cells expressing MCP-1 ($r_s = 0.63$, $p < 0.003$), and between the CD8$^+$ population and RANTES-expressing cells ($r_s = 0.6$, $p < 0.003$). A correlation was also found between CD68$^+$ macrophages and the number of cells expressing MCP-1 ($r_s = 0.50$, $p = 0.026$).

MCP-1 protein was detected by enzyme-linked immunosorbent assay in ascites from patients with ovarian cancer *(52)*. The mean level (4.28 ng/mL) was significantly higher than that in ascites from patients with cirrhosis (mean 0.76 ng/mL, $p < 0.00001$). Low but detectable levels were found in plasma from normal laboratory donors (mean 0.23 ng/mL), patients with benign gynecologic disease (mean 0.39 ng/mL), and patients with ovarian carcinoma (0.49 ng/mL); but in ovarian cancer patients, the ascites levels were significantly higher than plasma levels in any of these groups ($p < 0.00001$). In three patients, highly enriched TAMs and ovarian tumor cells were fractionated from ascites, and their capacity to release MCP-1 was assessed over 24 h. MCP-1 production was essentially confined to the ovarian carcinoma–enriched population. The tumor cell–enriched population produced 2.3, 40.9, and 47.2 ng/mL compared with 0.3, 0.2, and 0.1 ng/mL, respectively, produced by TAMs.

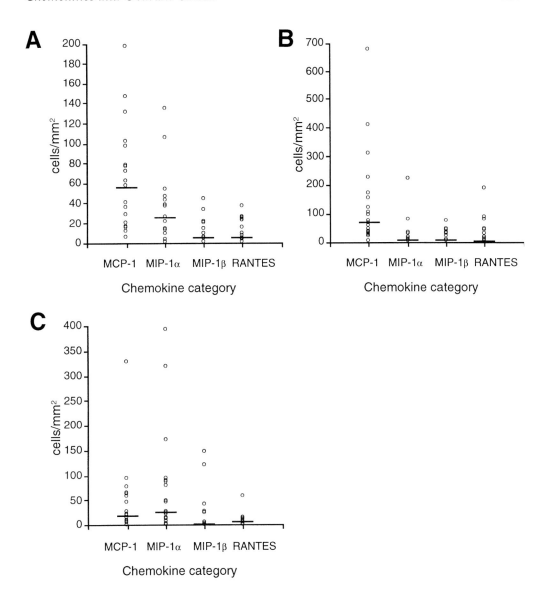

Fig. 3. The expression of C-C chemokines in ovarian carcinomas. Scatter plots of the calculated numbers of chemokine-expressing cells/mm^2 in whole tumor **(A)**, tumor parenchyma **(B)**, and stroma **(C)** for the chemokines MCP-1, MIP-1α, MIP-1β, and RANTES. The horizontal bars represent median values.

4.3. Regulation of MCP-1 Expression in Human Ovarian Cancer

One cytokine that appears to stimulate consistently MCP-1 production and that is present in ovarian cancers is TNF-α. mRNA and protein have both been detected in human ovarian tumors, and the amount of TNF-α produced correlated with tumor grade *(40)*. TNF-α expression has been found in other tumors, such as malignant melanoma *(53)*, some brain tumors *(54)*, and carcinoma of the breast *(55)*. In contrast to the destructive effect of high doses of exogenous TNF-α on methylcholanthrene-induced sarcomas in mice *(56)*, more recent evidence suggests a role for low doses of endogenous TNF-α in the growth of solid tumors. TNF-α stimulated the proliferation of several ovarian cancer cell lines *(42)*, and in a human tumor xenograft model of ovarian cancer, exogenous TNF-α caused malignant cells in ascites to adhere to the peritoneal surface and form solid tumors *(57)*.

TNF-α is a potent stimulus to the production of MCP-1 in ovarian tumor cell line cells and regulates the expression of MCP-1 at the level of mRNA *(58)*. Low doses of TNF-α can stimulate MCP-1 expression, and in the continued presence of TNF-α, MCP-1 mRNA levels can be sustained. As found in earlier studies on TDCF expression *(45)*, the constitutive expression of MCP-1 between cell lines is variable. The variation in the expression of MCP-1 by different cell lines and the stimulation of expression of MCP-1 by TNF-α helps explain the patchy pattern of MCP-1 expression that is seen in tumors, but since MCP-1 expression does not occur in or adjacent to areas of necrosis, another stimulus, hypoxia, was also examined.

Necrotic regions are likely to be anoxic. Nordsmark et al. *(59)* determined that the median oxygen tension in the majority of head and neck nodes from 14 patients with head and neck cancers was significantly lower (≤10 mmHg in 40% of nodes) than in the surrounding sc tissues (30–60 mmHg). Part of the reason for the observed low oxygen tensions may be the presence of tumor necrosis. In C3H mouse mammary carcinomas implanted into the feet of female mice, the percentage of oxygen tensions ≤5 mmHg increased with tumor size, but this increase was lost by taking into account the amount of the total tumor volume that was necrotic, implying that such regions make a significant contribution to low oxygen values *(60)*. Other studies provide evidence that oxygen tension adjacent to necrotic regions is very low. The gene for vascular endothelial growth factor (VEGF) is upregulated by hypoxia *(61)*, and *in situ* analysis of glioblastomas has shown that it is expressed immediately adjacent to necrotic foci *(62)*. In a human colonic carcinoma xenograft model in SCID mice *(63)*, oxygen tension declined away from blood vessels, such that values at ≥150 μm were nearly anoxic (0–0.5 mmHg). The distances in animal models are consistent with those in human tumors. In a histologic analysis of carcinoma of the esophagus, the mean distance between tumor capillaries and the onset of necrosis was 92 ± 34 μm *(64)*.

The effect of hypoxia on the proliferation of ovarian cell lines has also been studied. OW-1, SAU, and SKA cells cultured at ≤10 mmHG for 24 h remained viable as determined by trypan blue exclusion, but the decrease in the incorporation of [³H]thymidine indicated that there was an 80–90% inhibition of DNA synthesis *(65)*.

There is increasing evidence that in mammals a specific oxygen-sensing system mediates many of the responses to low oxygen tension. This system regulates the expression of genes, including enzymes involved in glucose metabolism, erythropoietin, and VEGF *(61)*. The effects of hypoxia can be mimicked by metal ions such as cobalt II *(66)*. Although the cytoplasmic oxygen-sensing protein remains to be determined, the involvement of the transcription factor hypoxia-inducible factor-1 (HIF-1) is now well established *(67)*.

We examined the effect of anoxia on MCP-1 expression in response to stimulation with TNF-α by three ovarian cancer cell lines *(58)*. In all three cell lines, anoxic culture resulted in a decrease in the expression of MCP-1. Cobalt chloride and desferrioxamine both mimicked the effect of anoxia on MCP-1 gene expression, whereas the metabolic inhibitor potassium chloride had no effect. These data are all consistent with the presence of a specific oxygen-sensing system in ovarian carcinoma cells acting through the transcription factor HIF-1. The effect of anoxia could be inhibited by cycloheximide (Scotton, C. J., personal communication), implying a requirement for *de novo* protein synthesis. Our results suggest that low oxygen tensions, particularly those that might occur in and around regions of necrosis, might switch off MCP-1 production, even in the presence of a potent stimulus such as TNF-α. Other genes have been identified that are downregulated in response to hypoxia *(68),* but this appears to be the first description of a chemokine gene that is hypoxically downregulated.

However, the downregulation of MCP-1 expression by hypoxia does present a paradox, since the sites at which macrophages accumulate in highest density are regions of necrosis. A second chemoattractant signal may be responsible. For instance, VEGF both is upregulated by hypoxia *(61)* and can act as a chemoattractant for macrophages. The details of exactly why macrophages become distributed as they do still remain to be unraveled, but a two-step paradigm for leukocyte migration has recently been proposed using IL-8 and formyl-methionine-leucine-proline, in which neutrophils responded to the second chemoattractant when the gradient of the first became saturated *(69).*

4.4. C-X-C Chemokines and Ovarian Cancer

The role of C-X-C chemokines has been much less thoroughly explored. In general, ovarian tumors appear to contain few neutrophils, those that are present being confined to the lumina of blood vessels. However, the potent neutrophil chemoattractant IL-8 can be detected in ascites from patients with ovarian tumors *(70),* and IL-8 mRNA has been detected in ovarian cancer cell lines *(71).* Of potential therapeutic interest is the observation that placlitaxel, used in chemotherapy of ovarian cancers, can stimulate IL-8 production by ovarian cancer cell lines *(72).*

5. SUMMARY

The potent monocyte/macrophage chemoattractant MCP-1 is expressed by tumor cells in human ovarian carcinomas and may be responsible for both the macrophage and T-cell infiltrate. TNF-α is a powerful stimulus to the production of MCP-1 by ovarian carcinoma cell lines. However, low oxygen tensions, such as may be found adjacent to necrotic regions, downregulate TNF-α-induced MCP-1 expression. A second chemoattractant may be responsible for attracting macrophages to necrotic sites. Whether chemokines can be harnessed to modify the host cell infiltrate in these tumors remains to be explored.

REFERENCES

1. Hornung, D., I. P. Ryan, V. A. Chao, J. L. Vigne, E. D. Schriock, and R. N. Taylor. 1997. Immunolocalization and regulation of the chemokine RANTES in human endometrial and endometriosis tissues and cells. *J. Clin. Endocrinol. Metab.* **82:** 1621–1628.
2. Tortolero-Luna, G., and M. F. Mitchell. 1995. The epidemiology of ovarian cancer. *J. Cell. Biochem.* **23 (Suppl.):** 200–207.
3. Parham, G., J. L. Phillips, M. L. Hicks, N. Andrews, W. B. Jones, H. M. Shingleton, and H. R. Menck. 1997. The National Cancer Data Base report on malignant epithelial ovarian carcinoma in African-American women. *Cancer* **80:** 816–826.

4. Westhoff, C. 1996. Ovarian cancer. *Annu. Rev. Pub. Health* **17:** 85–96.

5. Hoskins, W. J. 1995. Prospective on ovarian cancer: why prevent? *J. Cell. Biochem.* **23(Suppl.):** 189–199.

6. Jacobs, I. J., M. F. Kohler, R. W. Wiseman, J. R. Marks, R. Whitaker, B. A. Kerns, P. Humphrey, A. Berchuck, B. A. Ponder, and R. C. Bast, Jr. 1992. Clonal origin of epithelial ovarian carcinoma: analysis by loss of heterozygosity, p53 mutation, and X-chromosome inactivation. *J. Natl. Cancer Inst.* **84:** 1793–1798.

7. Scully, R. E. 1995. Pathology of ovarian cancer precursors. *J. Cell. Biochem.* **23(Suppl.):** 208–218.

8. Booth, M., V. Beral, and P. Smith. 1989. Risk factors for ovarian cancer: a case-control study. *Br. J. Cancer* **60:** 592–598.

9. Risch, H. A., L. D. Marrett, and G. R. Howe. 1994. Parity, contraception, infertility, and the risk of epithelial ovarian cancer. *Am. J. Epidemiol.* **140,** 585–597.

10. Rosenblatt, K. A., and D. B. Thomas. 1993. Lactation and the risk of epithelial ovarian cancer. The WHO Collaborative Study of Neoplasia and Steroid Contraceptives. *Int. J. Epidemiol.* **22:** 192–197.

11. Derman, S. G., and E. Y. Adashi. 1994. Adverse effects of fertility drugs. *Drug Safety* **11:** 408–421.

12. Underwood, J. C. 1974. Lymphoreticular infiltration in human tumours: prognostic and biological implications: a review. *Br. J. Cancer* **30:** 538–548.

13. Totterman, T. H., P. Hayry, E. Saksela, T. Timonen, and B. Eklund. 1978. Cytological and functional analysis of inflammatory infiltrates in human malignant tumors. II. Functional investigations of the infiltrating inflammatory cells. *Eur. J. Immunol.* **8:** 872–875.

14. Svennevig, J. L., M. Lovik, and H. Svaar. 1979. Isolation and characterization of lymphocytes and macrophages from solid, malignant human tumours. *Int. J. Cancer* **23:** 626–631.

15. Herrmann, G., P. M. Schumm Draeger, C. Muller, E. Atai, B. Wenzel, T. Fabian, K. H. Usadel, and K. Hubner. 1994. T lymphocytes, CD68-positive cells and vascularisation in thyroid carcinomas. *J. Cancer Res. Clin. Oncol.* **120:** 651–656.

16. Banner, B. F., L. Savas, S. Baker, and B. A. Woda. 1993. Characterization of the inflammatory cell populations in normal colon and colonic carcinomas. *Virchows Arch. B Cell Pathol. Incl. Mol. Pathol.* **64:** 213–220.

17. Scholl, S. M., C. Pallud, F. Beuvon, K. Hacene, E. R. Stanley, L. Rohrschneider, R. Tang, P. Pouillart, and R. Lidereau. 1994. Anti-colony-stimulating factor-1 antibody staining in primary breast adenocarcinomas correlates with marked inflammatory cell infiltrates and prognosis. *J. Natl. Cancer Inst.* **86:** 120–126.

18. Lwin, K. Y., O. Zuccarini, J. P. Sloane, and P. C. Beverley. 1985. An immunohistological study of leukocyte localization in benign and malignant breast tissue. *Int. J. Cancer* **36:** 433–438.

19. Yuh, K., M. Shimizu, S. Aoyama, I. Ichihara, H. Watanabe, M. Okumura, and M. Kikuchi. 1989. Immunological analysis and characterization of lymphocyte subsets in specimens of human hepatocellular carcinomas and metastatic liver cancers. *Cancer Immunol. Immunother.* **28:** 1–8.

20. Haskill, S., S. Becker, W. Fowler, and L. Walton. 1982. Mononuclear-cell infiltration in ovarian cancer. I. Inflammatory-cell infiltrates from tumour and ascites material. *Br. J. Cancer* **45:** 728–736.

21. Kabawat, S. E., R. C. Bast, Jr., W. R. Welch, R. C. Knapp, and A. K. Bhan. 1983. Expression of major histocompatibility antigens and nature of inflammatory cellular infiltrate in ovarian neoplasms. *Int. J. Cancer* **32:** 547–554.

22. Kooi, S., H. Z. Zhang, R. Patenia, C. L. Edwards, C. D. Platsoucas, and R. S. Freedman. 1996. HLA class I expression on human ovarian carcinoma cells correlates with T-cell infiltration in vivo and T-cell expansion in vitro in low concentrations of recombinant interleukin-2. *Cell Immunol.* **174:** 116–128.

23. van Ravenswaay Claasen, H. H., P. M. Kluin, and G. J. Fleuren. 1992. Tumor infiltrating cells in human cancer: on the possible role of CD16+ macrophages in antitumor cytotoxicity. *Lab. Invest.* **67**: 166–174.

24. Dietl, J., H. P. Horny, P. Ruck, and E. Kaiserling. 1993. Dysgerminoma of the ovary: an immunohistochemical study of tumor-infiltrating lymphoreticular cells and tumor cells. *Cancer* **71**: 2562–2568.

25. Lentz, S. S., D. J. McKean, J. S. Kovach, and K. C. Podratz. 1989. Phenotypic and functional characteristics of mononuclear cells in ovarian carcinoma tumors. *Gynecol. Oncol.* **34**: 136–140.

26. Reijnhart, R. M., M. M. Bieber, and N. N. Teng. 1994. FACS analysis of peritoneal lymphocytes in ovarian cancer and control patients. *Immunobiology* **191**: 1–8.

27. Negus, R. P. M., and F. R. Balkwill. 1997. The distribution of infiltrating cells and the regulation of chemokine expression in human ovarian cancer, in *Ovarian Cancer 5* (Sharp, F., A. D. Blackett, J. S. Berek, and R. C. Bast, eds.), Isis Medical Media, Oxford.

28. Canevari, S., G. Stoter, F. Arienti, G. Bolis, M. I. Colnaghi, E. M. Di Re, A. M. Eggermont, S. H. Goey, J. W. Gratama, C. H. Lamers, et al. 1995. Regression of advanced ovarian carcinoma by intraperitoneal treatment with autologous T lymphocytes retargeted by a bispecific monoclonal antibody. *J. Natl. Cancer Inst.* **87**: 1463–1469.

29. Ioannides, C. G., B. Fisk, K. R. Jerome, T. Irimura, J. T. Wharton, O. J. Finn. 1993. Cytotoxic T cells from ovarian malignant tumors can recognize polymorphic epithelial mucin core peptides. *J. Immunol.* **151**: 3693–3703.

30. Rabinowich, H., Y. Suminami, T. E. Reichert, P. Crowley-Nowick, M. Bell, R. Edwards, and T. L. Whiteside. 1996. Expression of cytokine genes or proteins and signaling molecules in lymphocytes associated with human ovarian carcinoma. *Int. J. Cancer* **68**: 276–284.

31. Lotzova, E. 1990. Role of human circulating and tumor-infiltrating lymphocytes in cancer defense and treatment. *Nat. Immun. & Cell Growth Reg.* **9**: 253–264 (review).

32. Gimmi, C. D., B. W. Morrison, B. A. Mainprice, J. G. Gribben, V. A. Boussiotis, G. J. Freeman, S. Y. Park, M. Watanabe, J. Gong, D. F. Hayes, D. W. Kufe, and L. M. Nadler. 1996. Breast cancer-associated antigen, DF3/MUC1, induces apoptosis of activated human T cells. *Nat. Med.* **2**: 1367–1370.

33. Strand, S., W. J. Hofmann, H. Hug, M. Muller, G. Otto, D. Strand, S. M. Mariani, W. Stremmel, P. H. Krammer, and P. R. Galle. 1996. Lymphocyte apoptosis induced by CD95 (APO-1/Fas) ligand-expressing tumor cells—a mechanism of immune evasion? *Nat. Med.* **2**: 1361–1366 (see comments).

34. Guinan, E. C., J. G. Gribben, V. A. Boussiotis, G. J. Freeman, and L. M. Nadler. 1994. Pivotal role of the B7:CD28 pathway in transplantation tolerance and tumor immunity. *Blood* **84**: 3261–3282.

35. Peng, L. M., S. Y. Shu, and J. C. Krauss. 1997. Monocyte chemoattractant protein inhibits the generation of tumor-reactive T-cells. *Cancer Res.* **57**: 4849–4854.

36. Haskill, S., H. Koren, S. Becker, W. Fowler, and L. Walton. 1982. Mononuclear-cell infiltration in ovarian cancer. III. Suppressor-cell and ADCC activity of macrophages from ascitic and solid ovarian tumours. *Br. J. Cancer* **45**: 747–753.

37. Richters, C. D., C. W. Burger, A. A. van de Loosdrecht, R. E. van Rijswijk, W. Calame, O. P. Bleker, J. B. Vermorken, P. Kenemans, and R. H. Beelen. 1993. The cellular composition in the peritoneal cavity and the cytotoxic function of the peritoneal cells from patients with ovarian cancer: effect of tumor necrosis factor-alpha treatment. *Cancer Lett.* **68**: 25–31.

38. Brunda, M. J., V. Sulich, R. B. Wright, and A. V. Palleroni. 1991. Tumoricidal activity and cytokine secretion by tumor-infiltrating macrophages. *Int. J. Cancer* **48**: 704–708.

39. Mantovani, A. 1981. In vitro effects on tumor cells of macrophages isolated from an early-passage chemically-induced murine sarcoma and from its spontaneous metastases. *Int. J. Cancer* **27**: 221–228.

40. Naylor, M. S., G. W. Stamp, W. D. Foulkes, D. Eccles, and F. R. Balkwill. 1993. Tumor necrosis factor and its receptors in human ovarian cancer: potential role in disease progression. *J. Clin. Invest.* **91:** 2194–2206.

41. Erroi, A., M. Sironi, F. Chiaffarino, Z. G. Chen, M. Mengozzi, and A. Mantovani. 1989. IL-1 and IL-6 release by tumor-associated macrophages from human ovarian carcinoma. *Int. J. Cancer* **44:** 795–801.

42. Wu, S., C. M. Boyer, R. S. Whitaker, A. Berchuck, J. R. Wiener, J. B. Weinberg, and R. C. Bast, Jr. 1993. Tumor necrosis factor alpha as an autocrine and paracrine growth factor for ovarian cancer: monokine induction of tumor cell proliferation and tumor necrosis factor alpha expression. *Cancer Res.* **53:** 1939–1944.

43. Sheid, B. 1992. Angiogenic effects of macrophages isolated from ascitic fluid aspirated from women with advanced ovarian cancer. *Cancer Lett.* **62:** 153–158.

44. Yoshida, S., M. Ono, T. Shono, H. Izumi, T. Ishibashi, H. Suzuki, and M. Kuwano. 1997. Involvement of interleukin-8, vascular endothelial growth factor, and basic fibroblast growth factor in tumor necrosis factor alpha-dependent angiogenesis. *Mol. Cell. Biol.* **17:** 4015–4023.

45. Bottazzi, B., N. Polentarutti, A. Balsari, D. Boraschi, P. Ghezzi, M. Salmona, and A. Mantovani. 1983. Chemotactic activity for mononuclear phagocytes of culture supernatants from murine and human tumor cells: evidence for a role in the regulation of the macrophage content of neoplastic tissues. *Int. J. Cancer* **31:** 55–63.

46. Bottazzi, B., P. Ghezzi, G. Taraboletti, M. Salmona, N. Colombo, C. Bonazzi, C. Mangioni, and A. Mantovani. 1985. Tumor-derived chemotactic factor(s) from human ovarian carcinoma: evidence for a role in the regulation of macrophage content of neoplastic tissues. *Int. J. Cancer* **36:** 167–173.

47. Graves, D. T., Y. L. Jiang, M. J. Williamson, and A. J. Valente. 1989. Identification of monocyte chemotactic activity produced by malignant cells. *Science* **245:** 1490–1493.

48. Yoshimura, T., E. A. Robinson, S. Tanaka, E. Appella, J. Kuratsu, and E. J. Leonard. 1989. Purification and amino acid analysis of two human glioma-derived monocyte chemoattractants. *J. Exp. Med.* **169:** 1449–1459.

49. Yoshimura, T., N. Yuhki, S. K. Moore, E. Appella, M. I. Lerman, and E. J. Leonard. 1989. Human monocyte chemoattractant protein-1 (MCP-1): full-length cDNA cloning, expression in mitogen-stimulated blood mononuclear leukocytes, and sequence similarity to mouse competence gene JE. *FEBS Lett.* **244:** 487–493.

50. Furutani, Y., H. Nomura, M. Notake, Y. Oyamada, T. Fukui, M. Yamada, C. G. Larsen, J. J. Oppenheim, and K. Matsushima. 1989. Cloning and sequencing of the cDNA for human monocyte chemotactic and activating factor (MCAF). *Biochem. Biophys. Res. Commun.* **159:** 249–255.

51. Bottazzi, B., F. Colotta, A. Sica, N. Nobili, and A. Mantovani. 1990. A chemoattractant expressed in human sarcoma cells (tumor-derived chemotactic factor, TDCF) is identical to monocyte chemoattractant protein-1/monocyte chemotactic and activating factor (MCP-1/MCAF). *Int. J. Cancer* **45:** 795–797.

52. Negus, R. P., G. W. Stamp, M. G. Relf, F. Burke, S. T. Malik, S. Bernasconi, P. Allavena, S. Sozzani, A. Mantovani, and F. R. Balkwill. 1995. The detection and localization of monocyte chemoattractant protein-1 (MCP-1) in human ovarian cancer. *J. Clin. Invest.* **95:** 2391–2396.

53. Mattei, S., M. P. Colombo, C. Melani, A. Silvani, G. Parmiani, and M. Herlyn. 1994. Expression of cytokine/growth factors and their receptors in human melanoma and melanocytes. *Int. J. Cancer* **56:** 853–857.

54. Merlo, A., A. Juretic, M. Zuber, L. Filgueira, U. Luscher, V. Caetano, J. Ulrich, O. Gratzl, M. Heberer, G. C. Spagnoli. 1993. Cytokine gene expression in primary brain tumours, metastases and meningiomas suggests specific transcription patterns. *Eur. J. Cancer* **29A:** 2118–2125.

55. Pusztai, L., L. M. Clover, K. Cooper, P. M. Starkey, C. E. Lewis, and J. O. McGee. 1994. Expression of tumour necrosis factor alpha and its receptors in carcinoma of the breast. *Br. J. Cancer* **70:** 289–292.

56. Carswell, E. A., L. J. Old, R. L. Kassel, S. Green, N. Fiore, and B. Williamson. 1975. An endotoxin-induced serum factor that causes necrosis of tumors. *Proc. Natl. Acad. Sci. USA* **72:** 3666–3670.

57. Malik, S. T., D. B. Griffin, W. Fiers, and F. R. Balkwill. 1989. Paradoxical effects of tumour necrosis factor in experimental ovarian cancer. *Int. J. Cancer* **44:** 918–925.

58. Negus, R. P. M., L. Turner, F. Burke, and F. R. Balkwill. 1998. Hypoxia downregulates MCP-1 expression: implications for macrophage distribution in tumors. *J. Leuk. Biol.* **63:** 758–765.

59. Nordsmark, M., S. M. Bentzen, and J. Overgaard. 1994. Measurement of human tumour oxygenation status by a polarographic needle electrode: an analysis of inter- and intratumour heterogeneity. *Acta Oncol.* **33:** 383–389.

60. Khalil, A. A., M. R. Horsman, and J. Overgaard. 1995. The importance of determining necrotic fraction when studying the effect of tumour volume on tissue oxygenation. *Acta Oncol.* **34:** 297–300.

61. Gleadle, J. M., B. L. Ebert, J. D. Firth, and P. J. Ratcliffe. 1995. Regulation of angiogenic growth factor expression by hypoxia, transition metals, and chelating agents. *Am. J. Physiol.* **268:** C1362–C1368.

62. Shweiki, D., A. Itin, D. Soffer, and E. Keshet. 1992. Vascular endothelial growth factor induced by hypoxia may mediate hypoxia-initiated angiogenesis. *Nature* **359:** 843–845.

63. Helmlinger, G., F. Yuan, M. Dellian, and R. Jain. 1997. Interstitial pH and pO_2 gradients in solid tumors *in vivo:* high-resolution measurements reveal a lack of correlation. *Nat. Med.* **3:** 177–182.

64. Porschen, R., S. Classen, M. Piontek, and F. Borchard. 1994. Vascularization of carcinomas of the esophagus and its correlation with tumor proliferation. *Cancer Res.* **54:** 587–591.

65. Krtolica, A., and J. W. Ludlow. 1996. Hypoxia arrests ovarian carcinoma cell cycle progression, but invasion is unaffected. *Cancer Res.* **56:** 1168–1173.

66. Goldberg, M. A., S. P. Dunning, and H. F. Bunn. 1988. Regulation of the erythropoietin gene: evidence that the oxygen sensor is a heme protein. *Science* **242:** 1412–1415.

67. Guillemin, K., and M. A. Krasnow. 1997. The hypoxic response: huffing and HIFing. *Cell* **89:** 9–12.

68. Ebert, B. L., J. M. Gleadle, J. F. O'Rourke, S. M. Bartlett, J. Poulton, and P. J. Ratcliffe. 1996. Isoenzyme-specific regulation of genes involved in energy metabolism by hypoxia: similarities with the regulation of erythropoietin. *Biochem. J.* **313:** 809–814.

69. Foxman, E. F., J. J. Campbell, and E. C. Butcher. 1997. Multistep navigation and combinatorial control of leukocyte chemotaxis. *J. Cell Biol.* **139:** 1349–1360.

70. Radke, J., D. Schmidt, M. Bohme, U. Schmidt, W. Weise, and J. Morenz. 1996. Cytokine level in malignant ascites and peripheral blood of patients with advanced ovarian carcinoma. *Geburtshilfe und Frauenheilkunde* **56:** 83–87.

71. Melani, C., S. M. Pupa, A. Stoppacciaro, S. Menard, M. I. Colnaghi, G. Parmiani, and M. P. Colombo. 1995. An in vivo model to compare human leukocyte infiltration in carcinoma xenografts producing different chemokines. *Int. J. Cancer* **62:** 572–578.

72. Lee, L. F., C. C. Schuerer-Maly, A. K. Lofquist, C. van Haaften-Day, J. P. Ting, C. M. White, B. K. Martin, and J. S. Haskill. 1996. Taxol-dependent transcriptional activation of IL-8 in a subset of human ovarian cancer. *Cancer Res.* **56:** 1303–1308.

12

The Possible Role of Chemokines in HPV-Linked Carcinogenesis

Frank Rösl, Kerstin Kleine-Lowinski, and Harald zur Hausen

1. INTRODUCTION

Specific types of human papillomaviruses (HPVs) (mostly HPV-16, HPV-18) are etiologically involved in the development of cervical cancer *(1,2)*. Although viral DNA induces immortalization of primary human keratinocytes in vitro, infection alone is not sufficient to cause malignant transformation *(3,4)*. In agreement with the multihit concept of many human neoplasias, additional damaging events are required to convert a cell toward malignancy and to induce cervical cancer *(5,6)*. Furthermore, the course of the disease is not only the result of failing intracellular surveillance mechanisms *(5,7)*, but is also determined by the immune status of the infected individual *(8,9)*. Epidemiologic studies have demonstrated that immunosuppressed patients or persons with impaired immunocompetence have a higher virus susceptibility and virus spread, and an increased incidence of preneoplastic lesions than age-matched controls *(9)*.

Apart from the immunoregulatory effector cells, a network of proinflammatory cytokines also exists *(10)*, which help control persistent viral infections. It has been shown by several in vitro studies that specific macrophage-derived cytokines, such as tumor necrosis factor-α (TNF-α) or transforming growth factor-β (TGF-β), can selectively suppress viral gene expression at the transcriptional level *(11–14)*. Since downregulation of viral gene expression in cervical carcinoma cells is regularly accompanied by a cessation of cellular growth *(15,16)*, it is reasonable to assume that immunoregulatory cytokines such as TNF-α or TGF-β may also play a pivotal role in the virus defense under in vivo conditions *(17)*.

Another important group of diffusible immunomodulators, the chemokines, belongs to a superfamily of structurally and functionally related proteins that are involved in the recruitment and chemotactic activation of cells within the immunologic compartment *(10,18,19)*. Disturbance of the cross talk between somatic and immunocompetent effector cells may also be an important aspect in HPV-linked carcinogenesis, since advanced intraepithelial cervical neoplasias are immunohistochemically characterized by a significant depletion of intraepithelial macrophages, Langerhans cells, and helper T-lymphocytes *(20–22)*.

Since little information exists about the function of chemokines during the development of cervical cancer, this chapter outlines some of our initial experimental attempts

From: *Chemokines and Cancer*
Edited by: B. J. Rollins © Humana Press Inc., Totowa, NJ

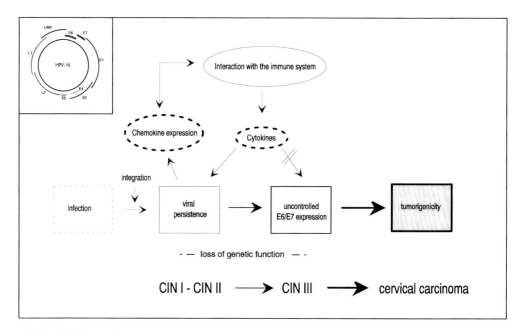

Fig. 1. Schematic overview of the different steps of HPV-linked carcinogenesis. The development of cervical cancer represents a multistep process, which is initiated by viral infection. Although integration of the viral DNA seems to occur very early, HPV-positive cells are nontumorigenic and still respond to growth-inhibitory cytokines ("viral persistence"). After longer periods of time and additional cell-damaging events, loss of genetic function leads to uncontrolled E6/E7 expression and finally to the progression of tumorigenicity. **(Inset)** Genome organization of HPV-16.

to understand such a relationship. To gain insight into this topic, we first briefly summarize some general properties of certain types of human pathogenic papillomaviruses and their etiologic role in the pathogenesis of cervical cancer. The second part mainly deals with the expression and transcriptional regulation of the monocyte chemoattractant protein-1 (MCP-1) gene, presently one of the best-characterized chemokines, in cervical carcinoma cells, somatic cell hybrids derived therefrom, and in primary human biopsy material.

2. THE ROLE OF HPVS IN THE DEVELOPMENT OF CERVICAL CANCER

2.1. Biologic Properties of HPVs

HPVs represent a group of small DNA tumor viruses that comprise, at present, 80 different genotypes *(6,23)* (for genome organization, *see* Fig. 1). Based on their presence in specific lesions, they were subdivided into "low"- and "high"-risk HPVs *(23)*. Low-risk types (HPV-6 and HPV-11) regularly produce benign lesions of the genital tract such as the exophytic condylomata acuminata *(6,23)*. Although more than 30 distinct HPV types have been isolated from anogenital precancerous and malignant biopsy specimens, only a restricted number, mainly HPV-16 but also HPV-18, -33, -45, -52,

-58, and a few others, belong to the high-risk group *(6,23)*. These specific types can be detected in approx 95% of cervical cancer biopsies *(6)*. Cancer of the uterine cervix, which is the second leading cause of cancer incidence in women worldwide, can be considered as a sexually transmitted disease, with a relationship between the onset of sexual activity, the number of sexual partners, and the prevalence of high-risk HPV positivity of histologically suspicious lesions *(9)*. Consequently, the distinction between high- and low-risk HPV types provides a significant gynecologic criteria for the prognostic risk assessment of a diagnosed HPV infection.

The primary targets of an HPV infection are keratinocytes of the stratum basale, which is the only cell layer within the cervical mucosa able to undergo cell division *(6,24)*. Furthermore, the availability of sensitive RNA/RNA *in situ* hybridization techniques have shown that the expression of the late open reading frames (ORFs) L1 and L2, encoding the capsid proteins necessary for DNA encapsidation and virus maturation, is closely linked to cell differentiation. Viral replication also increases toward the epithelial surface, with a maximum DNA synthesis rate confined to the superficial layers *(9,24,25)*. A classical histologic indication of an HPV infection is the appearance of koilocytic cells *(9)*.

Although the vast majority of viral infections normally occurs without any clinical symptoms, progression to cervical cancer is morphologically characterized by distinct histopathologic alterations of the squamous epithelium. Depending on the proportion of undifferentiated basaloid cells, emerging lesions are referred to as cervical intraepithelial neoplasia (CIN) grade I, II, and III *([6,9]; see* Fig. 1). Untreated CIN III lesions frequently proceed to carcinomas *in situ* and finally to invasively growing carcinomas with metastatic potential *(9)*. Since the production of infectious virus particles is tightly coupled with ongoing cell differentiation, it was not possible until now to propagate HPV under in vitro tissue culture conditions *(6)*. Nevertheless, DNA-mediated gene transfer experiments with various subgenomic HPV fragments have demonstrated that the oncogenic potential of high-risk viruses can be attributed to the E6 and E7 ORFs, a sequence stretch that is located adjacent to the upstream regulatory region (URR) *(see* Fig. 1) *(26)*. The URR harbors all promoter and enhancer elements necessary for efficient oncogene transcription. Continuous E6/E7 expression is not only responsible for immortalization of primary human keratinocytes and fibroblasts *(3,4,27)*, but is also required to maintain the proliferative capacity of established cervical carcinoma cells both in vitro (under tissue culture conditions) and in vivo (after heterotransplantation into nude mice) *(16,28)*.

Detailed Southern blot analyses have revealed that the viral DNA normally persists as an extrachromosomal element in a defined copy number in premalignant lesions, but is found to be integrated in the vast majority of cervical carcinomas *(29)*. Recombination of the viral DNA with host cellular sequences seems to be an early and important step in HPV-linked carcinogenesis *(see* Fig. 1), since it relieves the *trans*-repressing function of the E2 protein on its own promoter *(30,31)* and generates E6/E7 containing virus-cell fusion transcripts, which have a longer half-life than their authentic virus-specific counterparts *(32)*. Both events evidently provide a selective advantage for initiated cells, leading to an accumulation of the viral oncoproteins with a dose-responsive effect toward malignant transformation *(33)*.

2.2. Multistep Process of HPV-Linked Pathogenesis

There is substantial epidemiologic and molecular biologic evidence suggesting that the progression to cervical cancer is a multistep process *(2,17,34)*. The long latency period between primary viral infection and the final clinical manifestation of a tumor as well as the low number of HPV-positive individuals, who subsequently develop cancer, clearly indicate that virus infection is not sufficient to induce malignant transformation *(5,7)*. Indeed, as already shown by a number of in vitro transfection studies, constitutive E6/E7 expression merely results in cells with infinite life span, which are nontumorigenic after inoculation into nude mice *(3,27)*. Although the mechanism of E6/E7-induced cell immortalization is still poorly understood, both oncogenes apparently dysregulate the activity of those cellular proteins that play a central role in the cell-cycle control. In addition to an intrinsic *trans*-activator activity on heterologous promoters *(35)*, E6 seems to be mainly involved in the reduction of the biological half-life of p53 *(36,37)*, whose physiologic function is commonly considered as a guarantee for chromosomal stability after cellular DNA damage *(38)*. The other biologically relevant pathway concerns the interaction between E7 with the retinoblastoma protein Rb *(39)* and other members of the "pocket protein" family such as p107 and p130 *(40)*. E7 preferentially binds to the underphosphorylated form of Rb, leading to the illegitimate release of the transcription factor E2F and to premature induction of DNA synthesis *(41)*.

Apart from their effects on the cell cycle, long-term expression of E6/E7 also induces mutations of the host cell DNA and consequent labilization of the chromosomal complement *(42)*. This is an intriguing feature, since the development of most human cancers seems to be a recessive event, which is preceded by a segregation of specific alleles and loss of genetic functions *(43,44)*. Destabilization of the karyotype is not only restricted to E6/E7, but also occurs after expression of other viral oncogenes such as the SV40 large T-antigen *(45)* or the E1a protein of adenoviruses *(46)*.

During the past few years, it has become more and more evident that the loss of genetic information seems also to be a crucial event in the multistep progression to cervical cancer. This assumption was mainly deduced from somatic cell hybridization experiments, in which the malignant phenotype of cervical carcinoma cells can be completely suppressed after fusion with normal human fibroblasts or keratinocytes *(47)* (*see* Fig. 2). Detailed karyotypic and restriction enzyme fragment length polymorphism analyses of tumorigenic revertants derived from such hybrids have provided evidence for a nonrandom loss of specific chromosomes *(48)*. Moreover, taking advantage of individual chromosome-transfer techniques, it was demonstrated that only chromosome 11, but not other C-group chromosomes, exerts a tumor-suppressive effect on HPV-16- or HPV-18-positive cervical carcinoma cell lines. Reintroduction of only one normal copy of chromosome 11 in either HPV-16- or HPV-18-positive cervical carcinoma cells is sufficient to abrogate completely their in vivo growth in immunocompromised animals *(49,50)*.

It has been postulated that nontumorigenic HPV-positive cells possess an intracellular surveillance mechanism, which not only negatively interferes with the tumorigenic phenotype but also with the expression of the viral oncogenes E6 and E7 *(5,7)*. It was further hypothesized that the viral URR represents a major target for such an intracel-

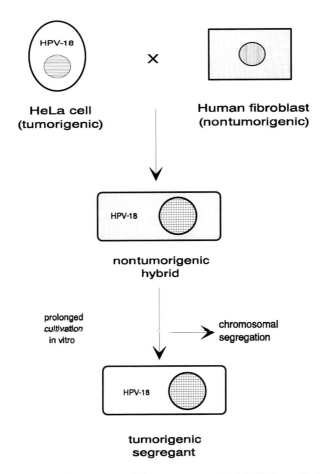

Fig. 2. Somatic cell hybrids as a model system to study MCP-1 regulation. Generation of nontumorigenic somatic cell hybrids after fusion with normal human fibroblasts (according to Stanbridge, *[47]*). Fusion of the HPV-18-positive cervical carcinoma cell line HeLa with normal human fibroblasts results in somatic cell hybrids, which were nontumorigenic in nude mice. Prolonged propagation of such cell under tissue culture conditions leads to the segregation of certain chromosomes and to the appearance of tumorigenic segregants.

lular control pathway, whose genetic loss during progression to cervical cancer is accompanied by increased cell proliferation and uncontrolled viral gene expression *(5,7,51)* (*see* Fig. 1).

RNA/RNA *in situ* hybridizations seem to support this notion, since there is very low transcriptional activity for E6/E7 RNA of high-risk HPV types in basal cells derived from low-grade CIN (CIN-I). Viral transcription, however, progressively increases in advanced lesions (CIN II and III) and is abundantly expressed in cervical cancer biopsy specimens *(24,25)*. Similar results can be obtained in heterotransplantation experiments of nonmalignant HPV-18-positive HeLa-fibroblast hybrids into nude mice. Although HeLa cells form rapidly growing tumors with an elevated viral expression rate ubiquitously distributed throughout the tissue section, viral transcription is found to be selectively downregulated in nontumorigenic hybrids between 2 and 3 d after inoculation

(52). Since the nonmalignant hybrids, their tumorigenic segregants, as well as the parental HeLa cells share similar in vitro growth properties, it is tempting to speculate that viral suppression in nonmalignant cells is mediated by diffusible growth-inhibitory factors (i.e., cytokines), which are present in the animal but absent under in vitro conditions *(5,17).*

2.3. The Effect of Cytokines on the Transcriptional Regulation of High-Risk HPV Types in Malignant and Nonmalignant Cells: Some General Aspects

The development of cervical cancer is not only the consequence of a failing intracellular surveillance mechanism *(7)* but can also be regarded as a result of an escape effect, which circumvents the immune response of the infected host. In addition to the HPV-specific T-cell-mediated immune response, depletion of intraepithelial macrophages and Langerhans cells in advanced CIN lesions may also favor malignant progression *(20,21,53),* since cells of the monocyte/macrophage lineage are known producers of growth-modulatory cytokines *(19,54).* Indeed, it has been well documented by a number of in vitro studies that particular cytokines such as TNF-α *(12,13),* interferon-α (IFN-α) (55), interleukin-1 (IL-1) (56), and TGF-β *(11,14)* can negatively interfere with both HPV transcription and cell proliferation. Interestingly, this biologic effect seems to be restricted to pre- or nonmalignant HPV-16/-18-positive cells, since cervical carcinoma cell lines are much less sensitive to cytokine treatment *(57–59)* (*see* also Fig. 1). Increased resistance can be mediated either by downregulation of the corresponding receptors or by an enhanced synthesis of soluble truncated receptors, which in both cases abrogate or diminish the cytokine response *(12,57).*

As demonstrated in the case of TNF-α and IL-1, cytokine-induced E6/E7 suppression is regulated at the level of initiation of transcription. Furthermore, a cytokine-responsive element was confined to the URR of HPV-16, which harbors multiple consensus sequences for the transcription factor NF-IL-6 *(56).* Overexpression of a cDNA encoding NF-IL-6 can substitute for cytokine function in negatively interfering with HPV-16 transcription. Since the NF-IL-6 sequences overlap with the binding sites for the activator protein-1 (AP-1), repression of the viral URR by NF-IL-6 is mainly owing to competition with AP-1, a transcription factor normally indispensable for efficient HPV-16 transcription *(60).* Hence, particular cytokines such as TNF-α and IL-1 fulfill exactly those criteria of in vivo factors, which were postulated to induce intracellular surveillance mechanism(s) *(17)* within nontumorigenic cells after heterografting them into nude mice.

To understand the mechanisms whereby growth-inhibitory cytokines reach their target cells and how these components of the immunologic network become activated, we focused our attention on the transcriptional regulation of the MCP-1 gene *(61),* which is currently one of the best-characterized members of the chemokine family *(19,62).* MCP-1 not only stimulates monocyte migration but also activates monocytes to secrete a variety of growth-modulatory cytokines *(63–65),* which in turn can exert their biologic functions on surrounding cells. An efficiently functioning cytokine network, which is built up by immunocompetent cells in their natural host, may also account for the spontaneous regression of papillomavirus-associated lesions, in which a strong infiltration of lymphocytes and high TNF-α-expressing mononuclear cells can be found *(66).*

Assuming that inappropriate chemokine expression may also be involved in HPV-linked carcinogenesis (Fig. 1), we set out to investigate the transcriptional regulation of the MCP-1 gene in malignant and nonmalignant HPV-positive cells.

3. CHEMOKINES AND CERVICAL CANCER

3.1. MCP-1 Gene Expression in Cervical Carcinoma Cells and Derived Somatic Cell Hybrids

The previously discussed studies have shown that all cervical carcinoma cell lines tested so far lack detectable levels of MCP-1 expression. Although cancer cells are characterized by instability of their karyotype, both Southern blot and polymerase chain reaction analyses gave no indications for deletions or gross genomic rearrangements of the MCP-1 gene or its promoter region. MCP-1 expression, however, can be restored in HPV-18-positive HeLa cells after fusion with normal human fibroblasts, in which case the resulting somatic cell hybrids were nontumorigenic in nude mice *(47)*. Tumorigenic segregants, which are derived from the same hybrids either after long-term propagation in tissue culture or after in vivo selection within the animal (see below), again lack MCP-1 expression *[13]* (*see* also Fig. 2). The absence of specific MCP-1 transcription without any detectable alterations at the DNA level in cervical carcinoma cells suggests that a correlation exists between the absence of MCP-1 expression and the appearance of a malignant phenotype.

This suggestion was mainly supported by earlier observations revealing that reconstituted chemokine expression has a tumor-suppressing function on certain malignant cell types under defined experimental conditions. This finding was initially reported by Rollins and colleagues *(67)*, who showed that the introduction of the MCP-1 gene in malignantly transformed hamster ovary cells completely prevents their tumor formation in nude mice, a phenomenon that is accompanied by a pronounced infiltration of monocytes at the site of injection *(67)*. However, MCP-1 *(68,69)* or other β-chemokines such as TCA3 *(70)*, cannot simply be considered as tumor-suppressing factors, because examples also exist in which the reexpression either has no effect or merely reduces the growth rate of the arising tumor *(71,72)*. Although these processes entail a cascade of one or more different signaling pathways, the genetic background of the individual cells probably determines how they respond to macrophage-derived cytokines, since tumor-associated macrophages can also induce the opposite effect, namely to promote cellular growth *(18,54,63)*.

The restoration of MCP-1 expression in somatic cell hybrids made between malignant HeLa cells and normal human fibroblast *(13)* is intriguing, especially with respect to the concomitant reappearance of a nontumorigenic phenotype *(47)*. Assuming that there is cross talk between nontumorigenic cells and the non T-cell-dependent immunologic compartment of the nude mouse, we could demonstrate that macrophage-derived cytokines such as TNF-α and IL-1 have a positive effect on the MCP-1 gene by strongly inducing its expression exclusively in the nonmalignant hybrids. Consistent with the notion that proteins involved in immunologic cell-cell communication should exert their biologic functions directly *(19)*, MCP-1 transcription was rapidly increased and independent from *de novo* protein synthesis *(13)*. This increase in MCP-1 expression is not restricted to species specificity of the cytokine, because identical results were obtained independently of whether human or mouse TNF-α was used (Finzer, P., and Rösl, F., unpublished results). The same cytokines, which induce chemokine expression in HeLa-fibroblast hybrids, also suppress endogenous HPV-18 transcription, whereas the expression of other reference genes such as β-actin remain unaffected *(13)*.

A direct functional relationship between the presence of cytokine-producing effector cells and the transcriptional control of viral gene expression was further demonstrated in cocultivation experiments between nontumorigenic hybrids, their tumorigenic counterparts, and enriched fractions of mononuclear cells from healthy human volunteers. Although increasing numbers of monocytes had no effect on HPV-18 E6/E7 expression in HeLa cells or in tumorigenic segregants, viral transcription was again selectively suppressed in the nontumorigenic hybrids under the same experimental conditions *(13)*.

Elevated MCP-1 expression probably triggers a feedback mechanism during which the physiologic response between chemokine-releasing (somatic cell hybrids and macrophages) and cytokine-producing cells (macrophages) becomes amplified. In other words, once a chemotactic gradient is established in vivo, enhanced monocyte migration may lead to higher secretion of growth-inhibitory cytokines, which in turn maintain the MCP-1 gene in an induced state. MCP-1 induction concomitant with the negative regulatory effect on the viral E6/E7 expression could therefore be considered as a reasonable explanation for the observed transcriptional suppression of HPV-18 after heterotransplantation of nonmalignant cells into nude mice *(52)*.

This assumption was further supported by a similar approach performed with HPV-16-immortalized human foreskin keratinocytes *(3)*. As already outlined, HPV-16-transfected cells were initially nontumorigenic in immunocompromised animals, but became malignantly transformed either after their long-term cultivation in tissue culture or after subsequent introduction of an additional oncogene *(27,73)*. Again, selective suppression of HPV-16 transcription after cocultivation was found only in nonmalignant keratinocytes, not in their malignant derivatives *(13)*.

On the other hand, transfection of an SV40 promoter/enhancer-driven MCP-1 expression vector in malignant HeLa cells is not accompanied by a nontumorigenic phenotype *(72)*, indicating that the simple reconstitution of a chemokine did not counterbalance the loss of genetic function complemented either by somatic cell hybridization *(47)* or via chromosome 11 microcell transfers *(49,50)*. MCP-1 reexpression in HeLa cells, however, is sufficient to restore their ability to attract human monocytes in an in vitro chamber migration assay *(72)*. Moreover, inoculation of such cells into immunocompromised animals results in a significant growth retardation, which is immunohistochemically characterized by an increased infiltration of macrophages into the inner tumor mass *(72)*.

Although HeLa cells were normally refractory to certain cytokines such as TNF-α and IL-1 *(13,58)*, invasion of activated mononuclear cells may create a microenvironmental situation, in which the secretion of locally high doses of growth-inhibitory cytokines can temporarily block the proliferation of the surrounding tumorigenic cells. A macrophage-derived growth factor that obviously can efficiently interfere with HPV-18 mRNA transcription in HeLa cells by arresting them in G1 of the cell cycle is IFN-α *(55)*. Which cytokines were actually involved in the in vivo growth control of HPV-positive cells is presently not known and awaits further elucidation.

It should be emphasized, however, that the absence of MCP-1 expression in HeLa cells and in tumorigenic segregants derived from nontumorigenic hybrids is not the result of a counterselection process against chemokine expression during long-term propagation of such cells under in vitro conditions, but can be directly correlated with an arising tumorigenic phenotype in vivo. If a sufficiently high number of injection sites inoculated with nonmalignant HeLa-fibroblast hybrids were challenged for growth in nude mice for longer periods of time (4 to 5 mo), rare tumorigenic segregants could be obtained. When monitoring MCP-1 expression within such nodules, transcription was either absent or only marginally detectable. Remarkably, the explanation of low-level MCP-1-expressing specimens in tissue culture revealed that the gene was no longer inducible by cytokine treatment. Moreover, the emergence of tumorigenic segregants can not only be correlated with a dysregulation in MCP-1 gene expression but also with the inability of TNF-α to suppress HPV-18 transcription, a property that previously characterized nonmalignant hybrids *(72)*. Outgrowing tumorigenic HeLa-fibroblast hybrids in nude mice may therefore represent a valid animal system to investigate immunologic escape processes from growth-inhibitory cytokines in greater detail.

3.2. Transcriptional Regulation of the MCP-1 Gene in HPV-Positive Cells

The JE gene, a rodent homolog of human MCP-1, was initially isolated as an immediate-early gene, which can be stimulated at the level of initiation of transcription by the platelet-derived growth factor *(75)*. Analyzing its transcriptional regulation in greater detail, it became clear that JE (MCP-1) expression can not only be induced by particular cytokines such as TNF-α *(13,76)*, TGF-β *(77)*, or IFN-γ *(76)*, but is also negatively controlled by antiinflammatory acting glucocorticoids *(78)* or even by hormones such as estrogen *(79)*.

One transcription factor that acts as a key regulator in a variety of immunologic control processes is NF-κB *(80,81)*. Cytokine-induced NF-κB activation is thought to be mediated by the generation of reactive oxygen intermediates (ROIs) *(82,83)*, which act as important second messengers to transduce the signal from the cell surface to the nucleus *(84)*. Intracellular ROIs trigger the phosphorylation and the release of the cytoplasmic inhibitor IκB, which leads to the translocation of the DNA-binding and *trans*-activating subunits p50/p65 of NF-κB to the nucleus *(85)*. The induction of a prooxidant state on cytokine binding to its receptor can be efficiently blocked by antioxidative drugs such as *N*-acetyl-L-cysteine or pyrrolidine-dithio-carbamate (PDTC) *(86)*.

The complete abrogation of TNF-α-mediated MCP-1 induction after pretreating cells with PDTC *(13)* suggests that NF-κB also plays a function in MCP-1 activation in nonmalignant HeLa-fibroblast hybrids. A direct role of NF-κB was further substantiated by band-shift and DNAse I footprinting analyses in other cell types *(87,88,89)*, leading to the identification of several distinct NF-κB binding sites within the 5′-regulatory region of both the rodent JE *(88)* and the human MCP-1 gene *(89)*.

The fact that HeLa cells contain functionally active forms of NF-κB *(81,91)* but lack detectable MCP-1 transcription is intriguing with respect to its reexpression in hybrid cells. NF-κB actually describes a family of transcription factors, which can form different sets of homo- or heterodimers via a conserved region called the *rel*-domain *(92)*.

Depending on their composition, these factors can either induce or suppress the expression of NF-κB-responsive genes *(80,91)*. As already shown for cells infected with adenovirus (Ad) types 5 and 12, modulation of *rel*-related protein function can affect the expression of genes involved in immune surveillance *(92)*. For example, disturbance of p50 subunit synthesis reduces the expression of the major histocompatibility complex class I in tumorigenic Ad 12, but not in nontumorigenic Ad 5–transformed rodent cells *(92)*. Whether an altered composition of NF-κB may also account for the differential regulation of MCP-1 in our somatic cell hybrid system is currently under investigation.

In this context, it is noteworthy that MCP-1 expression is not irreversibly downregulated in HeLa cells but can be reexpressed under certain experimental conditions. It has been demonstrated that viral transactivators such as the Tat protein of the human immunodeficiency virus can potentiate TNF-α-induced cytotoxicity. Increased TNF-α sensitivity was correlated with an enhanced binding affinity of NF-κB to its cognate recognition sequence in gel-retardation assays *(93)*. In stably transfected Tat-expressing HeLa cells, MCP-1 gene expression becomes reinducible after TNF-α or IL-1 treatment (P. Flurer and T. Rösl, unpublished results). Hence, comparative *in situ* hybridization studies on tissue sections of different progression states might provide insight on whether changes of NF-κB can be correlated with the absence of MCP-1 expression and other immunologic escape effects during the development of cervical cancer.

Another area of interest concerns the influence of viral oncogenes on chemokine expression. Since MCP-1 transcription is readily inducible by cytokines in both HPV-negative primary human keratinocytes *(75)* and human fibroblasts *(76)*, the question emerges, whether viral oncogenes such as E6/E7 can directly interfere with the JE (MCP-1) transcription in cervical carcinoma cells and can this be compensated by genetic complementation in somatic cell hybrids. Dysregulation of a chemokine by a viral oncogene is not without precedent. It has been reported that the E1a oncoprotein of Ad strongly reduces JE gene expression in transformed rodent cells. The decline was not caused by mRNA labilization nor by another posttranscriptional mechanism, but was found to be mediated at the level of initiation of transcription *(94)*. The region responsible for this suppression effect is confined to the N-terminal part of the protein, which is in close proximity to a stretch of amino acids conserved in all Ad E1a proteins *(95)*. Since the E7 oncoproteins from high-risk HPV types share homology to this specific region *(96,97)*, it is conceivable that a similar mechanism may influence MCP-1 transcription in HPV-positive cells. Cotransfection studies of MCP-1 promoter constructs together with HPV-16/-18 E7 expression vectors should provide an answer to this question.

3.3. MCP-1 Expression in Human Biopsy Specimens

The in vivo role of MCP-1 expression in the development of HPV-associated CIN and cervical carcinoma by RNA/RNA *in situ* hybridization has been examined in two independent studies *(98,99)*. Whereas Riethdorf and colleagues *(99)* report the detection of MCP-1 mRNA expression in normal, dysplastic, and neoplastic epithelia of the cervix uteri, our own hybridization and immunohistochemical experiments *(98)* revealed major differences in the expression pattern at different stages of disease pro-

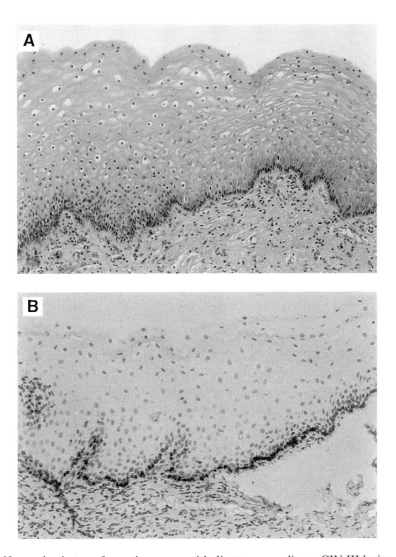

Fig. 3. Hyperplastic transformation zone epithelium surrounding a CIN III lesion. **(A)** Foci of moderate epithelial hyperplasia with parakeratosis in adjacent and distant areas at the edge of a CIN III lesion. Paraffin section, H&E staining; magnification × 200. **(B)** Detection of abundant MCP-1 expression over the basal cell layer of the focal hyperplastic epithelium after *in situ* hybridization with a ^{35}S-labeled antisense RNA. Paraffin section; magnification × 200. (Reproduced with permission from H. Kühne-Heid and R. Gillitzer.) **(C)** Pronounced infiltration of mononuclear cells (macrophages) in the subepithelial connective tissue. Immunostaining with a monoclonal CD68 antibody. Paraffin section; magnification × 200.

gression. Although normal basal keratinocyte layer normally lacks MCP-1 expression, RNA/RNA *in situ* hybridization showed abundant MCP-1-specific transcription signals in biopsies of cervical epithelium with erosive cervicitis, HPV-infected acanthotic but benign epithelium of the cervix, and over endothelial cells of capillaries and venules in the underlying stroma (Fig. 3A,B). MCP-1 hybridization signals did not consistently

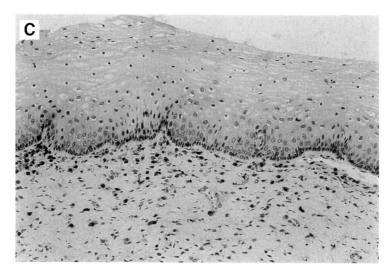

Fig. 3. (*continued*)

occur along the full length of squamous epithelium, but were preferentially observed at the metaplastic squamous epithelium of the transformation zone, where HPV infection seems to occur primarily (Fig. 3A,B). Here, MCP-1 transcripts were found abundantly in proliferating basal keratinocytes but not in suprabasal cell layers. The expression of MCP-1 mRNA was not always related to the presence of mononuclear infiltrates, but in some cases MCP-1 expression signals were accompanied by a characteristic pronounced infiltrate at the epidermo-mesenchymal junction (Fig. 3C). Langerhans cells within the epithelium, which also derive from the monocyte/macrophage cell lineage, were only scarcely detectable throughout the cervix.

In all biopsies of HPV-positive high-grade cervical dysplastic lesions, especially in CIN III, MCP-1 mRNA-expressing cells were not detectable at all, independently of whether the lesion was found in the ectocervix or the endocervical glands (Fig. 4A,B). On the other hand, although we also had HPV-positive squamous cell carcinomas of the cervix lacking MCP-1 expression, there were also cases that revealed scattered MCP-1-expressing cells at the invasion front of the tumor toward the fibromuscular septum. Correlating with MCP-1 mRNA expression, CD68-positive macrophages were detected around the tumor cell complexes.

The loss of MCP-1 expression in the progression of a hyperplastic lesion to low- and high-grade CIN lesions may partially account for the reduction of mononuclear cells during progression to cervical cancer *(20,21,53)*. On the other hand, we have no explanation for the occasional focal reexpression of the MCP-1 gene in the tumor tissue of cervical carcinomas with disintegration of the basal epithelial membrane. However, as already outlined, MCP-1 suppression in cervical carcinoma cells is not an irreversible phenomenon; it can be reactivated by certain external stimuli. We still know very little about the role of MCP-1 and other chemokines during HPV-linked carcinogenesis. Therefore, *in situ* hybridization studies on biopsy material using labeled probes from other chemokines should also provide a better understanding of this kind of immunologic defense mechanism during the development of cervical cancer.

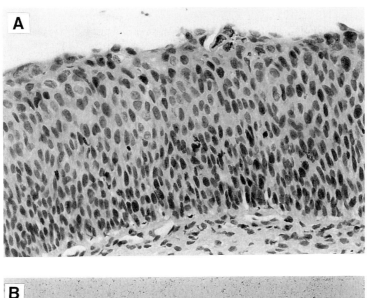

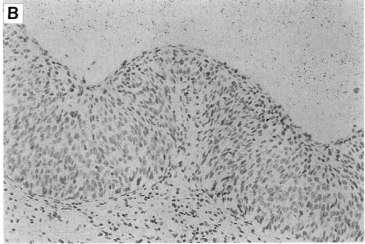

Fig. 4. High-grade squamous intraepithelial lesion (CIN III). **(A)** CIN III lesion with a full thickness replacement of the cervical epithelium by undifferentiated parabasal cells. Paraffin section, H&E staining; magnification × 400. **(B)** Lack of MCP-1 expression in CIN III lesions. *In situ* hybridization was carried out with a ^{35}S-labeled antisense RNA. Paraffin section; magnification × 200. (Reproduced with permission from H. Kühne-Heid and R. Gillitzer.)

ACKNOWLEDGMENTS

The authors are grateful to Dr. H. Kühne-Heid and to Dr. R. Gillitzer for their help with the *in situ* hybridization and immunohistologic staining methods of the biopsy material. The technical assistance of Atija Toksoy is also appreciated.

REFERENCES

1. zur Hausen, H. 1991. Viruses in human cancer. *Science* **254:** 1167–1173.
2. zur Hausen, H. 1991. Human papillomaviruses in the pathogenesis of anogenital cancer. *Virology* **184:** 9–13.

3. Dürst, M., R. T. Petrussevska, P. Boukamp, N. E. Fusenig, and L. Gissmann. 1987. Molecular and cytogenetic analysis of immortalized human primary keratinoytes obtained after transfection with human papillomavirus 16 DNA. *Oncogene* **1:** 251–256.

4. Kaur, P., and J. K. McDougall. 1989. HPV-18 immortalization of human keratinocytes. *Virology* **173:** 302–310.

5. zur Hausen, H. 1994. Disrupted dichotomous intracellular control of human papillomavirus infection in cancer of the cervix. *Lancet* **343:** 955–957.

6. zur Hausen, H. 1996. Papillomavirus infections—a major cause of human cancers. *BBA* **1288:** 55–78.

7. zur Hausen, H. 1986. Intracellular surveillance of persisting viral infections: human genital cancer results from deficient cellular control of papillomavirus gene expression. *Lancet* **ii:** 489–491.

8. Altmann, A., I. Jochmus, and F. Rösl. 1994. Intra- and extracellular control mechanisms of HPV infection. *Intervirology* **37:** 180–188.

9. Schneider, A., and L. A. Koutsky. 1992. Natural history and epidemiological features of genital HPV infection, in *The Epidemiology of Human Papillomavirus and Cervical Cancer* (N. Munoz, F. X. Borch, K. V. Shah, and A. Mekers, eds.), International Agency for Research on Cancer, pp. 25–52.

10. Balkwill, F. R., and F. Burke. 1989. The cytokine network. *Immunol. Today* **10:** 299–304.

11. Braun, L., M. Dürst, R. Mikumo, and P. Grupposo. 1990. Differential response of nontumorigenic and tumorigenic human papillomavirus type 16 positive epithelial cells to transforming growth factor β. *Cancer Res.* **50:** 7324–7332.

12. Malejczyk, J., M. Malejczyk, A. Köck, A. Urbanski, S. Majewski, N. Hunzelmann, S. Jablonska, G. Orth, and T. A. Luger. 1992. Autocrine growth limitation of human papillomavirus type 16-harboring keratinocytes by constitutively released tumor necrosis factor-α. *J. Immunol.* **149:** 2702–2708.

13. Rösl, F., M. Lengert, J. Albrecht, K. Kleine, R. Zawatzky, B. Schraven, and H. zur Hausen. 1994. Differential regulation of the JE gene encoding the monocyte chemoattractant protein (MCP-1) in cervical carcinoma cells and derived hybrids. *J. Virol.* **68:** 2142–2150.

14. Woodworth, C. D., V. Notario, and J. A. DiPaolo. 1990. Transforming growth factor beta 1 and 2 transcriptionally regulate human papillomavirus (HPV) type 16 early gene expression in HPV-immortalized human genital epithelial cells. *J. Virol.* **64:** 4767–4775.

15. Crook, C. P., J. P. Morgenstern, L. Crawford, and L. Banks. 1989. Continued expression of HPV 16 E7 protein is required for maintenance of the transformed phenotype of cells cotransformed by HPV 16 plus EJ-ras. *EMBO J.* **8:** 513–519.

16. von Knebel Doeberitz, M., T. Oltersdorf, E. Schwarz, and L. Gissmann. 1988. Correlation of modified human papillomavirus early gene expression with altered growth properties in C4-1 cervical carcinoma cells. *Cancer Res.* **48:** 3780–3786.

17. zur Hausen, H., and F. Rösl. 1994. *Pathogenesis of Cancer of the Cervix.* Cold Spring Harbor Symposia on Quantitative Biology, vol. **LIX.** Cold Spring Harbor Laboratory Press, NY, pp. 623–628.

18. Mantovani, A., B. Bottazzi, F. Colotta, S. Sozzani, and L. Ruco. 1992. The origin and function of tumor-associated macrophages. *Immunol. Today* **13:** 265–270.

19. Miller, M. D., and M. S. Krangel. 1992. Biology and biochemistry of the chemokines: a family of chemotactic and inflammatory cytokines. *Crit. Rev. Immunol.* **12:** 17–46.

20. Hughes, R. G., M. Norval, and S. E. M. Howie. 1988. Expression of major histocompatibility class II antigens by Langerhans' cells in cervical intraepithelial neoplasia. *J. Clin. Pathol.* **41:** 253–259.

21. Spinillo, A., P. Tenti, R. Zappatore, F. De Seta, E. Silini, and S. Guaschino. 1993. Langerhans' cell counts and cervical intraepithelial neoplasia in women with human immunodeficiency virus infection. *Gyn. Oncol.* **48:** 210–213.

22. Viac, J., I. Guerin-Reverchon, Y. Chardonnet, and A. Bremond. 1990. Langerhans cells and epithelial cell modifications in cervical intraepithelial neoplasia: correlation with human papillomavirus infection. *Immunobiology* **180:** 328–338.

23. de Villiers, E. M. 1989. Heterogeneity of the human papillomavirus group. *J. Virol.* **63:** 4898–4903.

24. Stoler, M. H., S. M. Wolinsky, A. Whitbeck, T. S. Broker, and L. T. Chow. 1989. Differentiation-linked human papillomavirus types 6 and 11 transcription in genital condylomata revealed by in situ hybridization with message-specific RNA probes. *Virology* **172:** 331–340.

25. Crum, C. P., G. Nuovo, D. Friedman, and S. J. Silverstein. 1988. Accumulation of RNA homologous to human papillomavirus type 16 opoen reading frames in genital precancers. *J. Virol.* **62:** 84–90.

26. Münger, K., W. C. Phelps, V. Bubb, P. M. Howley, and R. Schlegel. 1989. The E6 and E7 genes of the human papillomavirus type 16 are necessary and sufficient for transformation of primary human keratinocytes. *J. Virol.* **63:** 4417–4423.

27. Hurlin, P. J., P. Kaur, P. P. Smith, N. Perez-Reyes, R. A. Blanton, and J. K. McDougall. 1991. Progression of human papillomavirus type 18-immortalized human keratinocytes to a malignant phenotype. *Proc. Natl. Acad. Sci. USA* **88:**570–574.

28. von Knebel Doeberitz, M., C. Rittmüller, H. zur Hausen, and M. Dürst. 1992. Inhibition of tumorigenicity of cervical cancer cells in nude mice by HPV E6–E7 anti-sense RNA. *Int. J. Cancer* **51:** 831–834.

29. Cullen, A. P., R. Reid, M. Campion, and A. T. Lörinez. 1991. Analysis of the physical state of different human papillomavirus DNAs in intraepithelial and invasive cervical neoplasm. *J. Virol.* **65:** 606–612.

30. Bernard, B. A., C. Bailly, M.-C. Lenoir, M. Darmon, F. Thierry, and M. Yaniv. 1989. The human papillomavirus type 18 (HPV 18) E2 gene product is a repressor of the HPV 18 regulatory region in human keratinocytes. *J. Virol.* **63:** 4317–4324.

31. Daniel, B., G. Mukherjee, L. Seshadri, E. Vallikad, and S. Krishna. 1995. Changes in the physical state and expression of human papillomavirus type 16 in the progression of cervical intraepithelial neoplasia lesion analysed by PCR. *J. Gen. Virol.* **76:** 2589–2593.

32. Jeon, S., and P. F. Lambert. 1995. Integration of human papillomavirus type 16 into the human genome leads to increased stability of E6 and E7 mRNAs: implications for cervical carcinogenesis. *Proc. Natl. Acad. Sci. USA* **92:** 1654–1658.

33. Sang, B.-C., and M. S. Barbosa. 1992. Increased E6/E7 transcription in HPV 18 immortalized human keratinocytes results from inactivation of E2 and additional cellular events. *Virology* **189:** 448–455.

34. de Villiers, E.-M., D. Wagner, A. Schneider, H. Wesch, H. Miklaw, J. Wahrendorf, U. Papendick, and H. zur Hausen. 1992. Human papillomavirus DNA in women without and with cytological abnormalities: results of a five-year follow-up study. *Gynecol. Oncol.* **44:** 33–39.

35. Desaintes, C., S. Hallez, P. van Alphen, and A. Burny. 1992. Transcriptional activation of several heterologous promoters by E6 protein of human papillomavirus type 16. *J. Virol.* **66:** 325–333.

36. Scheffner, M., B. A. Werness, J. M. Huibregtse, A. J. Levine, and P. M. Howley. 1990. The E6 oncoprotein encoded by human papillomavirus types 16 and 18 promotes the degradation of p53. *Cell* **63:** 1129–1136.

37. Werness, B. A., A. Levine, and P. M. Howley. 1990. Association of human papillomavirus types 16 and 18 E6 proteins with p53. *Science* **248:** 76–79.

38. Lane, D. P. 1994. The regulation of p53 function. *Int. J. Cancer* **57:** 623–627.

39. Dyson, N., P. M. Howley, K. Münger, and E. Harlow. 1989. The human papillomavirus-16 E7 oncoprotein is able to bind to the retinoblastoma gene product. *Science* **243:** 934–937.

40. McIntyre, M. C., M. N. Ruesch, and L. A. Laimins. 1996. Human papillomavirus E7 oncoproteins bind a single form of cyclin E in a complex with cdk2 and p107. *Virology* **215:** 73–82.

41. Melillo, R. M., K. Helin, D. R. Lowy, and J. T. Schiller. 1994. Positive and negative regulation of cell proliferation by E2F-1: influence of protein level and human papillomavirus oncoproteins. *Mol. Cell. Biol.* **14:** 8241–8249.

42. Hashida, T., and S. Yasumoto. 1991. Induction of chromosome abnormalities in mouse and human epidermal keratinocytes by the human papillomavirus type 16 E7 oncogene. *J. Gen. Virol.* **72:** 1569–1577.

43. Chen, T. M., G. Pecoraro, and V. Defendi. 1993. Genetic analysis of in vitro progression of human papillomavirus-transfected human cervical cells. *Cancer Res.* **53:** 1167–1171.

44. Pereira-Smith, O. M., and J. R. Smith. 1988. Genetic analysis of indefinite division in human cells: identification of four complementation groups. *Proc. Natl. Acad. Sci. USA* **85:** 6042–6045.

45. Stewart, N., and S. Bacchetti. 1991. Expression of SV 40 large T antigen, but not small T antigen, is required for the induction of chromosomal aberrations in transformed human cells. *Virology* **180:** 49–57.

46. Caporossi, D., and S. Bacchetti. 1990. Definition of adenovirus type 5 functions involved in the induction of chromosomal aberrations in human cells. *J. Gen. Virol.* **71:** 801–808.

47. Stanbridge, E. 1984. Genetic analysis of tumorigenicity in human cell hybrids. *Cancer Surv.* **3:** 335–350.

48. Srivatsan, E. S., B. C. Misra, M. Venugopalan, and S. P. Wilczynski. 1991. Loss of heterozygosity for alleles on chromosome 11 in cervical carcinoma. *Am. J. Hum. Genetics* **49:** 868–877.

49. Koi, M., H. Morita, H. Yamada, H. Satoh, J. K. Barrett, and M. Oshimura. 1989. Normal human chromosome 11 suppresses tumorigenicity of human cervical tumor cell line SiHa. *Mol. Carcinog.* **2:** 12–21.

50. Saxon, P. J., E. S. Srivatsan, and E. J. Stanbridge. 1986. Introduction of human chromosome 11 via microcell transfer controls tumorigenic expression of HeLa cells. *EMBO J.* **5:** 3461–3466.

51. Rösl, F., T. Achtstätter, T. Bauknecht, G. Futterman, K. J. Hutter, and H. zur Hausen. 1991. Extinction of the HPV 18 upstream regulatory region in cervical carcinoma cells after fusion with non-tumorigenic human keratinocytes under non-selective condition. *EMBO J.* **10:** 1337–1345.

52. Bosch, F. X., E. Schwarz, P. Boukamp, N. E. Fusenig, D. Bartsch, and H. zur Hausen. 1990. Suppression *in vivo* of human papillomavirus type 18 E6–E7 gene expression in non-tumorigenic HeLa-fibroblast hybrid cells. *J. Virol.* **64:** 4743–4754.

53. Tay, S. K., D. Jenkins, P. Maddox, N. Hogg, and A. Singer. 1987. Tissue macrophage response in human papillomavirus infection and cervical intraepithelial neoplasia. *Brit. J. Obstet. Gynaecol.* **94:** 1094–1097.

54. Rappolee, D. A., and Z. Werb. 1992. Macrophage-derived growth factors. *Curr. Top. Microbiol. and Immunol.* **181:** 87–140.

55. Nawa, A., Y. Nishiyama, N. Yamamoto, K. Maeno, S. Goto, and Y. Tooda. 1990. Selective suppression of human papillomavirus type 18 mRNA level in HeLa cells by interferon. *Biochem. Biophys. Res. Commun.* **170:** 793–799.

56. Kyo, S., M. Inoue, Y. Nishio, K. Nakanishi, S. Akira, H. Inoue, M. Yutsudo, O. Tanizawa, and A. Hakura. 1993. NF-IL-6 represses early gene expression of human papillomavirus type 16 through binding to the noncoding region. *J. Virol.* **67:** 1058–1066.

57. Majewski, S., J. Malejczyk, and S. Jablonska. 1996. The role of cytokines and other factors in HPV infection and HPV-associated tumors. *Papillomavirus Rep.* **7:** 143–155.

58. Shepard, H. M., and G. D. Lewis. 1988. Resistance of tumor cells to tumor necrosis factor. *J. Clin. Immunol.* **8:** 333–341.

59. Sugarman, B. J., B. B. Aggarwal, P. E. Hass, I. S. Figari, M. A. Palladino, and H. M. Shepard. 1985. Recombinant human tumor necrosis factor-α: effects on proliferation of normal and transformed cells in vitro. *Science* **239:** 943–945.

60. Rösl, F., B. C. Das, M. Lengert, K. Geletneky, and H. zur Hausen. 1997. Antioxidant-induced changes of the AP-1 transcription complex are paralleled by a selective suppression of human papillomavirus transcription. *J. Virol.* **71:** 362–370.

61. Rollins, B. J., P. Stier, T. Ernst, and G. G. Wong. 1989. The human homolog of the JE gene encodes a monocyte secretory protein. *Mol. Cell. Biol.* **9:** 4687–4695.

62. Rollins, B. J. 1991. JE/MCP-1: an early-response gene encodes a monocyte-specific cytokine. *Cancer Cells* **3:** 517–524.

63. Celada, A., and C. Nathan. 1994. Macrophage activation revisited. *Immunol. Today* **15:** 100–103.

64. Colotta, F., A. Borre, J. M. Wang, M. Tattanelli, F. Maddalena, N. Polentarutti, G. Peri, and A. Mantovani. 1992. Expression of a monocyte chemotactic cytokine by human mononuclear phagocytes. *J. Immunol.* **148:** 760–765.

65. Jiang, Y., D. I. Beller, G. Frendl, and D. T. Graves. 1992. Monocyte chemoattractant protein-1 regulates adhesion molecule expression and cytokine production in human monocytes. *J. Immunol.* **148:** 2423–2428.

66. Hagari, Y., L. R. Budgeon, M. D. Pickel, and J. W. Kreider. 1995. Association of tumor necrosis factor-α gene expression and apoptotic cell death with regression of Shope papillomas. *J. Invest. Dermatol.* **104:** 526–529.

67. Rollins, B. J., and M. E. Sunday. 1991. Suppression of tumor formation in vivo by expression of the JE gene in malignant cells. *Mol. Cell. Biol.* **11:** 3125–3131.

68. Huang, S., K. Xie, R. K. Singh, M. Gutman, and M. Bar-Eli. 1995. Suppression of tumor growth and metastasis of murine renal adenocarcinoma by syngeneic fibroblasts genetically engineered to secrete the JE/MCP-1 cytokine. *J. Interferon Cytokine Res.* **15:** 655–665.

69. Huang, S., R. K. Singh, K. Xie, M. Gutman, K. K. Berry, C. D. Bucana, I. J. Fidler, and M. Bar-Eli. 1994. Expression of the JE/MCP-1 gene suppresses metastatic potential in murine colon carcinoma cells. *Cancer Immunol. Immunother.* **39:** 231–238.

70. Laning, J., H. Kawasaki, E. Tanaka, Y. Luo, and M. E. Dorf. 1994. Inhibition of in vivo growth by the β chemokine, TCA3. *J. Immunol.* **153:** 4625–4635.

71. Bottazzi, B., S. Walter, D. Govoni, F. Colotta, and A. Mantovani. 1992. Monocyte chemotactic cytokine gene transfer modulates macrophage infiltration, growth, and susceptibility to IL-2 therapy of a murine melanoma. *J. Immunol.* **148:** 1280–1285.

72. Kleine, K., G. König, J. Kreuzer, D. Komitowski, H. zur Hausen, and F. Rösl. 1995. The effect of the JE(MCP-1) gene, which encodes the monocyte chemoattractant protein-1 on the growth of HeLa cells and derived somatic cell hybrids in nude mice. *Mol. Carcinog.* **14:** 179–189.

73. Dürst, M., D. Gallahan, G. Jay, and J. S. Rhim. 1989. Glucocorticoid-enhanced neoplastic transformation of human keratinocytes by human papillomavirus type 16 and an activated ras oncogene. *Virology* **173:** 767–771.

74. Rollins, B. J., E. D. Morrison, and C. D. Stiles. 1988. Cloning and expression of JE, a gene inducible by platelet-derived growth factor and whose product has cytokine-like properties. *Proc. Natl. Acad. Sci. USA* **85:** 3738–3742.

75. Barker, J., V. Sarma, R. S. Mitra, V. M. Dixit, and B. J. Nickoloff. 1990. Marked synergism between tumor necrosis factor-α and interferon-γ in regulation of keratinocyte-derived adhesion molecules and chemotactic factors. *J. Clin. Invest.* **85:** 605–608.

76. Lee, T. H., G. W. Lee, E. B. Ziff, and J. Vilcek. 1990. Isolation and characterization of eight tumor necrosis factor-induced gene sequences from human fibroblasts. *Mol. Cell. Biol.* **10:** 1982–1988.

77. Hanazawa, S., A. Takeshita, Y. Tsukamoto, Y. Kawata, K. Takara, and S. Kitano. 1991.

Transforming-growth-factor-β induced gene expression of monocyte chemoattractant JE in mouse osteoblastic cells, MC3T3-E1. *Biochem. Biophys. Res. Commun.* **180:** 1130–1136.

78. Mukaida, N., C. C. O. Zachariae, G. L. Gusella, and K. Matsushima. 1991. Dexamethasone inhibits the induction of monocyte chemotactic-activating factor production by IL-1 or tumor necrosis factor. *J. Immunol.* **146:** 1212–1215.

79. Frazier-Jessen, M. R., and E. J. Kovacs. 1995. Estrogen modulation of JE/monocyte chemoattractant protein-1 mRNA expression in murine macrophages. *J. Immunol.* **154:** 1838–1845.

80. Baeuerle, P. A., and D. Baltimore. 1991. The physiology of the NF-κB transcription factor, in *Hormonal Control of Gene Expression* (Cohen, P., and J. G. Foulkes, eds.), Biomedical, Elsevier, Amsterdam, Holland.

81. Goossens, V., J. Grooten, K. deVos, and W. Fiers. 1995. Direct evidence for tumor necrosis factor-induced mitochondrial reactive oxygen intermediates and their involvement in cytotoxicity. *Proc. Natl. Acad. Sci. USA* **92:** 8115–8119.

82. Meier, B., H. H. Radeke, S. Selle, M. Younes, H. Sies, K. Resch, and G. G. Habermehl. 1989. Human fibroblasts release reactive oxygen species in response to interleukin-1 or tumor necrosis factor-α. *Biochem. J.* **263:** 539–545.

83. Meyer, M., R. Schreck, and P. A. Baeuerle. 1993. H_2O_2 and antioxidants have opposite effects on activation of NF-κB and AP-1 in intact cells: AP-1 as secondary antioxidant-responsive factor. *EMBO J.* **12:** 2005–2015.

84. Beg, A. A., T. S. Finco, P. V. Nantermet, and A. S. Baldwin. 1993. Tumor necrosis factor and interleukin-1 lead to phosphorylation and loss of IκBα: a mechanism for NF-κB activation. *Mol. Cell. Biol.* **13:** 3301–3310.

85. Schreck, R., P. Rieber, and P. A. Baeuerle. 1991. Reactive oxygen intermediates as apparently widely used messengers in the activation of the NF-κB transcription factor and HIV-1. *EMBO J.* **10:** 2247–2258.

86. Schreck, R., B. Meier, D. N. Männel, W. Dröge, and P. W. Baeuerle. 1992. Dithiocarbamates as potent inhibitors of nuclear factor κB activation in intact cells. *J. Exp. Med.* **175:** 1181–1194.

87. Freter, R. R., J. A. Alberta, K. K. Lam, and C. D. Stiles. 1995. A new platelet-derived growth factor-regulated genomic element which binds a serine/threonine phosphoprotein mediates induction of the slow immediate-early gene MCP-1. *Mol. Cell. Biol.* **15:** 315–325.

88. Ping, D., P. L. Jones, and J. M. Boss. 1996. TNF regulates the in vivo occupancy of both distal and proximal regulatory regions of the MCP-1/JE gene. *Immunity* **4:** 455–469.

89. Ueda, A., K. Okuda, S. Ohno, A. Shirai, T. Igarashi, K. Matsunaga, J. Fukushima, S. Kawamoto, Y. Ishigatsubo, and T. Okobo. 1994. NF-κB and Sp1 regulate transcription of the human monocyte chemoattractant protein-1 gene. *J. Immunol.* **153:** 2052–2063.

90. Baeuerle, P. A., and D. Baltimore. 1988. Activation of DNA binding activity in an apparent cytoplasmic precursor of the NF-κB transcription factor. *Cell* **53:** 211–217.

91. Thanos, D., and T. Maniatis. 1995. NF-κB: a lesson in family values. *Cell* **80:** 529–533.

92. Schouten, G. J., A. J. van der Eb, and A. Zantema. 1995. Downregulation of MHC class I expression due to interference with p105-NF-κB1 processing by Ad12E1A. *EMBO J.* **14:** 1498–1507.

93. Westendorp, M. O., V. A. Shatrov, K. Schulze-Osthoff, R. Frank, M. Kraft, M. Los, P. H. Krammer, W. Dröge, and V. Lehmann. 1995. HIV-1 Tat potentiates TNF-induced NF-kappa B activation and cytotoxicity by altering the cellular redox state. *EMBO J.* **14:** 546–554.

94. Timmers, H. T. M., H. van Dam, G. J. Pronk, J. L. Bos, and A. J. van der Eb. 1989. Adenovirus E1a represses transcription of the JE gene. *J. Virol.* **63:** 1470–1473.

95. Dorsman, J. C., B. M. Hagmeyer, J. Veenstra, P. Elfferich, N. Nabben, A. Zantema, and A. J. van der Eb. 1995. The N-terminal region of the adenovirus type 5 E1A protein can repress expression of cellular genes via two distinct but overlapping domains. *J. Virol.* **69:** 2962–2967.

96. Brokaw, J. L., C. L. Yee, and K. Münger. 1994. A mutational analysis of the amino terminal domain of the human papillomavirus type 16 E7 oncoprotein. *Virology* **205:** 603–607.

97. Phelps, W. C., C. L. Lee, K. Münger, and P. M. Howley. 1988. The human papillomavirus type 16 E7 gene encodes transactivation and transformation functions similar to those of adenovirus E1a. *Cell* **53:** 539–547.

98. Kleine-Lowinski, K., R. Gillitzer, H. Kühne-Heid, and F. Rösl. 1999. Monocyte chemoattractant protein-1 (MCP-1) gene expression in cervical intraepithelial neoplasia and cervical carcinomas. *Int. J. Cancer,* in press.

99. Riethdorf, L., S. Riethdorf, K. Gützlaff, F. Prall, and T. Löning. 1996. Differential expression of the monocyte chemoattractant protein-1 in human papillomavirus-16 infected squamous intraepithelial lesions and squamous cell carcinomas of the cervix uteri. *Am. J. Pathol.* **149:** 1469–1476.

13

Chemokines and Central Nervous System Malignancies

Teizo Yoshimura and Jun-ichi Kuratsu

1. INTRODUCTION

Tumors in the central nervous system (CNS) arise from different cell components of the CNS and are classified as shown in Table 1 (see also ref. *1*). It is well known that the tumors in the CNS, especially glioma, produce various cytokines including interleukins (ILs), tumor necrosis factor-α (TNF-α), and colony-stimulating factors [recently reviewed by van Meir *(2)*]. Although the significance of cytokine production by the tumors may not be biologically clear, these cytokines could affect the biology of the tumors.

The infiltration of macrophages into certain types of tumors (tumor-associated macrophages [TAMs]) is an established fact *(3,4)*. TAMs can be recruited by chemoattractants produced by host cells or tumor cells (*see* Chapters 3 and 6). Tumors that arise in the CNS, such as malignant glioma or meningioma, are often infiltrated by macrophages. The infiltration of macrophages is one of the histologic characteristics of malignant glioma. In 1989 we succeeded in purifying a chemoattractant for human monocytes from the culture supernatant of a human malignant glioma cell line and subsequently cloned the cDNA *(5–8)*. This chemoattractant is now known as monocyte chemoattractant protein-1 (MCP-1), the human orthologue of the product of the mouse gene, *JE (9)*. MCP-1 is also identical to previously reported factors such as lymphocyte-derived chemotactic factor (LDCF), smooth muscle cell–derived chemotactic factor, and tumor-derived chemotactic factor, and also to monocyte chemotactic and activating factor *(8)*. After the discovery of MCP-1 in human malignant glioma cell lines, we continued our investigation on the roles of MCP-1 in the recruitment of TAM into malignant glioma. In this chapter, we present our data on MCP-1 production by malignant glioma and meningioma. We also introduce data on the production of another chemokine, IL-8, by malignant glioma and discuss the possible effects of these chemokines on tumor biology.

2. MCP-1 AND CNS MALIGNANCIES

2.1. Identification, Purification, and Cloning of MCP-1 from Malignant Glioma Cells

Malignant glioma is of astrocytic origin and is the second most common brain tumor in humans *(10)*. One of the histopathologic characteristics of malignant glioma is the

From: *Chemokines and Cancer*
Edited by: B. J. Rollins © Humana Press Inc., Totowa, NJ

Table 1
Histologic Typing of CNS Tumors[a]

1. Tumors of neuroepithelial tissues
    1.1. Astrocytic tumors
    1.2. Oligodendroglial tumors
    1.3. Ependymal tumors
    1.4. Mixed gliomas
    1.5. Choroid plexus tumors
    1.6. Neuroepithelial tumors of uncertain origin
    1.7. Neuronal and mixed neuronal-glial tumors
    1.8. Pineal parenchymal tumors
    1.9. Embryonal tumors
2. Tumors of cranial and spinal nerves
3. Tumors of the meninges
4. Lymphomas and hemopoietic neoplasms
5. Germ cell tumors
6. Cysts and tumor-like lesions
7. Tumors of the sellar region
8. Local extensions from regional tumors
9. Metastatic tumors
10. Unclassified tumors

[a]Modified from ref. *1*.

infiltration of TAMs *(11–13)*. To account for the infiltration of TAMs into malignant glioma, we postulated that malignant glioma cells produced a chemoattractant that attracted blood monocytes.

Several human malignant glioma cell lines produced monocyte chemotactic activity (MCA), which we called glioma-derived monocyte chemotactic factor (GDCF) *(5)*. Among the cell lines, U-105MG cells produced the largest amount of MCA. This activity was eluted around 17 kDa from a gel-filtration column, which was similar to the molecular mass of MCA derived from lipopolysaccharide- or phytohemagglutinin (PHA)-stimulated peripheral blood mononuclear cells (PBMCs) *(14)*. Two forms of GDCF were subsequently purified from serum-free U-105MG culture fluid in three steps: column chromatography on orange-A agarose, carboxymethyl high-performance liquid chromatography (HPLC), and reversed phase-HPLC. The cation exchange column divided the MCA into two well-separated peaks. On sodium dodecyl sulfate-polyacrylamide gel electrophoresis (SDS-PAGE) gels, they migrated as 15- and 13-kDa proteins (GDCF-1 and -2) (Fig. 1). GDCFs were indistinguishable from LDCF-1 and -2 isolated from the culture fluid of PHA-stimulated human PBMCs. The cDNA encoding MCP-1 was later cloned from a cDNA library constructed from U-105MG cells. The amino acid sequence of GDCF-2 was completely analyzed *(15)*. The two GDCFs/LDCFs represent a single gene product, and thus the difference between GDCF-1/LDCF-1 and GDCF-2/LDCF-2 is owing to a posttranslational modification. A generic name, MCP-1, is now used for the protein. The protein identical to MCP-1 was purified from other cell sources by various investigators *(8,9)*.

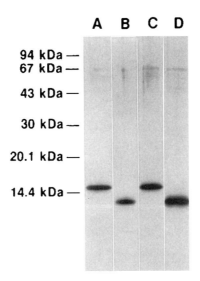

Fig. 1. SDS-PAGE of GDCF-1 and -2 purified from the culture supernatant of U-105MG human malignant glioma cell cells. GDCF-1 and -2 **(C,D)** were identical to LDCF-1 and -2 **(A,B)** purified from the culture supernatant of PHA-stimulated PBMCs *(6,14)*.

MCP-1 attracts 30–40% of input human blood monocytes in chemotaxis chambers in vitro. The MCA was also shown in vivo by expressing MCP-1 in transgenic mice and directly injecting recombinant MCP-1 into the skin of animals *(16–21)*. Despite the existence of redundant monocyte chemotactic chemokines, MCP-1 appears to play a major role in the recruitment of monocytes in vivo *(22)*. MCP-1 also attracts T-cells both in vitro and in vivo *(23,24)*. However, MCP-1 does not attract tissue macrophages such as peritoneal resident macrophages or neutrophils in vitro and in vivo.

2.2. Production of MCP-1 by Malignant Glioma Cell Lines In Vitro

A number of malignant glioma cell lines investigated to date express MCP-1 mRNA or produce MCP-1 to some degree in the absence of stimulus (Fig. 2) *(25–27)*. The basal level expression of MCP-1 mRNA or production of MCP-1 protein can be significantly enhanced by stimulating the cells with different cytokines such as IL-1, TNF-α, platelet-derived growth factor (PDGF), or interferons *(28)*.

The mechanisms of the human *MCP-1* gene transcription were investigated in a malignant glioma cell line as well as other cell lines *(29,30)*. In A172 cells, an Sp1 site (GC-box) located between –64 and –59 in the proximal 5′-flanking region of the gene was responsible for basal transcription, whereas an NF-κB site located between –2612 and –2603 in the distal region (A2 site) was responsible for the enhanced *MCP-1* gene transcription induced by IL-1β, TNF-α, or PMA. Recently, we have shown that another NF-κB site (A1 site) located between –2640 and –2632, upstream of the A2 site, cooperates with the A2 site, and that the binding of NF-κB/Rel protein dimers such as $(p65)_2$ and/or c-Rel/p65, but not p50/p65, c-Rel/p50, or $(p50)_2$, to both A1 and A2 sites selectively enhances the transcription of this gene in different types of cells, including A172 cells *(30)*. In addition to the enhanced *MCP-1* gene transcription after stimula-

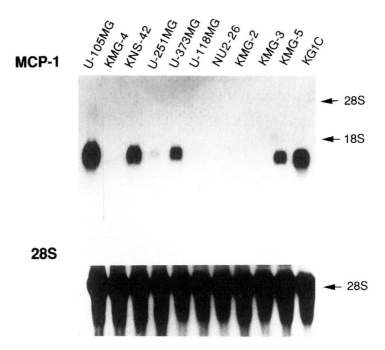

Fig. 2. Expression of MCP-1 mRNA in various human glioma cell lines. MCP-1 mRNA was detected in 6 of 11 cell lines examined by Northern blot analysis *(26)*. Arrows show the position of 28S and 18S rRNA.

tion, prolonged MCP-1 mRNA stability is also responsible for the elevated MCP-1 mRNA expression by stimulated glioma cells *(25)*. In unstimulated U-373MG cells, the half-life of MCP-1 mRNA was approx 6 h. By contrast, the half-life of MCP-1 mRNA was greatly prolonged in IL-1-stimulated U-373MG cells. A protein synthesis inhibitor, cycloheximide, also caused elevated MCP-1 mRNA expression in both unstimulated and IL-1-stimulated U-373MG cells. Thus, elevated MCP-1 mRNA expression in malignant glioma cell lines is owing to the enhanced *MCP-1* gene transcription and prolonged MCP-1 mRNA stability.

2.3. Production of MCP-1 by Malignant Glioma In Vivo

MCP-1 mRNA expression and production were investigated by using tumor specimens from malignant glioma patients *(26,27)*. In our study, MCP-1 mRNA was detected in all of eight tumor specimens by Northern blot analysis (Fig. 3). Both MCP-1 mRNA and protein were found predominantly in large glioma cells with pleomorphic nuclei, but not in the areas of small glioma cells, by *in situ* hybridization and immunohistochemistry. Vascular endothelium in the glioma tissues was also weakly stained positively by immunohistochemistry. Adjacent brain tissue did not show a significant level of MCP-1 mRNA or protein. Infiltration of macrophages into the glioma tissues was also detected by immunohistochemistry with an antimacrophage antibody, and the degree of macrophage infiltration correlated with the level of MCP-1 expression. This study suggested that glioma cell–derived MCP-1 induced the infiltration of macrophages into the glioma tissues *(26)*. Similar results were also reported by Desbaillets et al. *(27)*. In

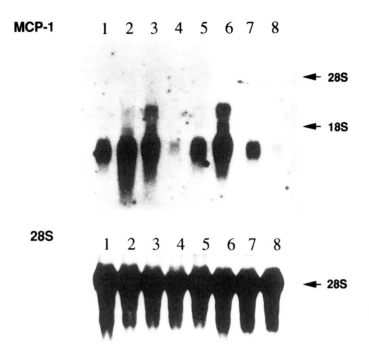

Fig. 3. Expression of MCP-1 mRNA in malignant gliomas *(26)*. MCP-1 mRNA was detected in all tumor specimens by Northern blot analysis. Arrows show the position of 28S and 18S rRNA.

their study, MCP-1 mRNA was detected in 17 of 17 glioblastomas, 3 of 6 anaplastic astrocytomas, and 6 of 6 low-grade astrocytomas by reverse transcriptase polymerase chain reaction and Northern blot analysis. MCP-1 mRNA was located in neoplastic astrocytes and endothelial cells by *in situ* hybridization.

The presence of MCP-1 in cerebrospinal fluid and cyst fluid was investigated. We measured MCP-1 concentrations in the cerebrospinal fluids from 19 patients with malignant gliomas, 9 patients with benign gliomas, and 7 patients with nontumor disorders of the CNS by sandwich enzyme-linked immunosorbent assay (ELISA) *(31)*. As shown in Figure 4, the MCP-1 concentrations in the cerebrospinal fluid samples from malignant glioma patients were significantly higher than those from patients with benign glioma or with no tumor. Furthermore, cerebrospinal fluid samples from malignant glioma patients with subarachnoid dissemination contained significantly higher amounts of MCP-1 than those from patients without dissemination. These results suggest that measuring MCP-1 concentration in cerebrospinal fluids by ELISA may lead to more accurate diagnosis of malignant glioma and the detection of subarachnoid dissemination of the tumor cells for prognosis and appropriate therapy. Cyst fluids from malignant glioma patients also contained high concentrations of MCP-1 *(27,31)*.

2.4. Production of MCP-1 by Meningioma

Meningiomas are the most common tumors in the CNS and contain large numbers of macrophages *(11,32)*. Wood and Morantz *(13)* reported that meningiomas had a

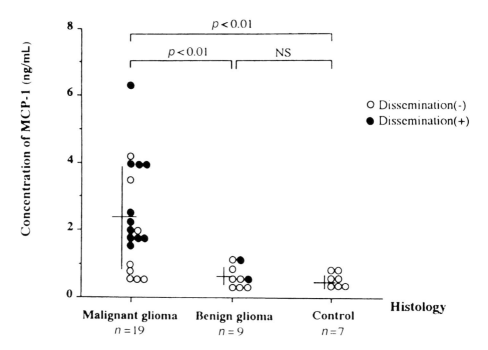

Fig. 4. MCP-1 concentrations in cerebrospinal fluids obtained from 19 patients with malignant glioma, 9 patients with benign glioma, and 7 patients with nontumor disorders of the CNS *(31)*. The data were analyzed by Student's *t*-test.

mean macrophage content of 42% (range 50–80%), whereas glioblastomas had 41% (range 5–78%). To investigate whether MCP-1 plays a role in the infiltration of macrophages into meningiomas, we investigated the expression and localization of MCP-1 in meningiomas by Northern blot analysis and immunohistochemistry *(33)*. MCP-1 mRNA was detected in 7 of 16 meningiomas obtained by surgery (Fig. 5). The intensity of the signal determined by densitometry differed among specimens by a factor of 10. MCP-1 protein was detected in the same 7 cases that were positive by Northern blot analysis and located in the cytoplasm of meningioma cells by immunohistochemistry. The degree of macrophage infiltration correlated with the level of MCP-1 expression. This study suggests that meningioma cell–derived MCP-1 induces monocyte infiltration into meningioma tissues.

PDGF has been shown to stimulate MCP-1 expression in fibroblasts *(34)*. Since meningioma cells secrete PDGF-like molecules that stimulate their own growth in an autocrine manner *(35)*, MCP-1 expression may be regulated by PDGF-like molecules produced by the meningioma. However, the mechanisms involved in MCP-1 mRNA expression and production by meningioma cells remain unknown.

Cerebral edema results from the disruption of the blood-brain barrier with increased vascular permeability and excessive interstitial fluid accumulation. Bruce et al. *(36)* reported that brain tumors produced and released a specific substance that evoked cerebral edema by increasing vascular permeability. In addition to its MCA, MCP-1 also induces the release of superoxide and lysosomal protease from monocytes *(8)*. Furthermore, MCP-1 is capable of directly inducing histamine release from basophils *(8)*. It is

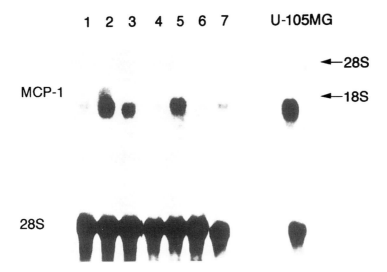

Fig. 5. Expression of MCP-1 in meningiomas *(33)*. Seven cases with positive expression of MCP-1 are shown. Total RNA from U-105MG cells was used as a positive control. The intensity of the signal determined by densitometry differed among specimens by a factor of 10. Arrows show the position of 28S and 18S rRNA.

known that some meningiomas are accompanied by perifocal edema. Shinonaga et al. *(37)* suggested that infiltrating macrophages may play an important role in the pathogenesis of peritumoral edema in meningiomas. Therefore, we speculated that the perifocal edema might be attributed to the release of vascular permeability factors released by macrophages accumulating in meningioma tissues. We examined the extent of peritumoral edema (1) as the ratio of the low-density area around the tumor to the enhanced high-density area by contrast-enhanced computed tomography scans, and (2) as the ratio of the high-intensity area around the tumor to the gadolinium-enhanced high-intensity area in T1-weighted images by T2-weighted images on magnetic resonance imaging. There was no significant correlation between the MCP-1 mRNA expression level and the extent of perifocal edema. Thus, the production of MCP-1 by meningioma cells does not appear directly related to the extent of perifocal edema in meningioma. Many other factors including tumor size, tumor location, and the extent of vascularity must be examined to understand the pathogenesis of perifocal edema in brain tumors.

2.5. Infiltration of Monocytes into Transplanted MCP-1-Producing Malignant Gliomas

Macrophages consist of heterogenous subpopulations differing in location, morphology, phenotype, and function *(38)*. The production of macrophage-specific monoclonal antibodies (MAb) with different specificities has made it possible to detect each macrophage subpopulation in normal tissues *(39)* and also in various diseased tissues *(40–42)*. Various mouse MAbs against rat macrophages such as RM-1, ED1, ED2, ED3, TRPM-3, and Ki-M2R are useful to discriminate macrophage subpopulations in rats. ED2 and Ki-M2R react with resident macrophage, whereas TRPM-3 reacts with monocyte-derived exudate macrophages and their activated forms *(43,44)*.

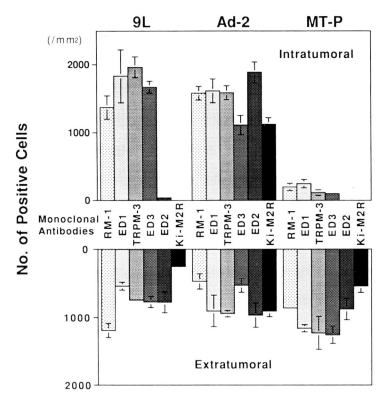

Fig. 6. Macrophage subpopulations infiltrating into 9L (MCP-1-producing rat gliosarcoma), Ad-2 (MCP-1-producing rat mammary carcinoma), and MT-P (MCP-1-nonproducing rat malignant fibrous histiocytoma) tumors *(45)*. Numbers of the cells positive for 6 anti-rat macrophage MAbs were counted inside and peripheral to the area of each tumor. The specificity of each antibody is as follows: RM-1, monocytes and most macrophages; ED1, monocytes and most macrophages; ED2, resident or tissue-fixed macrophages; ED3, certain macrophage subpopulations in lymphoid organs; TRPM-3, exudate or monocyte-derived macrophages and certain macrophage subpopulations in lymphoid organs; Ki-M2R, resident or tissue-fixed macrophages.

We first investigated the distribution pattern of macrophage subpopulations inside and in the surrounding area of rat tumors produced by injection of tumor cells into the sc space of syngeneic rats *(45)*. A large number of TRPM-3-positive cells were detected inside 9L, MCP-1-producing rat gliosarcoma with few ED2-positive and no Ki-M2R-positive cells inside the tumors (Fig. 6). There was no significant infiltration of macrophages inside MT-P, non-MCP-1-producing rat malignant fibrous histiocytoma. A similar pattern was observed when MCP-1-transfected MT-P (MT-P/MCP-1) cells were transplanted. Four MT-P/MCP-1 cell lines were cloned based on different MCP-1 production levels. When these cell lines were transplanted, there was a significant correlation between the levels of MCP-1 production and the numbers of intratumorally infiltrating TRPM-3-positive macrophages. Takeshima et al. previously suggested that the majority of infiltrating macrophages into human glioma tissues were derived from blood monocytes rather than proliferating microglia cells contained in brain tissues *(26)*. As described previously, MCP-1 attracts blood monocytes. The data from our studies with a rat transplanted tumor model and human malignant glioma tissues indicate that tumor-derived MCP-1 can induce intratumoral infiltration of blood monocytes. Recently, Zhang et al. *(46)* presented data indicating that injections of anti-MCP-1 neutralizing antibody inhibited intratumoral monocyte infiltration into MCP-1-producing transplanted tumors.

Matsushima et al. *(47)* previously reported that MCP-1 stimulated human monocytes to be growth inhibitory for tumor cells. Thus, MCP-1 not only attracts monocytes but also stimulates them to acquire anti-tumor function. In our transplanted tumor model, MT-P/MCP-1-transplanted tumors exhibited lower growth rates than parental MT-P-transplanted tumors *(45)*.

2.6. Effects of MCP-1 Overexpression in Experimental Malignant Glioma in Rats

Since the growth of transplanted tumor cells producing high levels of MCP-1 was inhibited, we speculated that the induction of high-level MCP-1 expression in tumors might be useful to suppress the growth of tumors in vivo. We injected rat glioma cell line cells, C6 cells, into rat brain tissues and induced MCP-1 mRNA expression and MCP-1 production by two methods: (1) a high-efficiency in vivo gene transfer using intraarterial plasmid DNA injection following in vivo electroporation *(48)*, and (2) direct intratumoral injection of an MCP-1-inducing cytokine, TNF-α *(28)*. In both cases, we detected MCP-1 production and infiltration of TRPM-3-positive monocytes into the tumors after the procedures. However, the production of MCP-1 and infiltration of monocytes were transient, and the growth of the tumors was not affected. These results indicate that transient induction of high-level MCP-1 production in tumor cells can cause infiltration of monocytes in vivo, but that it is not sufficient to retain those monocytes inside the tumors and to stimulate monocytes to acquire anti-tumor activity. Prolonged MCP-1 expression and combinations with other monocyte-stimulating agents may result in the infiltration of monocytes and local stimulation of infiltrating monocytes.

In contrast to our studies, Manome et al. *(49)* used irradiated MCP-1-producing rat gliosarcoma cells (9L-JE cells) to generate immune response against 9L cells in their syngeneic brain tumor model. The vaccination of animals with intradermal injection of 9L-JE cells increased the antitumor response against intradermally inoculated 9L cells but not against intracerebrally inoculated 9L cells. This study suggests that chemokine-based immunotherapy may not be effective against intracranial tumors including gliomas.

2.7. MCP-1 Production after Intracranial Administration of TNF-α in Human Malignant Glioma Patients

TNF-α was administered into the tumors of patients with recurrent supratentorial malignant gliomas that were refractory to the standard therapy (multiinstitutional phase 2 clinical trial, MHR-24) *(50)*. The patients underwent surgical removal of the tumor and placement of a reservoir/catheter system in the residual-tumor cavity at least 2 wk prior to the local TNF-α administration. The cavity fluids from two patients were analyzed for MCP-1 concentration *(28)*. All cavity fluids obtained after TNF-α administration contained high amounts of MCP-1. The concentration of MCP-1 was increased 8- and 27-fold after 24 and 38 h following TNF-α administration, respectively (case 1 was 44.5–357.3 ng/mL and case 2 was 31.8–850.5 ng/mL). Although the origin of MCP-1 was not investigated in the study, the administration of TNF-α appeared to stimulate the production of MCP-1 in glioma tissues. However, the overall effects of this clinical trial were disappointing.

3. IL-8 AND CNS MALIGNANCIES

3.1. Production of IL-8 by Malignant Glioma Cell Lines In Vitro

Various tumor cell lines of the CNS produce IL-8 in vitro. Kasahara et al. *(25)* investigated IL-8 mRNA expression in four human cell lines. Two glioblastoma cell lines, U-373MG and T98G, expressed significant amounts of IL-8 mRNA after IL-1α or TNF-α stimulation. The production of IL-8 by IL-1α-stimulated U-373MG cells was also confirmed by radioimmunoassay. One glioblastoma cell line, A172, and two neuroblastoma cell lines, IMR32 and GOTO, did not express significant amounts of IL-8 mRNA after stimulation. Dexamethasone inhibited IL-8 mRNA expression and production by IL-1α-stimulated T98G cells *(51)*. Transcription of the *IL-8* gene requires either the combination of NF-κB and C/EBP/NF-IL-6 or that of NF-κB and activator protein-1 that bind to the promoter region of the *IL-8* gene, depending on the type of cells *(52)*. Mukaida et al. *(52)* reported that dexamethasone appeared to interfere with the binding of the most essential transcription factor, NF-κB, to its cognate *cis*-element, resulting in the suppressive effect on the *IL-8* gene transcription in T98G cells. Recently, Scheinman et al. *(53)* and Auphan et al. *(54)* have reported that glucocorticoid induces the transcription of the *IκB* gene, which results in an increased rate of IκB protein synthesis. In the study by Scheinman et al. *(53)*, TNF-α stimulation caused the release of NF-κB from IκB in HeLa cells. However, in the presence of glucocorticoid, this newly released NF-κB quickly reassociated with newly synthesized IκB, thus markedly reducing the amount of NF-κB that translocates to the nucleus. The same mechanism may be applied to the inhibitory effect of dexamethasone on the *IL-8* gene transcription in T98G cells.

van Meir et al. *(55)* detected IL-8 mRNA expression in 11 of 12 glioblastoma cell lines without any stimulus. Five of the 6 cell lines expressing IL-8 mRNA secreted biologically active IL-8 into the culture supernatants. Both the expression of IL-8 mRNA and the secretion of IL-8 were augmented with IL-1 or TNF-α. Tada et al. *(56)* also investigated IL-8 production by malignant glioma cell lines in vitro and purified the 77-amino acid form of IL-8 from the culture supernatants of 2 TNF-α-stimulated malignant glioma cell lines *(56,57)*.

3.2. Production of IL-8 by Tumors of the CNS In Vivo

van Meir et al. *(55)* detected IL-8 mRNA in 2 of 2 low-grade astrocytomas, 1 of 2 anaplastic astrocytomas, and 6 of 6 glioblastomas. IL-8 was present in the cyst fluids of 1 of 4 low-grade astrocytomas, 1 anaplastic astrocytoma, 2 of 2 glioblastomas, 1 oligodendroglioma grade III, and 1 metastatic tumor of cervical cancer. Cerebrospinal fluids of 3 of 4 metastatic lymphomas, 2 of 16 glioblastomas, 1 of 2 low-grade astrocytomas, but none of 3 anaplastic astrocytomas and none of 9 meningiomas contained IL-8. Neutrophil infiltration is not common in gliomas but lymphocyte infiltration is. Since IL-8 attracts T-lymphocytes in vitro, glioma-derived IL-8 may play a role in lymphocyte infiltration in gliomas. It is also possible that IL-8 may participate in neo-vascularization in gliomas *(55)*.

Neutrophil chemotactic activity was increased in the cavity fluids of malignant glioma patients of the phase I clinical trial previously described *(50)*. This increased neutrophil chemotactic activity was associated with leukocytosis in the cavity fluids. Some cavity fluids with high neutrophil chemotactic activity were analyzed by reversed-phase chromatography on HPLC. The peak activity was found in the fraction where the reference IL-8 eluted, suggesting that the increased neutrophil chemotactic activity found in the cavity fluids was owing to the production of IL-8.

4. CONCLUSION

As described in this chapter, it is now clear that malignant gliomas produce chemokines such as MCP-1 and IL-8. Although the biologic significance of IL-8 production by gliomas is not clear, glioma-derived MCP-1 is, at least in part, responsible for the infiltration of blood monocytes into the tumors. The effect of MCP-1 production on the biology of malignant gliomas, however, remains unclear. As reviewed in Chapter 3, the roles of TAMs are still not known. From our study in a rat transplanted malignant glioma model, infiltrating monocytes could suppress the growth of the tumor if the production of MCP-1 is high. The suppressed growth rate of MCP-1-producing tumor cells compared with non-MCP-1-producing cells was also shown by others in other transplanted tumor models *(58,59)*. In contrast to the experimental tumor models, naturally occurring malignant gliomas continue to grow and subsequently kill patients. This may be owing to insufficient production of MCP-1 by the tumors. Further investigation is necessary to clarify the roles of MCP-1 in tumor biology.

We performed experiments to study whether MCP-1 can be used for the treatment of glioma patients. Although we were able to induce MCP-1 production in rat transplanted gliomas by in vivo electroporation or direct injection of MCP-1-inducing cytokine, TNF-α, MCP-1 production and monocyte infiltration were transient, and we did not observe antitumor effects by infiltrating monocytes. If we can induce long-term MCP-1 production in malignant gliomas and can stimulate the infiltrating monocytes for anti-tumor activity, it might be possible to use MCP-1 as a method to treat malignant glioma in combination with other treatments. One substantial advantage of using MCP-1 to other cytokines is its rather specific monocyte-recruiting activity of MCP-1 in contrast to the multiple functions of other cytokines that result in severe side effects.

ACKNOWLEDGMENT

The authors are indebted to their colleagues, without whom much of the presented work could not have been done.

REFERENCES

1. Kleihues, P. C. Burger, and B. W. Scheithauer. 1993. The new WHO classification of brain tumours. *Brain Pathol.* **3:** 255–268.
2. van Meir, E. G. 1995. Cytokines and tumors of central nervous system. *Glia* **15:** 264–288.
3. Evans, R. 1972. Macrophages in syngeneic tumors. *Transplantation* **14:** 468–473.
4. Evans, R., and S. Haskill. 1983. Activities of macrophages within and peripheral to the

tumor mass, in *The Reticuloendothelial System* (Herberman, R. B., ed.), Plenum, New York, pp. 155–176.

5. Kuratsu, J., E. J. Leonard, and T. Yoshimura. 1989. Production and characterization of human glioma cell-derived monocyte chemotactic factor. *J. Natl. Cancer Inst.* **81:** 347–351.

6. Yoshimura, T., E. A. Robinson, S. Tanaka, E. Appella, J. Kuratsu, and E. J. Leonard. 1989. Purification and amino acid analysis of two human glioma-derived monocyte chemoattractants. *J. Exp. Med.* **169:** 1449–1459.

7. Yoshimura, T., N. Yuhki, S. K. Moore, E. Appella, M. I. Lerman, and E. J. Leonard. 1989. Human monocyte chemoattractant protein-1 (MCP-1): full-length cDNA cloning, expression in mitogen-stimulated blood mononuclear leukocytes, and sequence similarity to mouse competence gene JE. *FEBS Lett.* **244:** 487–493.

8. Yoshimura, T., and A. Ueda. 1996. Structure, function, and mechanism of action of monocyte chemoattractant protein-1, in *Human Cytokines: Handbook for Basic and Clinical Research, Vol. II* (Aggarwal, B. B., and J. U. Gutterman, eds.), Blackwell, Cambridge, MA, pp. 198–221.

9. Rollins, B. J. 1991. JE/MCP-1: an early-response gene encodes a monocyte-specific cytokine. *Cancer Cells* **3:** 517–524.

10. Kuratsu, J., and Y. Ushio. 1996. Epidemiological study of primary intracranial tumors: a regional survey in Kumamoto Prefecture in the southern part of Japan. *J. Neurosurg.* **84:** 946–950.

11. Phillips, J. P., O. Eremin, and J. R. Anderson. 1982. Lymphoreticular cells in human brain tumors and in normal brain. *Br. J. Cancer* **45:** 61–69.

12. von Hanwehr, R. I., F. Hofman, C. Taylor, and M. L. J. Apuzzo. 1984. Mononuclear lymphoid population infiltrating the microenvironment of primary CNS tumors: characterization of cell subsets with monoclonal antibodies. *J. Neurosurg.* **60:** 1138–1147.

13. Wood, G. W., and R. A. Moranz. 1979. Immunological evaluation of the lymphoreticular infiltrate of human central nervous system tumors. *J. Natl. Cancer Inst.* **62:** 485–491.

14. Yoshimura, T., E. A. Robinson, S. Tanaka, E. Appella, and E. J. Leonard. 1989. Purification and amino acid analysis of two human monocyte chemoattractants produced by phytohemagglutinin-stimulated human blood mononuclear leukocytes. *J. Immunol.* **142:** 1956–1962.

15. Robinson, E. A., T. Yoshimura, E. J. Leonard, S. Tanaka, P. R. Griffin, J. Shabanowitz, D. F. Hunt, and E. Appella. 1989. Complete amino acid sequence of a human monocyte chemoattractant, a putative mediator of cellular immune reactions. *Proc. Natl. Acad. Sci. USA* **86:** 1850–1854.

16. Rutledge, B. J., H. Rayburn, R. Rosenberg, R. J. North, R. P. Gladue, C. L. Cordless, and B. J. Rollins. 1995. High level of monocyte chemoattractant protein-1 expression in transgenic mice increases their susceptibility to intracellular pathogens. *J. Immunol.* **155:** 4838–4843.

17. Fuentes, M. E., S. K. Durham, M. R. Swerdel, A. C. Lewin, D. S. Barton, J. R. Megill, R. Bravo, and S. A. Lira. 1995. Controlled recruitment of monocytes and macrophages to specific organs through transgenic expression of monocyte chemoattractant protein-1. *J. Immunol.* **155:** 5769–5776.

18. Nakamura, K., I. R. Williams, and T. S. Kupper. 1996. Keratinocyte-derived monocyte chemoattractant protein-1 (MCP-1): analysis in a transgenic model demonstrates MCP-1 can recruit dendritic and Langerhans cells to skin. *J. Invest. Dermatol.* **105:** 635–643.

19. Gunn, M. D., N. A. Nelken, X. Liao, and L. T. Williams. 1997. Monocyte chemoattractant protein-1 is sufficient for the chemotaxis of monocytes and lymphocytes in transgenic mice but requires an additional stimulus for inflammatory activation. *J. Immunol.* **158:** 376–383.

20. Yoshimura, T. 1993. cDNA cloning of guinea pig monocyte chemoattractant protein-1 and expression of the recombinant protein. *J. Immunol.* **150:** 5025–5032.

21. Yamashiro, S., M. Takeya, J. Kuratsu, Y. Ushio, K. Takahashi, and T. Yoshimura. 1998. Intradermal injection of monocyte chemoattractant protein-1 induces emigration and differentiation of blood monocytes in rat skin. *Int. Arch. Allergy Immunol.* **115:** 15–23.

22. Kuziel, W. A., S. J. Morgan, T. C. Dawson, S. Griffin, O. Smithies, K. Ley, and N. Maeda. 1997. Severe reduction in leukocyte adhesion and monocyte extravasation in mice deficient in CC chemokine receptor 2. *Proc. Natl. Acad. Sci. USA* **94:** 12,053–12,058.

23. Carr, M. W., S. J. Roth, E. Luther, S. S. Ross, and T. A. Springer. 1994. Monocyte chemoattractant protein-1 acts as a T-lymphocyte chemoattractant. *Proc. Natl. Acad. Sci. USA* **91:** 3652–3656.

24. Rand, M. L., J. S. Warren, M. K. Mansour, W. Newman, and D. J. Ringler. 1996. Inhibition of T cell recruitment and cutaneous delayed-type hypersensitivity-induced inflammation with antibodies to monocyte chemoattractant protein-1. *Am. J. Pathol.* **148:** 855–864.

25. Kasahara, T., N. Mukaida, K. Yamada, H. Yagisawa, T. Akahoshi, and K. Matsushima. 1991. IL-1 and TNF-α induction of IL-8 and monocyte chemotactic and activating factor (MCAF) mRNA expression in a human astrocytoma cell line. *Immunology* **74:** 60–67.

26. Takeshima, H., J. Kuratsu, M. Takeya, T. Yoshimura, and Y. Ushio. 1994. Expression and localization of messenger RNA and protein for monocyte chemoattractant protein-1 in human malignant glioma. *J. Neurosurg.* **80:** 1056–1062.

27. Desbaillets, I., M. Tada, N. de Trobolet, A.-C. Diserens, M.-F. Hamou, and E. G. van Meir. 1994. Human astrocytomas and glioblastomas express monocyte chemoattractant protein-1 (MCP-1) in vivo and in vitro. *Int. J. Cancer* **58:** 240–247.

28. Yoshizato, K., J. Kuratsu, H. Takeshima, T. Nishi, T. Yoshimura, and Y. Ushio. 1996. Tumor necrosis factor-α-induced macrophage infiltration in gliomas is mediated by the production of monocyte chemoattractant protein-1. *Int. J. Oncol.* **8:** 493–497.

29. Ueda, A., K. Okuda, S. Ohno, A. Shirai, T. Igarashi, K. Matsunaga, J. Fukushima, S. Kawamoto, Y. Ishigatsubo, and T. Okubo. 1994. NF-κB and Sp1 regulate transcription of human monocyte chemoattractant protein-1 gene. *J. Immunol.* **153:** 2052–2063.

30. Ueda, A., Y. Ishigatsubo, T. Okubo, and T. Yoshimura. 1997. Transcriptional regulation of the human monocyte chemoattractant protein-1 gene: cooperation of two NF-kB sites and NF-kB/rel subunit specificity. *J. Biol. Chem.* **272:** 31,092–31,099.

31. Kuratsu, J., K. Yoshizato, T. Yoshimura, E. J. Leonard, H. Takeshima, and Y. Ushio. 1993. Quantitative study of monocyte chemoattractant protein-1 (MCP-1) in cerebrospinal fluids and cyst fluids from patients with malignant glioma. *J. Natl. Cancer Inst.* **85:** 1836–1839.

32. Morantz, R. A., G. W. Wood, M. Foster, M. Clark, and K. Gollahon. 1979. Macrophages in experimental and human brain tumors. *J. Neurosurg.* **50:** 305–311.

33. Sato, K., J. Kuratsu, H. Takeshima, T. Yoshimura, and Y. Ushio. 1995. Expression of monocyte chemoattractant protein-1 in meningioma. *J. Neurosurg.* **82:** 874–878.

34. Cochran, B. H., A. C. Reffel, and C. D. Stiles. 1983. Molecular cloning of gene sequences regulated by platelet-derived growth factor. *Cell* **33:** 939–947.

35. Todo, T., E. Adams, and R. Fahlbusch. 1993. Inhibitory effect of trapidil on human meningioma cell population via interruption of autocrine growth stimulation. *J. Neurosurg.* **78:** 463–469.

36. Bruce, J. N., G. R. Criscuolo, M. J. Merrill, R. R. Moquin, J. B. Blacklock, and E. H. Oldfield. 1987. Vascular permeability induced by protein product of malignant brain tumors: inhibition by dexamethasone. *J. Neurosurg.* **67:** 880–884.

37. Shinonaga, M., C. C. Chan, N. Suzuki, M. Sato, and T. Kawabara. 1988. Immunohistological evaluation of macrophage infiltrates in brain tumors. *J. Neurosurg.* **68:** 259–265.

38. Morahan, P., A. Volkman, M. Melnicoff, and W. Dempsey. 1988. Macrophage heterogeneity, in *Macrophages and Cancer* (Hepper, G. H., and A. M. Fulton, eds.), CRC, Boca Raton, FL, pp. 2–25.

39. Dijkstra, C., E. Döpp, P. Joling, and G. Kraal. 1985. The heterogeneity of mononuclear

phagocytes in lymphoid organs: distinct macrophage subpopulations in the rat recognized by monoclonal antibodies, ED1, ED2, and ED3. *Immunology* **54:** 580–598.

40. Polman, C. H., C. D. Dijkstra, T. Sminia, and J. C. Koetsier. 1986. Immunohistological analysis of macrophages in the central nervous system of Lewis rats with acute experimental allergic encephalomyelitis. *J. Neuroimmunol.* **11:** 215–222.

41. Verschure, P. J., J. F. van Noorden, and C. D. Dijkstra. 1989. Macrophages and dendritic cells during the early stages of antigen-induced arthritis in rats: immunohistochemical analysis of cryostat sections of the whole knee joint. *Scand. J. Immunol.* **29:** 371–381.

42. Dijkstra, C. D., E. A. Döpp, I. M. C. Vogels, and C. J. F. van Noorden. 1987. Macrophages and dendritic cells during antigen-induced arthritis: an immunohistochemical study using cryostat sections of the whole knee joint of rat. *Scand. J. Immunol.* **26:** 513–523.

43. Miyamura, S., M. Naito, M. Takeya, H. Okumura, and K. Takahashi. 1988. Analysis of rat peritoneal macrophages with combined ultrastructural peroxidase cytochemistry and immunoelectron microscopy using anti-rat macrophage monoclonal antibodies. *J. Clin. Electron Microsc.* **21:** 545–546.

44. Takeya, M., L. Hsiao, and K. Takahashi. 1987. A new monoclonal antibody, TRPM-3, binds specifically to certain rat macrophage populations: immunohistochemical and immunelectron microscopic analysis. *J. Leukoc. Biol.* **41:** 187–195.

45. Yamashiro, S., M. Takeya, T. Nishi, J. Kuratsu, T. Yoshimura, Y. Ushio, and K. Takahashi. 1994. Tumor-derived monocyte chemoattractant protein-1 induces intratumoral infiltration of monocyte-derived macrophage subpopulation in transplanted rat tumors. *Am. J. Pathol.* **145:** 913–921.

46. Zhang, L., T. Yoshimura, and D. T. Graves. 1997. Antibody to Mac-1 or MCP-1 inhibits monocyte recruitment and promotes tumor growth. *J. Immunol.* **158:** 4855–4861.

47. Matsushima, K., C. G. Larsen, G. C. DuBois, and J. J. Oppenheim. 1989. Purification and characterization of a novel monocyte chemotactic and activating factor produced by a human myelomonocytic cell line. *J. Exp. Med.* **169:** 1485–1490.

48. Nishi, T., K. Yoshizato, S. Yamashiro, H. Takeshima, K. Sato, K. Hamada, I. Kitamura, T. Yoshimura, H. Saya, J. Kuratsu, and Y. Ushio. 1996. High-efficiency in vivo gene transfer using intra-arterial plasmid DNA injection following in vivo electroporation. *Cancer Res.* **56:** 1050–1055.

49. Manome, Y., P. Y. Wen, A. Hershowitz, T. Tanaka, B. J. Rollins, D. W. Kufe, and H. A. Fine. 1995. Monocyte chemoattractant protein-1 (MCP-1) gene transduction: an effective tumor vaccine strategy for non-intracranial tumors. *Cancer Immunol. Immunother.* **41:** 227–235.

50. Tada, M., Y. Sawamura, S. Sakuma, K. Suzuki, H. Ohta, T. Aida, and H. Abe. 1993. Cellular and cytokine responses of the human central nervous system to intracranial administration of tumor necrosis factor α for the treatment of malignant gliomas. *Cancer Immunol. Immunother.* **36:** 251–259.

51. Mukaida, N., M. Morita, Y. Ishikawa, N. Rice, S. Okamoto, T. Kasahara, and K. Matsushima. 1994. Novel mechanism of glucocorticoid-mediated gene repression: nuclear factor-κB is target for glucocorticoid-mediated interleukin 8 gene expression. *J. Biol. Chem.* **269:** 13,289–13,295.

52. Mukaida, N., S. Okamoto, Y. Ishikawa, and K. Matsushima. 1994. Molecular mechanism of interleukin-8 gene expression. *J. Leukoc. Biol.* **56:** 554–558.

53. Scheinman, R. I., P. C. Cogswell, A. K. Lofquist, and A. S. Baldwin, Jr. 1995. Role of transcriptional activation of IκBα in mediation of immunosuppression by glucocorticoids. *Science* **270:** 283–286.

54. Auphan, N., J. A. DiDonato, C. Rosette, A. Helberg, and M. Karin. 1995. Immunosuppression by glucocorticoids: inhibition of NF-κB activity through induction of IκB synthesis. *Science* **270:** 286–289.

55. van Meir, E., M. Ceska, F. Effenberger, A. Walz, E. Grouzmann, I. Desbaillets, K. Frei, A. Fontana, and N. de Tribolet. 1992. Interleukin-8 is produced in neoplastic and infectious diseases of the human central nervous system. *Cancer Res.* **52:** 4297–4305.

56. Tada, M., K. Suzuki, Y. Yamakawa, Y. Sawamura, S. Sakuma, H. Abe, E. van Meir, and N. de Tribolet. 1993. Human glioblastoma cells produce 77 amino acid interleukin-8 (IL-8 (77)). *J. Neurooncol.* **16:** 25–34.

57. Yoshimura, T., E. A. Robinson, E. Appella, K. Matsushima, S. D. Showalter, A. Skeel, and E. J. Leonard. 1989. Three forms of monocyte-derived neutrophil chemotactic factor (MDNCF) distinguished by different lengths of the amino terminal sequence. *Mol. Immunol.* **26:** 87–93.

58. Rollins, B. J., and M. Sunday. 1991. Suppression of tumor formation in vivo by expression of the JE gene in malignant cells. *Mol. Cell Biol.* **11:** 3125–3131.

59. Walter, S., B. Bottazzi, D. Govoni, F. Colotta, and A. Mantovani. 1991. Macrophage infiltration and growth of sarcoma clones expressing different amounts of monocyte chemotactic protein/JE. *Int. J. Cancer* **49:** 431–435.

14

Chemokines and *Helicobacter pylori* Infection

Jean E. Crabtree and Ivan J. D. Lindley

1. INTRODUCTION

Helicobacter pylori is a spiral Gram-negative bacterium that chronically infects the gastroduodenal mucosal surface of humans (Fig. 1). Since the initial successful culture of *H. pylori* in the early 1980s, and the appreciation that this bacterium is the causative agent of chronic gastritis *(74,111),* the major role this organism plays in gastroduodenal disease has become apparent. Although many infected subjects remain asymptomatic, the very strong association with peptic ulcer disease was quickly established, and bacterial eradication markedly reduces the incidence of ulcer recurrence *(18).* Subsequent studies detailed an association between *H. pylori* infection and gastric mucosa–associated lymphoid tissue–type lymphoma *(6,56,84,115)* and gastric adenocarcinoma *(4,25,50,83,86,106).*

Given these disease associations, an understanding of host-bacterial interactions and the immunopathology of infection is obviously of major clinical relevance. Infection of the gastroduodenal mucosa with *H. pylori* is invariably associated with chronic inflammation *(26,44).* The inflammation, which in part reflects the bacterial density of infection *(7),* is characterized by mononuclear and polymorphonuclear cell infiltration. The recruitment of inflammatory cells is of major importance for host defense against pathogens at mucosal sites; however, in chronic *H. pylori* infection, leukocyte infiltration may be pivotal to the pathogenesis of gastroduodenal disease *(26).* Thus, understanding the molecular and cellular events leading to leukocyte extravasation and transepithelial migration in response to *H. pylori* is important not only for unraveling the role of *H. pylori* in gastroduodenal disease, but also for facilitating our understanding of other chronic infectious and idiopathic diseases associated with neutrophil infiltration and activation.

2. *H. PYLORI:* A TYPE I CARCINOGEN

Several diverse malignancies are known to arise from a background of chronic inflammation. Cholangiocarcinoma and bladder cancer are strongly associated with infection with the Digeneans *Opisthorchis sinensis* and *Schistosoma haematobium.* The viral infections hepatitis B and C and human papillomavirus have been causally linked with hepatocellular carcinoma and cervical carcinoma. *H. pylori* is the first bacterium to be linked with the development of human neoplasia. Prospective epidemiologic stud-

From: *Chemokines and Cancer*
Edited by: B. J. Rollins © Humana Press Inc., Totowa, NJ

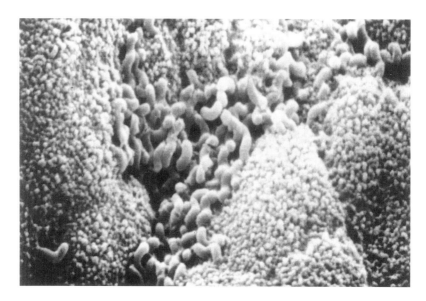

Fig. 1. Scanning electron micrograph of *H. pylori* on human gastric mucosa (kindly provided by Dr. N. Figura).

ies in ethnically diverse populations have shown a three- to sixfold increased risk of gastric cancer in *H. pylori*–infected subjects *(50,83,86)*. Additionally, worldwide studies show that the prevalence of infection with *H. pylori* correlates with gastric cancer mortality *(106)*. In 1994 a Working Party of the International Agency for Cancer Research considered the association between *H. pylori* and gastric cancer sufficient to classify the bacterium as a type 1 carcinogen *(57)*. Approximately 80–90% of gastric cancers are now considered to be associated with long-term chronic infection with *H. pylori (4,25)*.

It has long been established that gastric cancer occurs particularly in patients with chronic atrophic gastritis. Correa et al. *(18)* proposed that gastric carcinogenesis was a multistep process involving a progression from chronic gastritis to gastric atrophy, intestinal metaplasia, dysplasia, and adenocarcinoma (Fig. 2). Prospective studies have now documented that *H. pylori* infection increases the risk of developing the gastric cancer precursor conditions of atrophy and intestinal metaplasia *(65)*. The progression to atrophic gastritis may vary with *H. pylori* strain type *(66)* and may be increased by pharmacologic suppression of acid *(67,68)*. With the identification of *H. pylori* as the causative agent of chronic gastritis, it is likely that the inflammatory steps initiated by *H. pylori* infection are an essential prerequisite for the multiple genotypic and phenotypic alterations that lead to neoplasia *(21)*. This area is currently the focus of intense investigation, and the relevance and importance of the chemokines (especially interleukin-8 [IL-8]) to gastric pathology has been the subject of much recent interest.

The autonomy of mucosal surfaces as sites of chemokine production has recently been emphasized. The epithelium, the primary microbial-host interface, is an important source of chemokines *(10,11,28,33,41,60,75,90,96,107)*, with both viral and bacterial infections stimulating epithelial cells to secrete chemokines. The epithelium thus

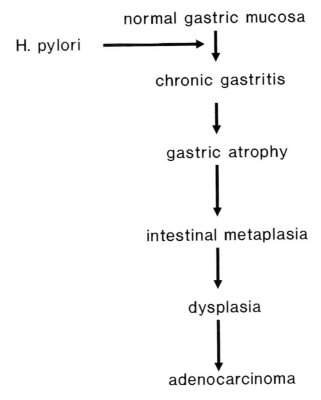

Fig. 2. The multistep process of gastric carcinogenesis as proposed by Correa et al. *(20)*.

makes an active contribution to regulating cellular responses to pathogens. Recent studies on *H. pylori* have focused on the mucosal chemokine response to infection and the identification of bacterial virulence factors involved in the induction of chemokines.

3. MUCOSAL CHEMOKINES IN *H. PYLORI* INFECTION: IN VIVO STUDIES

Infection with *H. pylori* is associated with elevated gastric mucosal IL-8 protein and IL-8 mRNA expression *(29,80,87,118,119)*, and also increased expression of other C-X-C and C-C chemokines *(97,98,105,120)*. Antral biopsies from patients with active gastritis (characterized by the intraepithelial infiltration of polymorphonuclear cells) secrete higher levels of IL-8 during short-term in vitro culture than biopsies from patients with inactive gastritis or histologically normal mucosa, demonstrating a direct association between mucosal IL-8 and polymorphonuclear cell infiltration *(2,29)*. Assessment of IL-8 protein concentrations in homogenates of gastric biopsies *(87)* and IL-8 mRNA expression in gastric mucosa *(97,118)* has also confirmed this direct association between IL-8 and neutrophil infiltration. Both polymorphonuclear cell infiltration and IL-8 mRNA in the antral mucosa decline rapidly after *H. pylori* eradication, indicating the direct effect of infection on IL-8 gene transcription *(80)*. Gastric expression of mRNA for the C-X-C chemokines growth-related oncogene-α (GRO-α) and epithelial cell–derived neutrophil-activating factor-78 (ENA-78) and C-C chemokines

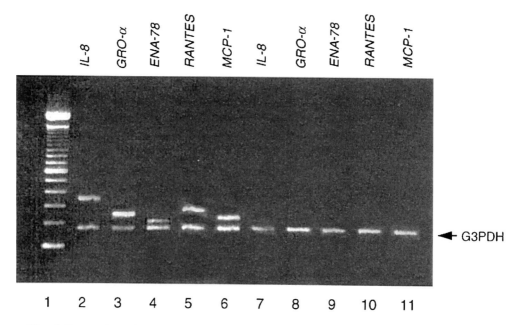

Fig. 3. Expression of IL-8, GRO-α, ENA-78, RANTES, and MCP-1 mRNA in gastric antral mucosa. Gastric biopsy from an *H. pylori*–positive patient **(lanes 2–6)** and a -negative patient **(lanes 7–11)** analyzed for the expression of chemokine and G3PDH (control) mRNA by reverse transcriptase polymerase chain reaction **(Lane 1)** 100-bp DNA ladder. (Reproduced with permission from ref. *98.*)

monocyte chemoattractant protein-1 (MCP-1) and RANTES is also increased in *H. pylori* infection *(97,98)* (Fig. 3). The relationship between these chemokines and the histopathology of chronic gastritis has not been determined.

As with other epithelia *(60,90,107)*, the gastric epithelium is a recognized source of IL-8 *(28)* and GRO-α *(105)*. *H. pylori* infection is associated with increased IL-8 immunoreactivity in the gastric epithelium *(28)* (Fig. 4). IL-8 secretion from polarized intestinal epithelial monolayers in vitro is primarily basolateral *(46,76)*. The binding of IL-8 and other C-X-C chemokines to glycosaminoglycans in the tissue matrix is thought to result in bioactive gradients for polymorphonuclear cell migration *(76,112)*. Recent studies using a novel immunochemiluminescence technique to localize IL-8 in the gastric mucosa have demonstrated high concentrations of IL-8 within the lamina propria with concentrations decreasing from the epithelial layer *(27)*.

Chemokines such as IL-8 are also present in gastric juice *(30,48)*. This suggests that some luminal release occurs through epithelial erosion or cell shedding. IL-8, although acid stable, is rapidly broken down by pepsin, but this process is pH dependent, and when gastric pH is above 5.0 enzymatic degradation does not occur *(30)*. As a consequence of this proteolytic degradation, gastric juice concentrations of IL-8 in *H. pylori*–positive and -negative patients with gastric pH below 4.0 are very low, and not specifically elevated in relation to *H. pylori* infection *(30)*. However, in patients with hypochlorhydria, whether atrophy associated or pharmacologically induced, gastric juice IL-8 concentrations are markedly increased relative to subjects with normal gastric physiologic responses, and can be as high as 1–8 ng/mL *(30)*. As gastric cancer

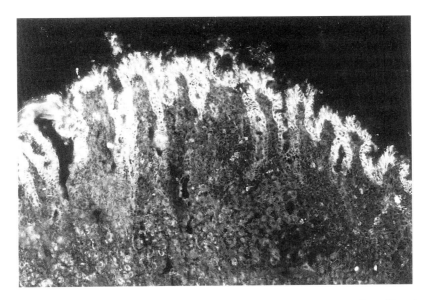

Fig. 4. Immunofluorescent localization of IL-8 in the corpus mucosa of an *H. pylori*–positive patient with chronic gastritis. (Reproduced with permission from ref. *28.*)

arises often against a background of gastric atrophy and associated hypochlorhydria, the marked increases in chemokines in hypochlorhydric subjects may be relevant to gastric neoplasia (*see* Subheading 6.).

The gastric chemokine response may be particularly important in the early stages of *H. pylori* infection, and the epithelium is likely to act as a crucial first line of defense. In humans the initial immunologic events following gastric colonization have rarely been documented. Isolated histologic studies of acute *H. pylori* infection suggest that there is a marked neutrophilic component *(73,101)* that may be effective in bacterial clearance in some instances. The long-term persistence of a neutrophilic response in chronic *H. pylori* infection suggests that these cells play a major role in inflammatory reactions to the bacterium. An understanding of the various roles of chemokines in *H. pylori*–induced inflammation and the virulence factors stimulating these peptides may provide important clues as to the mechanisms by which infection produces clinical disease.

4. *H. PYLORI* VIRULENCE FACTORS AND THE INDUCTION OF GASTRODUODENAL CHEMOKINES: IN VITRO STUDIES

4.1. Direct and Proinflammatory Cytokine-Induced Chemokine Responses

The pathways by which *H. pylori* stimulates mucosal chemokines are the subject of active investigation. In vitro studies with a range of gastric epithelial cell lines have shown that epithelial chemokines such as IL-8 can be induced following direct interaction with *H. pylori* (*see* Subheading 4.2) *(31–33,42,55,95)* and following exposure to the endogenous proinflammatory mediators IL-1 and tumor necrosis factor-α (TNF-α) *(122)* (Fig. 5). The secretion of these proinflammatory cytokines from lamina propria mononuclear cells following stimulation with *H. pylori* lipopolysaccharide (LPS) *(70)* and LPS-free bacterial components such as the urease *(54,70)* will therefore contribute

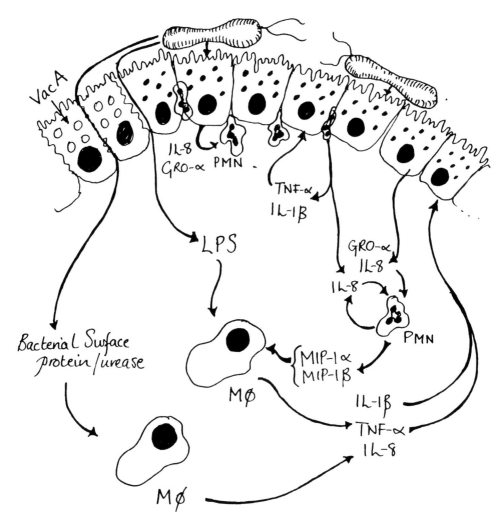

Fig. 5. Possible pathways of epithelial chemokine induction with *H. pylori* infection.

to increased epithelial chemokine expression in *H. pylori* infection. Increased gastric mucosal TNF-α *(34,80,118)* and IL-1 *(82,87)* mRNA expression and protein have been documented in infected subjects. Although in vivo the source of IL-1 and TNF-α is likely to be mainly macrophages, both neutrophils *(15)* and *H. pylori*–specific gastric T-cells *(47)* will also be a source of TNF-α.

Neutrophils are an important cellular source of both C-X-C and C-C chemokines, secreting IL-8, macrophage inflammatory protein-1α (MIP-1α) and MIP-1β *(15,62,104)*. Following initial attraction to the site of infection, the release of chemokines from neutrophils may further amplify the cellular response to infection (Fig. 5). Whole-cell preparations of *H. pylori* stimulate neutrophil IL-8 secretion *(35)*. This response is likely to be, in part, mediated by LPS. Purified *H. pylori* LPS induces both human peripheral blood neutrophil *(35)* and monocyte *(13)* preparations to secrete IL-8. *H. pylori* LPS has a low biologic activity relative to LPS of other bacterial species *(79)*. The regulation of the chemokine inflammatory cascades in mononuclear and polymorphonuclear cells is mediated by IL-10 *(36,62)*, probably by inhibition of the nuclear localization of the transcription factor NF-κB *(110)*. IL-10 is increased in the gastric mucosa in *H. pylori* infection *(87,118)*, and studies in IL-10-deficient mice have shown the essential role of this cytokine in downregulating inflammatory responses to enteric flora *(64)*.

4.2. H. Pylori cag *Pathogenicity Island and the Induction of Epithelial Chemokines*

The interaction of *H. pylori* with gastric epithelial cells in vitro induces a range of intracellular changes, including reorganization of cytoskeletal actin *(94,100)*, tyrosine phosphorylation of epithelial cell proteins *(94)*, and associated increases in chemokine secretion *(31–33,42,55,95,105)*. The induction of chemokines in gastric epithelial cells is dependent on viable bacterial preparations *(31,95)*. In addition, conversion from the spiral to the coccoid form results in the loss of the ability to induce IL-8 *(19)*, suggesting that complex bacterial-epithelial interactions are involved. The chemokine response of gastric epithelial cells is not specific for *H. pylori;* IL-8 secretion can also be induced by other pathogenic organisms such as *Salmonella typhimurium (42)*, *Pseudomonas aeruginosa, Campylobacter jejuni*, and *Escherichia coli* DH5α, but not *Campylobacter fetus (95)*, *Helicobacter mustelae (31)*, or *Helicobacter felis* (unpublished observations). IL-8 secretion from gastric epithelial cells is not induced by LPS as coculture of viable *H. pylori* with polymyxins B and E has no inhibitory effect on the IL-8 stimulatory capacity of the bacterium *(55)*.

The secretion of chemokines induced by *H. pylori* can be blocked by protein tyrosine kinase inhibitors such as genistein and herbimycin A *(1,37)*. Recent studies show that induction of IL-8 by *H. pylori* in gastric epithelial cells is associated with NF-κB activation *(1)* and that transcriptional regulation involves both NF-κB and activator protein-1 binding regions in the promoting region of the IL-8 gene *(1)*. The ability of *H. pylori* to activate signal transduction in gastric epithelial cells with resulting chemokine secretion is strain specific and occurs only in response to *H. pylori* strains with the CagA⁺ phenotype *(31,32,95)*. CagA-negative strains induce minimal chemokine secretion. Semiquantitative analysis of mRNA expression in gastric epithelial cells after bacterial coculture shows that the expression of IL-8 mRNA increases only in response to wild-type strains of the CagA phenotype *(31,32)*. It is clear from several studies with *H. pylori* that the VacA cytotoxin, which is often coexpressed in CagA-positive strains *(22,109)*, is not the inducer of chemokines in gastric epithelial cells. Viable wild-type variant strains that are cytotoxic but lack CagA *(32)* and crude cytotoxin preparations *(95)* do not induce IL-8 in gastric epithelial cells. In addition, *vacA* isogenic mutant strains stimulate similar IL-8 responses to parental strains *(55,95)*.

Mutational studies have recently identified specific *H. pylori* gene products involved in epithelial cell activation. Initial studies with isogenic mutants showed that CagA is not the direct inducer of IL-8 *(33,95)*. The genetic locus containing *cagA* (*cag*) is part of a pathogenicity island spanning 40 kb, which encodes more than 40 putative proteins *(16,23)*. Proteins encoded by genes within this pathogenicity island form a secretion system that may function to export molecules involved in bacterial-epithelial interactions *(23)*. Transposon inactivation of several genes in the left half of the pathogenicity island abolishes the ability of *H. pylori* to induce IL-8 in gastric epithelial cells

(16). Mutations in *cagE* (also described as *picB [108]*, *cagG, cagH, cagI, cagL,* and *cagM*) all significantly reduce the ability of *H. pylori* both to induce epithelial IL-8 *(16)* and to activate NF-κB *(81)*. Inactivation of genes in the right half of the *cag* pathogenicity island also impairs IL-8 secretion *(38)*. It appears, therefore, that genes throughout the whole *cag* pathogenicity island are essential for the induction of epithelial chemokine expression. It is currently unclear whether the IL-8-inducing molecule is the product of one of the inactivated genes, or whether the secretory system encoded by *cag* genes is responsible for the export of a molecule that induces IL-8 after bacterial–host cell interaction.

Recent studies have shown that many enteric pathogens will induce intestinal epithelial cells to secrete chemokines *(46,60,69,75–77,92,96)*. This cellular response parallels the ability of epithelial cells to chemotactically imprint subepithelial matrices in vitro and to support the directional transmatrix migration of polymorphonuclear cells to the subepithelial space *(76)*. Induction of epithelial chemokines by *H. pylori (31,42)* and some enteric pathogens *(75)* is not dependent on epithelial invasion. Studies with *Salmonella* serotypes have shown the ability of a pathogen to induce epithelial chemokines and to stimulate polymorphonuclear cell migration in a virulence determinant associated with enteritis *(75)*. It is therefore of particular interest that in *H. pylori,* there is a dichotomy in the ability of strains to induce epithelial chemokine responses similar to those observed with enteritis-inducing pathogens. Epithelial chemokine responses have clearly evolved to protect the host against pathogens; however, long-term activation of such responses in chronic infections may have pathogenic consequences. Although current studies have focused on investigating the induction of IL-8 *(31–33,42,55,95)* and GRO-α *(105)*, numerous other host genes are likely to be transcriptionally activated following the interaction of *cag*⁺ *H. pylori* with the gastric epithelium.

5. IN VIVO EVIDENCE FOR *H. PYLORI* STRAIN-SPECIFIC INDUCTION OF CHEMOKINES AND RELEVANCE TO GASTRIC NEOPLASIA

The CagA protein is immunodominant and the presence of antibodies to this protein is a good determinant of the *cag* status of the infecting *H. pylori* strain. Mucosal IgA recognition of CagA in patients with chronic gastritis is significantly associated with the activity of gastritis (i.e., intraepithelial neutrophil infiltration) *(39)*, an observation confirmed at the microbiologic level *(87,118)*. These histopathologic observations are consistent with an enhanced C-X-C chemokine response in patients infected with *cagA*⁺ *H. pylori.* Recent studies have confirmed both increased gastric mucosal IL-8 mRNA expression and IL-8 protein content in *cagA*-positive compared to *cagA*-negative infection *(87,118,121)*. Interestingly, mRNA for IL-10 is also more frequently observed in *cagA*-positive infection *(87,118)* and active gastritis *(118)*, suggesting that the transcription of this cytokine that downregulates inflammatory responses may relate to the extent of mucosal damage.

Current evidence shows that human infection with *cag*⁺ *H. pylori,* which stimulates epithelial chemokine responses in vitro, is associated with increased mucosal chemokine and cellular responses in vivo. Murine studies also indicate that *cag*⁺ *H. pylori* strains induce enhanced inflammation compared to *cag*⁻ strains *(52,71)*. Although many studies have documented an association between infection with *cag*⁺

strains and peptic ulceration *(24,39,114)*, there is now increasing evidence that *cag*⁺ infection increases the risk of developing the gastric cancer precursor conditions of atrophic gastritis and intestinal metaplasia *(8,40,66)* and gastric cancer *(12,25,85)*. There are diverse reports regarding *cag*⁺ infection and the incidence of gastric B-cell lymphomas *(45,49,59);* however, the development of gastric lymphoid follicles is an ubiquitous response to infection *(51)*.

In *H. pylori*–infected nonulcer patients, CagA seropositivity is associated with a highly significant risk of intestinal metaplasia, a histologic feature rarely observed in those infected with *cag*⁻ strains *(40)*. This suggests that the *cag* locus genes, or the immunopathologic events and chemokine responses induced by *cag* locus gene products, are essential factors initiating the development of gastric intestinal metaplasia. *H. pylori* infection is associated with both intestinal and diffuse types of gastric cancer. Only the former arises against a background of atrophic gastritis and intestinal metaplasia *(20)*. Recent prospective epidemiologic studies have shown that only the intestinal type of gastric cancer is associated with infection with *cag*⁺ strains *(12,85)*. The importance of the *cag* locus gene products in gastric neoplasia has been further reinforced by the recent observations that the worldwide variation in gastric cancer mortality is associated more strongly with a variation in infection with *cag*⁺ strains than *cag*⁻ strains of *H. pylori (113)*. Interestingly, in vivo studies indicate that *cag*⁺ infection may be associated with increased antral epithelial proliferation and reduced apoptosis relative to *cag*⁻ infection *(88)*. Preliminary studies with gastric epithelial cell lines suggest that *cag*⁺ strains upregulate *bc12,* a known inhibitor of apoptosis *(5)*.

6. CHEMOKINES AND GASTRIC HYPOCHLORHYDRIA

In patients who develop atrophic gastritis and hypochlorhydria, colonization of the gastric environment with other bacterial flora can result in the loss of *H. pylori* infection *(61,117)*. There has been considerable debate regarding the etiologic importance of bacterial overgrowth in the hypochlorhydric stomach in the development of gastric cancer. The original Correa et al. *(18)* hypothesis proposed that nitrate-reducing bacteria would result in increased luminal nitrite and potential formation of mutagenic and carcinogenic N-nitroso compounds following nitrosation of dietary/endogenous amines and amides *(20)*. A role for N-nitroso compounds in hypochlorhydria-associated gastric carcinogenesis is unproven.

Hypochlorhydria is associated with high concentrations of IL-8 in the gastric juice *(30)*, and other chemokines are likely to be similarly increased. Gastric juice concentrations of growth factors such as epidermal growth factor are also elevated *(72)*, or show increased bioactivity *(89)* at elevated pH owing to decreased peptic activity *(89)*. It is important to question the potential functional role of chemokines in gastric juice on gastric physiologic responses and epithelial cell proliferation and differentiation. Hypochlorhydria is associated with hypergastrinemia. The increased risk of noncardia gastric cancer in *H. pylori* infection is strongly related to the degree of hypergastrinemia *(53)*. Interestingly, in vitro studies with isolated canine G-cells have shown that IL-8 stimulates gastrin release *(9)*, but whether elevated gastric juice IL-8 contributes to the hypergastrinemia in vivo is unknown. However, gastric lavage at pH 7.0 in patients with pernicious anemia results in a significant decrease in plasma gastrin levels, suggesting that luminal factors do have a contributory role in hypergastrinemia *(43)*.

Furthermore, studies in germ-free and conventional rats have shown that achlorhydria-induced hypergastrinemia is dependent on the presence of microbial flora *(14)*. A possible explanation of the latter two studies is that chemokines induced by gastric bacterial flora contribute to the hypergastrinemia associated with gastric achlorhydria.

In vitro studies suggest that IL-1α may act as an autocrine growth factor for gastric cancer cells *(58)*. Although a similar role has been proposed for IL-8 with some tumor cells *(93)*, IL-8 does not appear to be an autocrine growth factor of gastric cancer cell lines (unpublished observations). One area in which elevated chemokines in gastric juice may be relevant to gastric tumorigenesis is their important role in mediating *(63,99,102)* or inhibiting *(102,103)* angiogenesis. The C-X-C chemokines with the ELR (Glu-Leu-Arg) sequence have been reported to have angiogenic effects, whereas the non-ELR members of the C-X-C subfamily (e.g., platelet factor 4) inhibit angiogenesis *(102,103)*. The composition of chemokines in hypochlorhydric gastric juice may be important in the regulation of tumor neovascularization and therefore the initiation and maintenance of tumor growth. Local production of IL-8 by gastric cancer cells *(28)* may also be relevant to angiogenesis and thus metastatic potential. Inhibition of IL-8 has been shown to decrease tumorigenesis of human non-small cell lung cancer in SCID mice by blocking angiogenic activity *(3)*. The importance of achlorhydria in the development of gastric cancer may relate not to the potential for the generation of N-nitroso compounds *(20)*, but to the decreased peptic activity resulting in increased luminal exposure to biologically active chemokines, cytokines, and growth factors. If this hypothesis is correct, the implications of long-term pharmacologic suppression of acid should be addressed.

7. CONCLUSION

Since the identification of *H. pylori* in the early 1980s *(74,111)*, the importance of this organism in gastroduodenal disease has become fully appreciated. *H. pylori* provides a unique unibacterial system for examining human mucosal responses and the association between inflammation and malignancy. It is interesting that other agents associated with malignancy, such as asbestos, trigger similar epithelial chemokine responses *(91)*. Mucosal irritants, whether infectious or chemical, stimulate similar epithelial signaling cascades that are likely to be relevant to the subsequent association with neoplasia. Differences in the production of chemokine mediators by *H. pylori* strains may, in part, explain the spectrum of clinical disease manifestations.

ACKNOWLEDGMENTS

Work conducted in the laboratory of J.E.C. was undertaken with financial support from the Yorkshire Cancer Research, European Commission (contract number 18CT95002A), and the Northern and Yorkshire Regional Health Authority.

REFERENCES

1. Aihara, M., D. Tsuchimoto, H. Takizawa, A. Azuma, H. Wakebe, Y. Ohmoto, K. Imagawa, M. Kikuchi, N. Mukaida, and K. Matsushima. 1997. Mechanisms involved in *Helicobacter pylori*-induced interleukin-8 production by a gastric cancer cell line, MKN 45. *Infect. Immun.* **65:** 3218–3224.
2. Ando, T., K. Kusugami, M. Ohsuga, M. Shinoda, M. Sakakibara, H. Saito, A. Fukatsu,

S. Ichiyama, and M. Ohta. 1996. Interleukin-8 activity correlates with histological severity in *Helicobacter pylori*-associated antral gastritis. *Am. J. Gastroenterol.* **91:** 1150–1156.

3. Arenberg, D. A., S. L. Kunkel, P. J. Polverini, M. Glass, M. D. Burdick, and R. M. Strieter. 1996. Inhibition of interleukin-8 reduces tumorigenesis of human non-small cell lung cancer in SCID mice. *J. Clin. Invest.* **97:** 2792–2802.

4. Asaka, M., T. Kimura, M. Kato, M. Kudo, K. Miki, K. Ogoshi, T. Kato, M. Tatsuta, and D. Y. Graham. 1994. Possible role of *Helicobacter pylori* infection in early gastric cancer development. *Cancer* **73:** 2691–2694.

5. Ashktorab, H., C. R. Allen, B. Reeves, and D. T. Smoot. 1997. Regulation of apoptosis by differential expression of waf1, p53 and bcl2 in gastric cells exposed to *H. pylori. Gastroenterology* **112:** A534.

6. Bayerdörffer, E., A. Neubauer, B. Rudolph, C. Thiede, N. Lehn, S. Eidt, and M. Stolte. 1995. Regression of primary gastric lymphoma of mucosa-associated lymphoid tissue type after cure of *Helicobacter pylori* infection. *Lancet* **345:** 1591–1594.

7. Bayerdorffer, E., N. Lehn, R. Hatz, G. A. Mannes, H. Oertel, T. Sauerbruch, and M. Stolte. 1992. Differences in expression of *Helicobacter pylori* gastritis in antrum and body. *Gastroenterology* **102:** 1575–1582.

8. Beales, I. L. P., J. E. Crabtree, D. Scunes, A. Covacci, and J. Calam. 1996. Antibodies to CagA are associated with gastric atrophy in *Helicobacter pylori* infection. *Eur. J. Gastroenterol. Hepatol.* **8:** 645–649.

9. Beales, I., S. Srinivasan, M. Blaser, J. Scheiman, J. Calam, J. Park, T. Yamada, and J. DelValle. 1995. Effect of *Helicobacter pylori* constituents and inflammatory cytokines on gastrin release from isolated canine G cells. *Gastroenterology* **108:** A779.

10. Becker, S., H. S. Koren, and D. C. Hencke. 1993. Interleukin-8 expression in normal nasal epithelium and its modulation by infection with respiratory syncytial virus and cytokines tumour necrosis factor, interleukin-1 and interleukin-6. *Am. J. Respir. Cell. Mol. Biol.* **8:** 20–27.

11. Berkman, N., A. Robichaud, V. L. Krishnan, et al. 1996. Expression of RANTES in human airway epithelial cells: effect of corticosteroids and interleukin-4, -10 and -13. *Immunology* **87:** 599–603.

12. Blaser, M. J., G. I. Perez-Perez, H. Kleanthous, T. L. Cover, R. M. Peek, P. H. Chyou, G. N. Stemmermann, and A. Nomura. 1995. Infection with *Helicobacter pylori* strains possessing *cagA* associated with an increased risk of developing adenocarcinoma of the stomach. *Cancer Res.* **55:** 2111–2115.

13. Bliss, C. M., D. T. Golenboock, S. Keates, J. K. Linevsky, and C. P. Kelly. 1996. *Helicobacter pylori* lipopolysaccharide stimulates the release of chemotactic cytokines from human monocytes. *Gastroenterology* **110:** A867.

14. Calam, J., R. A. Goodlad, C. Y. Lee, B. Ratcliffe, M. E. Coates, G. W. H. Stamp, and N. A. Wright. 1991. Achlorhydria-induced hypergastrinaemia: the role of bacteria. *Clin. Sci.* **80:** 281–284.

15. Cassatella, M. A. 1995. The population of cytokines by polymorphonuclear neutrophils. *Immunol. Today* **16:** 21–26.

16. Censini, S., C. Lange, Z. Xiang, J. E. Crabtree, P. Ghiara, M. Borodovsky, R. Rappuoli, and A. Covacci. 1996. *cag,* a pathogenicity island of *Helicobacter pylori,* encodes Type I-specific and disease-associated virulence factors. *Proc. Natl. Acad. Sci. USA* **93:** 14,648–14,653.

17. Choi, A. M. K., and D. B. Jacoby. 1992. Influenza virus A infection induces interleukin-8 gene expression in human airway epithelial cells. *FEBS Lett.* **309:** 327–329.

18. Coglhan, J. D., D. Gilligan, H. Humphries, et al. 1987. *Campylobacter pylori* and recurrence of duodenal ulcers. *Lancet* **ii:** 1109–1111.

19. Cole, S., D. Cirillo, M. F. Kagnoff, D. G. Guiney, and L. Eckmann. 1997. Coccoid and

spiral *Helicobacter pylori* differ in their abilities to adhere to gastric epithelial cells and induce interleukin-8 secretion. *Infect. Immun.* **65:** 843–846.

20. Correa, P., W. Haenszel, C. Cuello, S. Tannenbaum, and M. Archer. 1975. A model for gastric cancer epidemiology. *Lancet* **ii:** 58–60.

21. Correa, P. 1992. Human gastric carcinogenesis: a multistep and multifactorial process. *Cancer Res.* **52:** 6735–6740.

22. Covacci, A., S. Censini, M. Bugnoli, R. Petracca, D. Burroni, G. Macchia, A. Massone, E. Papini, Z. Xiang, N. Figura, and R. Rappuoli. 1993. Molecular characterization of the 128-kDa immunodominant antigen of *Helicobacter pylori* associated with cytotoxicity and duodenal ulcer. *Proc. Natl. Acad. Sci. USA* **90:** 5791–5795.

23. Covacci, A., S. Falkow, D. E. Berg, and R. Rappuoli. 1997. Did the inheritance of a pathogenicity island modify the virulence of *Helicobacter pylori? Trends Microbiol.* **5:** 205–208.

24. Cover, T. L., C. P. Dooley, and M. J. Blaser. 1990. Characterisation of and human serologic response to proteins in *Helicobacter pylori* broth culture supernatants with vacuolising cytotoxin activity. *Infect. Immun.* **58:** 603–610.

25. Crabtree, J. E., J. I. Wyatt, G. M. Sobala, G. Miller, D. S. Tompkins, J. N. Primrose, and A. G. Morgan. 1993. Systemic and mucosal humoral responses to *Helicobacter pylori* in gastric cancer. *Gut* **34:** 1339–1343.

26. Crabtree, J. E. 1996. Gastric mucosal inflammatory responses to *Helicobacter pylori*. *Aliment Pharmacol. Ther.* **10(Suppl. 1):** 29–37.

27. Crabtree, J. E., P. Pasini, F. Bazzoli, J. I. Wyatt, S. Perry, I. J. D. Lindley, E. Roda, and A. Roda. 1996. Chemiluminescent imaging of IL-8 in the gastric mucosa. *Gut* **39(Suppl. 2):** A105.

28. Crabtree, J. E., J. I. Wyatt, L. K. Trejdosiewicz, P. Peichl, P. N. Nichols, N. Ramsay, J. N. Primrose, and I. J. D. Lindley. 1994. Interleukin-8 expression in *Helicobacter pylori,* normal and neoplastic gastroduodenal mucosa. *J. Clin. Pathol.* **47:** 61–66.

29. Crabtree, J. E., P. Peichl, J. I. Wyatt, U. Stachl, and I. J. D. Lindley. 1993. Gastric IL-8 and IL-8 IgA autoantibodies in *Helicobacter pylori* infection. *Scand. J. Immunol.* **37:** 65–70.

30. Crabtree, J. E., G. R. Davies, S. Perry, J. I. Wyatt, P. Peichl, and I. J. D. Lindley. 1995. Gastric juice IL-8 and IL-8 autoantibodies: relationship to gastric pH. *Gut* **37(Suppl. 1):** A33.

31. Crabtree, J. E., S. M. Farmery, I. J. D. Lindley, N. Figura, P. Peichl, and D. S. Tompkins. 1994. CagA/cytotoxic strains of *Helicobacter pylori* and interleukin-8 in gastric epithelial cells. *J. Clin. Pathol.* **47:** 945–950.

32. Crabtree, J. E., A. Covacci, S. M. Farmery, Z. Xiang, D. S. Tompkins, S. Perry, I. J. D. Lindley, and R. Rappuoli. 1995. *Helicobacter pylori* induced interleukin-8 expression in gastric epithelial cells is associated with CagA positive phenotype. *J. Clin. Pathol.* **48:** 41–45.

33. Crabtree, J. E., Z. Xiang, I. J. D. Lindley, D. S. Tompkins, R. Rappuoli, and A. Covacci. 1995. Induction of interleukin-8 secretion from gastric epithelial cells by *cagA* negative isogenic mutant of *Helicobacter pylori. J. Clin. Pathol.* **48:** 967–969.

34. Crabtree, J. E., T. M. Shallcross, R. V. Heatley, and J. I. Wyatt. 1991. Mucosal tumour necrosis factor-alpha and interleukin-6 in patients with *Helicobacter pylori*-associated gastritis. *Gut* **44:** 768–771.

35. Crabtree, J. E., S. Perry, A. Moran, P. Peichl, D. S. Tompkins, and I. J. D. Lindley. 1994. Neutrophil IL-8 secretion induced by *Helicobacter pylori. Am. J. Gastroenterol.* **89:** 1337.

36. Crabtree, J. E., S. Perry, and I. J. D. Lindley. 1996. IL-10 inhibits *H. pylori* induced neutrophil but not epithelial chemokine secretion. *Gut* **39(Suppl. 2):** A42.

37. Crabtree, J. E. 1997. Virulence factors of *H. pylori* and their effect on chemokine produc-

tion, in *The Immunobiology of H. pylori* (Ernst, P. B., P. Michetti, and P. D. Smith, eds.), Lippincott-Raven, Philadelphia, pp. 101–112.

38. Crabtree, J. E., D. Kersulyte, V. Hernandez, I. J. D. Lindley, and D. E. Berg. 1997. *Helicobacter pylori* induction of IL-8 synthesis in gastric epithelial cells depends on genes throughout the *cag* pathogenicity island. *Gut* **40(Suppl. 1):** A69.

39. Crabtree, J. E., J. E. Taylor, J. I. Wyatt, R. V. Heatley, T. M. Shallcross, D. S. Tompkins, and B. J. Rathbone. 1991. Mucosal IgA recognition of *Helicobacter pylori* 120 kDa protein, peptic ulceration and gastric pathology. *Lancet* **338:** 332–335.

40. Crabtree, J. E., J. I. Wyatt, S. Perry, G. R. Davies, A. Covacci, and A. G. Morgan. 1996. CagA seropositive *Helicobacter pylori* infected non-ulcer patients have increased frequency of intestinal metaplasia. *Gastroenterology* **110:** A85.

41. Cromwell, O., Q. Hamid, C. J. Corrigan, J. Barkans, Q. Meng, P. D. Collins, and A. B. Kay. 1992. Expression and generation of interleukin-8, IL-6 and granulocyte-macrophage colony-stimulating factor by bronchial epithelial cells and enhancement by IL-1β and tumour necrosis factor-α. *Immunology* **77:** 7–12.

42. Crowe, S. E., L. Alvarez, M. Dytoc, R. H. Hunt, M. Muller, P. Sherman, J. Patel, Y. Jin, and P. B. Ernst. 1995. Expression of interleukin-8 and CD45 by human gastric epithelium after *Helicobacter pylori* infection in vitro. *Gastroenterology* **108:** 65–74.

43. Deprez, P. H., P. Ghosh, R. A. Goodlad, S. L. Lacey, S. Millership, R. J. Playford, C. Y. Lee, and J. Calam. 1991. Hypergastrinaemia: a new mechanism. *Lancet* **338:** 410, 411.

44. Dixon, M. F., R. M. Genta, J. H. Yardley, and P. Correa. 1996. Classification and grading of gastritis: the updated Sydney System. *Am. J. Surg. Pathol.* **20:** 1161–1181.

45. Eck, M., B. Schmaußer, R. Haas, A. Greiner, S. Czub, and H. K. Muller-Hermelink. 1997. MALT-type lymphoma of the stomach is associated with *Helicobacter pylori* strains expressing the CagA protein. *Gastroenterology* **112:** 1482–1486.

46. Eckmann, L., M. F. Kagnoff, and J. Fierer. 1993. Epithelial cells secrete the chemokine interleukin-8 in response to bacterial entry. *Infect. Immun.* **61:** 4569–4574.

47. D'Elios, M. M., M. Manghetti, M. De Carli, F. Costa, C. T. Baldari, D. Burroni, J. L. Telford, S. Romagnani, and G. Del Prete. 1997. T helper 1 effector cells specific for *Helicobacter pylori* in gastric antrum of patients with peptic ulcer disease. *J. Immunol.* **158:** 962–967.

48. Fan, X. G., A. Chua, X. J. Fan, and P. W. N. Keeling. 1995. Increased gastric production of interleukin-8 and tumour necrosis factor in patients with *Helicobacter pylori* infection. *J. Clin. Pathol.* **48:** 133–136.

49. Foerster, E. C., P. Koch, O. Koch, M. Tiemann, W. Domschke, and J. E. Crabtree. 1995. Serum response to *Helicobacter pylori* in primary B-cell gastric lymphoma. *Gut* **37(Suppl. 2):** A6.

50. Forman, D., D. G. Newell, F. Fullerton, J. W. G. Yarnell, A. R. Stacey, N. Wald, and F. Sitas. 1991. Association between infection with *Helicobacter pylori* and risk of gastric cancer: evidence from a prospective investigation. *BJM* **302:** 1302–1305.

51. Genta, R. M., H. W. Hammer, and D. Y. Graham. 1993. Gastric lymphoid follicles in *Helicobacter pylori* infection. *Hum. Pathol.* **24:** 577–583.

52. Ghiara, P., M. Marchetti, M. J. Blaser, et al. 1995. Role of the *Helicobacter pylori* virulence factors vacuolating cytotoxin, CagA and urease in a mouse model of disease. *Infect. Immun.* **63:** 4154–4160.

53. Hansen, S., S. E. Vollset, J. E. S. Ardill, E. El-Omar, K. Melby, S. Aase, E. Jellum, and K. E. L. McColl. 1997. Hypergastrinaemia is a strong predictor of distal gastric adenocarcinoma among *Helicobacter pylori* infected persons. *Gastroenterology* **112:** A575.

54. Harris, P. R., H. L. T. Mobely, G. I. Perez-Perez, M. J. Blaser, and P. D. Smith. 1996. *Helicobacter pylori* urease is a potent stimulus of mononuclear phagocyte activation and inflammatory cytokine production. *Gastroenterology* **111:** 419–425.

55. Huang, J., P. W. O'Toole, P. Doig, and T. J. Trust. 1995. Stimulation of interleukin-8 production in epithelial cell lines by *Helicobacter pylori*. *Infect. Immun.* **63:** 1732–1738.

56. Hussell, T., P. G. Isaacson, J. E. Crabtree, and J. Spencer. 1993. The response of cells from low grade B cell gastric lymphomas of mucosa-associated lymphoid tissue to *Helicobacter pylori*. *Lancet* **342:** 571–574.

57. Anonymous. 1994. *Schistosomes, Liver Flukes and Helicobacter pylori*. IARC Monographs on the Evaluation of Carcinogenic Risks to Humans, vol. 61. IARC, Lyon, France.

58. Ito, R., Y. Kitadai, E. Kyo, H. Yokozaki, W. Yasui, U. Yamashita, H. Nikaia, and E. Tahara. 1993. Interleukin 1α acts as an autocrine growth stimulator for human gastric carcinoma cells. *Cancer Res.* **53:** 4102–4106.

59. de Jong D., R. W. M. van der Hulst, G. Pals, W. C. van Dijk, A van der Ende, G. N. J. Tytgatt, B. G. Taal, and H. Boot. 1996. Gastric non-Hodgkins lymphoma of mucosa-associated lymphoid tissue are not associated with more aggressive *Helicobacter pylori* strains as identified by CagA. *Am. J. Clin. Pathol.* **106:** 670–675.

60. Jung, H. C., L. Eckmann, S. K. Yang, A. Panja, J. Fierer, E. Morzycka-Wroblewska, and M. F. Kagnoff. 1995. A distinct array of proinflammatory cytokines is expressed in human colon epithelial cells in response to bacterial invasion. *J. Clin. Invest.* **95:** 55–65.

61. Karnes, W. E., I. M. Samloff, M. Siurala, M. Kekki, P. Sipponen, S. W. R. Kim, and J. H. Walsh. 1991. Positive serum antibody and negative tissue staining for *Helicobacter pylori* in subjects with atrophic body gastritis. *Gastroenterology* **101:** 167–174.

62. Kasama, T., R. M. Strieter, N. W. Lukacs, M. D. Burdick, and S. L. Kunkel. 1994. Regulation of neutrophil-derived chemokine expression by IL-10. *J. Immunol.* **152:** 3559–3569.

63. Koch, A. E., P. J. Polverini, S. L. Kunkel, L. A. Harlow, L. A. Pietra, V. M. Elner, S. G. Elner, and R. M. Strieter. 1992. Interleukin-8 as a macrophage-derived mediator of angiogenesis. *Science* **258:** 1798–1801.

64. Kuhn, R., J. Lohler, D. Rennick, K. Rajewsky, and W. Muller. 1993. Interleukin-10-deficient mice develop chronic enterocolitis. *Cell* **75:** 263–274.

65. Kuipers, E. J., A. M. Uyterlinde, A. S. Pena, R. Roosendaal, G. Pals, G. F. Nelis, H. P. M. Festen, and S. G. M. Meuwissen. 1995. Long-term sequelae of *Helicobacter pylori* gastritis. *Lancet* **345:** 1525–1528.

66. Kuipers, E. J., G. I. Perez-Perez, S. G. M. Meuwissen, and M. J. Blaser. 1995. *Helicobacter pylori* and atrophic gastritis: importance of cagA status. *J. Natl. Cancer Inst.* **87:** 1777–1780.

67. Kuipers, E. J., L. Lundell, E. C. Klinkenberg-Knol, N. Havu, H. P. M. Festen, B. Leidman, C. B. H. W. Lamers, J. B. M. J. Jansen, J. Dalenback, P. Snel, G. F. Nelis, and S. G. M. Meuwissen. 1996. Atrophic gastritis and *Helicobacter pylori* infection in patients with reflux esophagitis treated with omeprazole or fundoplication. *N. Engl. J. Med.* **334:** 1018–1022.

68. Logan, R. P. H., M. M. Walker, J. J. Misiewicz, P. A. Gummett, Q. N. Karim, and J. H. Baron. 1995. Changes in the intragastric distribution of *Helicobacter pylori* during treatment with omeprazole. *Gut* **36:** 12–16.

69. Mahida, Y. R., S. Makh, S. Hyde, T. Gray, and S. P. Borriello. 1996. Effect of *Clostridium difficile* toxin A on human intestinal epithelial cells: induction of interleukin 8 production and apoptosis after cell detachment. *Gut* **38:** 337–347.

70. Mai, U. E. H., G. I. Perez-Perez, L. M. Wahl, S. M. Wahl, M. J. Blaser, and P. D. Smith. 1991. Soluble surface proteins from *Helicobacter pylori* activate monocytes/macrophages by Lipopolysaccharide-independent mechanism. *J. Clin. Invest.* **87:** 894–900.

71. Marchetti, M., B. Arico, D. Burroni, N. Figura, R. Rappuoli, and P. Ghiara. 1995. Development of a mouse model of *Helicobacter pylori* infection that mimics human disease. *Science* **267:** 1655–1658.

72. Marcinkiewicz, M., B van der Linden, D. A. Peura, G. Goldin, S. Parolisi, and J. Sarosiek. 1996. Impact of *Helicobacter pylori* colonization on immunoreactive epidermal growth factor and transforming growth factor-α in gastric juice. *Dig. Dis. Sci.* **41:** 2150–2155.

73. Marshall, B., J. Armstrong, D. McGechie, and R. Glancy. 1985. Attempt to fulfil Koch's postulate for pyloric *Campylobacter. Med. J. Aust.* **152:** 436–439.

74. Marshall, B. J. 1983. Unidentified curved bacilli on gastric epithelium in active chronic gastritis. *Lancet* **i:** 1273–1275.

75. Massion, P. P., H. Inoue, J. Richman-Eisenstat, D. Grunberg, P. G. Jorens, B. Housset, J. F. Pittet, J. P. Wiener-Kronish, and J. A. Nadel. 1994. Novel *Pseudomonas* product stimulates interleukin-8 production in airway epithelial cells in vitro. *J. Clin. Invest.* **93:** 26–32.

76. McCormick, B. A., P. M. Hofman, J. Kim, D. K. Carnes, S. I. Miller, and J. L. Madara. 1995. Surface attachment of *Salmonella typhimurium* to intestinal epithelia imprints the subepithelial matrix with gradients chemotactic for neutrophils. *J. Cell. Biol.* **131:** 1599–1608.

77. McCormick, B. A., S. P. Coglan, C. Delp-Archer, S. I. Miller, and J. L. Madara. 1993. *Salmonella typhimurium* attachment to human intestinal epithelial monolayers: transcellular signalling to subepithelial neutrophils. *J. Cell. Biol.* **123:** 895–907.

78. McCormick, B. A., S. I. Miller, D. Carnes, and J. L. Madara. 1995. Transepithelial signalling to neutrophils by *Salmonellae:* a novel virulence mechanism for gastroenteritis. *Infect. Immun.* **63:** 2302–2309.

79. Moran, A. P. 1996. The role of lipopolysaccharide in *Helicobacter pylori* pathogenesis. *Aliment. Pharmacol. Ther.* **10(Suppl. 1):** 39–50.

80. Moss, S. F., S. Legon, J. Davies, and J. Calam. 1994. Cytokine gene expression in *Helicobacter pylori* associated antral gastritis. *Gut* **35:** 1567–1570.

81. Müntzenmaier, A., E. Glocker, A. Covacci, S. Bereswill, P. Baeuerle, M. Kist, and H. Pahl. 1997. *Helicobacter pylori* mediated activation of NFκB in epithelial cells: the influence of genes located in the *cag*-pathogenicity island. *Ir. J. Med. Sci.* **166(Suppl. 3):** 11.

82. Noach, L. A., N. B. Bosma, J. Jansen, F. J. Hoek, S. J. H. van Deventer, and G. N. J. Tytgat. 1994. Mucosal tumour necrosis factor-alpha, interleukin-1 beta, and interleukin-8 production in patients with *Helicobacter pylori* infection. *Scand. J. Gastroenterol.* **29:** 425–429.

83. Nomura, A., G. N. Stemmerman, P. H. Chyou, I. Kato, G. I. Perez-Perez, and M. J. Blaser. 1991. *Helicobacter pylori* infection and gastric cancer among Japanese Americans in Hawaii. *N. Engl. J. Med.* **325:** 1132–1136.

84. Parsonnet, J., S. Hansen, L. Rodriguez, A. B. Gleb, R. A. Warnke, E. Jellum, N. Orentreich, J. H. Vogelman, and G. D. Friedman. 1994. *Helicobacter pylori* infection and gastric lymphoma. *N. Engl. J. Med.* **330:** 1267–1271.

85. Parsonnet, J., G. D. Friedman, N. Orentreich, and H. Vogelman. 1997. Risk for gastric cancer in people with CagA positive and CagA negative *Helicobacter pylori* infection. *Gut* **40:** 297–301.

86. Parsonnet, J., G. D. Friedman, D. P. Vandersteen, Y. Chang, J. H. Vogelman, N. Orentreich, and R. K. Sibley. 1991. *Helicobacter pylori* infection and risk of gastric carcinoma. *N. Engl. J. Med.* **325:** 1127–1131.

87. Peek, R. M. Jr., G. G. Miller, K. T. Tham, G. I. Perez-Perez, X. Zhao, J. C. Atherton, and M. J. Blaser. 1995. Heightened inflammatory response and cytokine expression *in vivo* to CagA+ *Helicobacter pylori* strains. *Lab. Invest.* **73(6):** 760–770.

88. Peek, R. M., S. F. Moss, K. T. Tham, G. P. Perez-Perez, S. Wang, G. G. Miller, J. C. Atherton, P. R. Holt, and M. J. Blaser. 1997. Infection with *H. pylori cagA+* strains dissociates gastric epithelial cell proliferation from apoptosis. *J. Natl. Cancer Inst.* **89:** 863–868.

89. Playford, P. J., T. Marchbank, D. P. Calnan, J. Calam, P. Royston, J. J. Batten, and H. F. Hansen. 1995. Epidermal growth factor is digested to smaller, less active forms in acidic gastric juice. *Gastroenterology* **108:** 92–101.

90. Raqib, R., A. A. Lindberg, B. Wretland, P. K. Bardham, U. Andersson, and J. Andersson. 1995. Persistence of local cytokine production in Shigellosis in acute and convalescent stages. *Infect. Immun.* **63:** 289–296.

91. Rosenthal, G. J., D. R. Germolec, M. E. Blazka, et al. 1994. Asbestos stimulates IL-8 production from human lung epithelial cells. *J. Immunol.* **153:** 3237–3244.

92. Savkovic, S. D., A. Koutsouris, and G. Hecht. 1996. Attachment of a noninvasive enteric pathogen, enteropathogenic *Escherichia coli,* to cultured human intestinal epithelial monolayers induces transmigration of neutrophils. *Infect. Immun.* **64:** 4480–4487.

93. Schadendorf, D., A. Moller, B. Algermissen, M. Worm, M. Sticherling, and B. M. Czarnetzki. 1993. IL-8 produced by human malignant melanoma cells *in vitro* is an essential autocrine growth factor. *J. Immunol.* **151:** 2667–2675.

94. Segal, E. D., S. Falkow, and D. S. Tompkins. 1996. *Helicobacter pylori* attachment to gastric cells induces cytoskeletal rearrangements and tyrosine phosphorylation of host cell proteins. *Proc. Natl. Acad. Sci. USA* **93:** 1259–1264.

95. Sharma, S. A., M. K. R. Tummura, G. G. Miller, and M. J. Blaser. 1995. Interleukin-8 response of gastric epithelial cell lines to *Helicobacter pylori* stimulation in vitro. *Infect Immun.* **63:** 1681–1687.

96. Sheth, R., J. Anderson, T. Sato, B. Oh, J. Scott, S. J. Hempson, E. Rollo, E. R. Mackow, and R. D. Shaw. 1996. Rotavirus stimulates IL-8 secretion from cultured epithelial cells. *Virology* **221:** 251–259.

97. Shimoyama, T., S. M. Everett, M. F. Dixon, A. T. R. Axon, and J. E. Crabtree. 1998. Chemokine mRNA expression in gastric mucosa is associated with *Helicobacter pylori cagA* positivity and severity of gastritis. *J. Clin. Pathol.* **51:** 765–770.

98. Shimoyama, T., and J. E. Crabtree. 1997. Mucosal chemokines in *Helicobacter pylori* infection. *J. Physiol. Pharmacol.* **48:** 315–323.

99. Smith, D. R., P. J. Polverini, S. L. Kunkel, M. B. Orringer, R. I. Whyte, M. D. Burdick, C. A. Wilke, and R. M. Strieter. 1994. Inhibition of interleukin-8 attenuates angiogenesis in bronchogenic carcinoma. *J. Exp. Med.* **179:** 1409–1415.

100. Smoot, D. T., J. H. Resau, T. Naab, B. C. Desbordes, T. Gilliam, K. Bull-Henry, S. B. Curry, J. Nidiry, J. Sewchand, K. Mills-Robertson, K. Frontin, E. Abebe, M. Dillon, G. R. Chippendale, P. C. Phelps, V. F. Scott, and H. L. T. Mobley. 1993. Adherence of *Helicobacter pylori* to cultured gastric epithelial cells. *Infect. Immun.* **61:** 350–355.

101. Sobala, G. M., J. E. Crabtree, M. F. Dixon, C. J. Scorah, J. D. Taylor, B. J. Rathbone, R. V. Heatley, and A. T. R. Axon. 1991. Acute *Helicobacter pylori* infection: clinical features, local and systemic immune responses, gastric mucosal histology and gastric juice ascorbic acid concentrations. *Gut* **32:** 1415–1418.

102. Strieter, R. M., P. J. Polverini, D. A. Arenberg, A. Walz, G. Opdenakker, J. Van Damme, and S. L. Kunkel. 1995. Role of C-X-C chemokines as regulators of angiogenesis in lung cancer. *J. Leukoc. Biol.* **57:** 752–762.

103. Strieter, R. M., S. L. Kunkel, D. A. Arenberg, M. D. Burdick, and P. J. Polverini. 1995. Interferon gamma inducible protein 10 (HP10), a member of the C-X-C-chemokine family, is an inhibitor of angiogenesis. *Biochem. Biophys. Res. Commun.* **210:** 51–57.

104. Strieter, R. M., K. Kasahara, R. M. Allen, T. J. Standiford, M. W. Rolfe, F. S. Becker, S. W. Chensue, and S. L. Kunkel. 1992. Cytokine-induced neutrophill-derived interleukin-8. *Am. J. Pathol.* **141:** 397–407.

105. Takizawa H., A. Azuma, M. Aihara, T. Doi, Y. Funakoshi, K. Imagawa, and M. Kikuchi. 1996. *Helicobacter pylori* induced chemokine production in human gastric carcinoma cell lines: effects of rebamipide. *Gastroenterology* **110:** A272.

106. The Eurogast Study Group. 1993. An international association between *Helicobacter pylori* and gastric cancer. *Lancet* **341:** 1359–1362.

107. Tonetti, M. S., M. A. Imboden, L. Gerber, N. P. Lang, J. Laissue, and C. Mueller. 1994. Localised expression of mRNA for phagocyte-specific chemotactic cytokines in human periodontal infections. *Infect. Immun.* **62:** 4005–4014.

108. Tummuru, M. K. R., S. A. Sharma, and M. J. Blaser. 1995. *Helicobacter pylori picB,* a homologue of the *Bordetella pertussis* toxin secretion protein, is required for induction of IL-8 in gastric epithelial cells. *Mol. Microbiol.* **18:** 867–876.

109. Tummuru, M. K. R., T. L. Cover, and M. J. Blaser. 1993. Cloning and expression of a high-molecular-mass major antigen of *Helicobacter pylori:* evidence for linkage to cytotoxin production. *Infect. Immun.* **61:** 1799–1809.

110. Wang, P., P. Wu, M. I. Siegel, R. W. Egan, and M. M. Billah. 1995. Interleukin (IL)-10 inhibits nuclear factor kB (NFkB) activation in human monocytes. *J. Biol. Chem.* **270:** 9558–9563.

111. Warren, J. R. 1983. Unidentified curved bacilli on gastric epithelium in active chronic gastritis. *Lancet* **i:** 1273.

112. Webb, L. M. C., M. U. Ehrengruber, I. Clark-Lewis, M. Baggiolini, and A. Rot. 1993. Binding to heparin sulfate or heparin enhances neutrophil responses to interleukin-8. *Proc. Natl. Acad. Sci. USA* **90:** 7158–7162.

113. Webb, P. M., D. Forman, D. Newell, A. Covacci, and J. E. Crabtree. 1996. An international association between prevalence of infection with CagA positive strains of *H. pylori* and mortality from gastric cancer. *Gut* **39(Suppl. 2):** A1.

114. Weel, J. F. L., R. W. M. van der Hulst, Y. Gerrits, P. Roorda, M. Feller, J. Dankert, G. N. J. Tytgat, and A. van der Ende. 1996. The interrelationship between cytotoxin-associated gene A, vacuolating cytotoxin, and *Helicobacter pylori*-related diseases. *J. Infect. Dis.* **173:** 1171–1175.

115. Wotherspoon A. C., C. Oritz-Hidalgo, M. R. Falzon, and P. G. Isaacson. 1991. *Helicobacter pylori*-associated gastritis and primary B-cell gastric lymphoma. *Lancet* **338:** 1175–1176.

116. Wotherspoon, A. C., C. Doglioni, T. C. Diss, L. Pan, A. Moschini, M. de Bone, and P. G. Isaacson. 1993. Regression of low grade B-cell gastric lymphoma of MALT type following eradication of *Helicobacter pylori. Lancet* **342:** 575–577.

117. Wyatt, J. I., T. M. Shallcross, J. E. Crabtree, and R. V. Heatley. 1992. *Helicobacter pylori* gastritis and peptic ulceration in the elderly. *J. Clin. Pathol.* **45:** 1070–1074.

118. Yamaoka, Y., M. Kita, T. Kodama, N. Sawai, and J. Imanishi. 1996. *Helicobacter pylori cagA* gene and expression of cytokine messenger RNA in gastric mucosa. *Gastroenterology* **110:** 1744–1752.

119. Yamaoka, Y., M. Kita, T. Kodama, N. Sawai, K. Kashima, and J. Imanishi. 1995. Expression of cytokine mRNA in gastric mucosa with *Helicobacter pylori* infection. *Scand. J. Gastroenterol.* **30:** 1153–1159.

120. Yamaoka, Y., M. Kita, T. Kodama, N. Sawai, and J. Imanishi. 1996. Expression of chemokine mRNA in gastric mucosa with *Helicobacter pylori* infection. *Gastroenterology* **110:** A1049.

121. Yamaoka, Y., M. Kita, T. Kodama, N. Sawai, K. Kashima, and J. Imanishi. 1997. Induction of various cytokines and development of severe mucosal inflammation by *cagA* gene positive *Helicobacter pylori* strains. *Gut* **41:** 442–451.

122. Yashimoto, K., S. Okamoto, N. Mukaida, S. Murakami, M. Mai, and K. Matsushima. 1992. Tumour necrosis factor-α and interferon-gamma induce interleukin-8 production in human gastric cancer cell line through acting concurrently on AP-1 and NF-κB-like binding sites of the IL-8 gene. *J. Biol. Chem.* **267:** 22,506–22,511.

VI
Chemokines and Stem Cell Proliferation

15

Chemokines and Hematopoiesis

Hal E. Broxmeyer and Chang H. Kim

1. HEMATOPOIESIS

Hematopoiesis refers to the production of blood cells, a dynamic process that supplies and replenishes the mature blood cell elements necessary to sustain life *(1–4)*. The homeostatic mechanisms that maintain blood cell levels within defined limits under normal conditions and the accelerated production of these cells under stress-induced conditions, such as infection or after cytotoxic drug therapy, reflect a balance between cell-cell and cytokine-cell interactions.

A simplified version of the hierarchy of blood cell production is shown in Figure 1, with an emphasis on the myeloid system. The assays used to quantitate cells within the morphologically nonrecognizable hematopoietic stem and progenitor cell compartments are inserted into Fig. 1 *(4–6)*.

The earliest, most immature cells, which give rise to the circulating blood elements, are termed *hematopoietic stem cells (1,2)*. These cells can self-renew, make more of themselves, and engraft recipients with resultant long-term marrow repopulation. The assay for this earliest stem cell population utilizes repopulation of blood cells in mice that have received a lethal dose of irradiation. This repopulation is long term. Presently, there is no assay available that is believed to definitively detect this early cell in humans, although investigators are evaluating the effects of injecting human cells into mice as a possible assay for these cells. Within the stem cell population are also cells that are more mature than the long-term marrow repopulating cells in that they have some degree of self-renewal capacity, but they do not necessarily have the capacity for long-term marrow repopulation. There are assays believed to detect these more mature subsets of stem cells for mice in vivo and for mouse or human cells in vitro. Blood cell production is considered to be a catenated system with stem cells giving rise to progenitor cells of different blood lineages, which, ultimately, give rise to the first morphologically recognizable cells within a blood cell lineage—the precursor cells (e.g., myeloblasts, proerythroblasts, promonocytes).

Understanding the proliferation, differentiation, and self-renewal capacity of hematopoietic stem and progenitor cells and modulation of these events under normal conditions, after stress or during disease, is the focus of the efforts of a large number of laboratories. What is clear is that this regulation and the abnormalities of it that are associated with disease reflect the effects of stromal cells, other accessory cells, and

From: *Chemokines and Cancer*
Edited by: B. J. Rollins © Humana Press Inc., Totowa, NJ

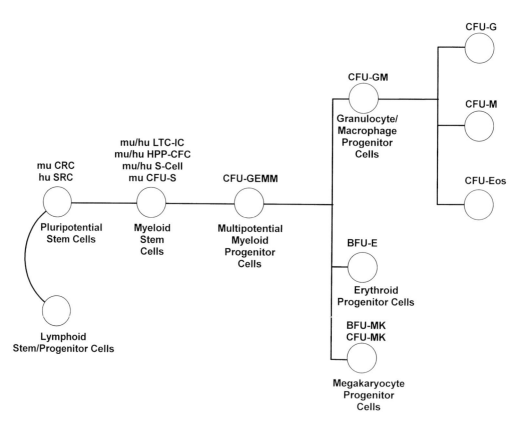

Fig. 1. Simplified schematic representation of the catenated flow of blood cell production, with a focus on the myeloid cells, from the pluripotential hematopoietic stem cells with long-term marrow repopulating capacity to the more mature myeloid stem cells, with less repopulating capacity, to the multipotential and then more lineage-restricted progenitor cells. Note that each category within the stem and progenitor cells probably contains populations of less mature to more mature subsets. As an example, cells within the different progenitor cell categories that respond to the proliferative effects of multiple growth-stimulating cytokines (such as colony-stimulating factor[s] plus potent costimulating cytokines that synergize) are considered to be more immature progenitors than those within the category that respond to stimulation by one growth-stimulating cytokine. hu, human; mu, murine; CRC, competitive repopulating cell (an in vivo mouse assay); SRC, SCID repopulating cell: the human cell that repopulates a sublethally irradiated mouse with severe combined immunodeficiency; LTC-IC, long-term culture-initiating cell; HPP-CFC, high proliferative potential colony-forming cell; CFU (colony-forming unit)-S (spleen); S-cell, stem cell; GEMM, granulocyte erythroid macrophage megakaryocyte; GM, granulocyte macrophage; G, granulocyte; M, macrophage; BFU-E, burst-forming unit erythroid; MK, megakaryocyte. Information on these assays can be found in refs. *4* and *6.*

the cytokines produced by these cells on the stem and progenitor cells *(4–6)*. In the adult, the main source of stem and progenitor cells is the bone marrow, but these cells can be found circulating in the blood, although at extremely low concentrations unless these cells are mobilized from the marrow in response to exogenously administered cytokines, or during recovery from chemotherapy. High concentrations of stem and progenitor cells can also be found normally in the umbilical cord and placental blood

(7,8). Adult bone marrow, mobilized peripheral blood, and cord blood have each served as sources of transplantable stem and progenitor cells. The mechanisms involved in the mobilization of stem and progenitor cells to the blood or in the relatively high frequency of these cells noted in cord blood is currently not known, but probably reflects the homing and migration properties of these cells; this capacity for movement most likely reflects the movement of these cells in early embryonic and fetal life *(9)*. During embryonic and fetal development, hematopoietic stem and progenitor cells are found first in the caudal intraembryonic splanchnopleura/yolk sac area, next in fetal liver, and then in fetal bone marrow *(9–14)*. The regulation of stem/progenitor cell movement and the mechanisms involved in these events are also intense areas of investigation. This no doubt involves specific adhesive properties of these cells and the responses of these cells to cytokines and accessory cells.

This chapter reviews information on the roles of a family of cytokine molecules, called chemokines (so named for their <u>chemo</u>tactic cyto<u>kine</u> properties) in the modulation of the proliferation, differentiation, and movement of hematopoietic stem and progenitor cells.

2. CHEMOKINES AND THEIR RECEPTORS

Although chemokines are a relatively new family of proteins in terms of our understanding of the actual numbers of these cytokines and their receptors, more than 50 chemokines have been reported to date *(15–19)*. Table 1 gives frequently used abbreviations for these chemokines; Table 2 lists those chemokines evaluated for activity by the authors. Chemokines fall into at least four different subgroups, which include position-invariant cysteine cysteine (C-C), C-X-C (where X can be any amino acid), C, or CX_3C motifs near the N-terminal portion of the molecule *(15,17,19,20)*. Currently, nine receptors have been identified for the C-C chemokines; these have been termed CCR1–CCR9. Five receptors have been identified for C-X-C chemokines, and these have been termed CXCR1–CXCR5. One receptor has been identified for the CX_3C chemokine and termed CX_3CR1. There is redundancy in chemokine–chemokine receptor interactions. Many chemokine receptors bind more than one chemokine and some chemokines bind to more than one receptor. Table 3 gives examples of chemokines that bind chemokine receptors. Chemokine receptors are G protein linked, but not much is known regarding how specific chemokine functions link to intracellular signals transmitted through the specific chemokine receptor, especially when more than one chemokine can bind a receptor, yet not all chemokines that bind that receptor elicit the same functional activity. Additionally, CCR9 is a promiscuous receptor for C-C chemokines, but there is no evidence yet that this is a signaling receptor *(21)*. Moreover, the Duffy antigen receptor for chemokines (DARC) is a unique receptor in that it binds members of both the C-C and C-X-C chemokine families *(22–24)*. DARC may also not be a signaling receptor. There are still chemokines in search of a receptor, and receptors in search of a chemokine. Added to this complexity are virally encoded chemokine-like molecules, and receptors *(25–30)*. It will be interesting to see what future research unravels about this complex area of chemokines and chemokine receptors, e.g., how specificity is maintained, how the actions of these molecules and receptors are mechanistically mediated intracellularly, how these effects/events mediate

Table 1
Chemokine Abbreviations[a]

Abbreviation	Full name
BLC/BCA-1	B-lymphocytes chemoattractant/B-cell-attracting chemokine
CKβ	Chemokine β
ELC	EBI (EBV-induced gene) 1-ligand chemokine
ENA	Epithelial cell–derived neutrophil attractant
GCP	Granulocyte chemotactic protein
GRO	Growth-related oncogene
HCC	HCC
I-309	I-309
IL-8	Interleukin-8
IP	Interferon-γ-inducible protein
LARC	Liver and activation-regulated chemokine
LKN	Leukotactin
LMC	Lymphocyte and monocyte chemoattractant
MCIF	Macrophage colony inhibitor factor
MCP	Monocyte chemoattractant protein
MDC	Macrophage-derived chemokine
MIG	Monokine induced by interferon-γ
MIP	Macrophage inflammatory protein
MPIF	Myeloid progenitor inhibitor factor
MRP	MIP-1α related protein
NAP	Neutrophil-activating peptide
NCC	Novel CC chemokine
PF4	Platelet factor 4
RANTES	Regulated on activation of normal T-cell expressed and secreted
SDF	Stromal cell–derived factor
SLC	Secondary lymphoid-tissue chemokine
TARC	Thymus and activation-regulated chemokine
TCA	T-cell activation gene
TECK	Thymus-expressed chemokine

[a] Although this table lists abbreviations, note that there are many different MIPs (e.g., MIP-1α, MIP-1β, MIP-2α, MIP-2β, MIP-3α, MIP-3β, MIP-4, and MIP-5) and MCPs (MCP-1 to MCP-5). Additionally, there are a number of other chemokines such as eotaxin-1 and eotaxin-2, lymphotactin and fractalkine/neurotactin, exodus, and 6CKine, which are not usually abbreviated.

normal cellular regulatory interactions, what role they play in disease, and how this information can be utilized clinically to enhance the efficacy of various treatments.

3. CHEMOKINE EFFECTS IN VITRO ON THE PROLIFERATION OF HEMATOPOIETIC STEM AND PROGENITOR CELLS

3.1. Enhancing Effects of Murine Macrophage Inflammatory Proteins on Proliferation of Progenitor Cells

The first biologic activity demonstrated for chemokine family members in the area of blood cell production was enhancement of proliferation of more mature members of the colony-forming unit–granulocyte-macrophage (CFU-GM) and CFU-macrophage (CFU-M) progenitor cell subsets *(31,32)*. These relatively more mature progenitor cell subsets *(see* Fig. 1) respond to the proliferative signal of a single cytokine such as

Table 2
Chemokine Family Members[a]

Position-invariant C-C motif: β-subfamily	*Position-invariant C-X-C motif: α-subfamily*
Suppressive	*Suppressive*
MIP-1α (macrophage inflammatory protein) = LD78	GRO-β = MIP-2α
MCP-1 (monocyte chemoattractant protein-1) = MCAF	IL-8 (Interleukin-8) = NAP-1
MCP-4/CKβ-10	PF4 (platelet factor 4)
LKN-1 (leukotactin-1) MIP-5/HCC2	IP-10 (interferon-γ-inducible protein-10)
CKβ-4/MIP-3α/LARC/Exodus-1	MIG (monokine induced by interferon-γ)
Exodus-2/6Ckine/CKβ9	GCP-2
Exodus-3/CKβ11/MIP-3β/ELC	ENA-78
CKβ7/MIP-4	
CKβ8/MPIF-1	*Nonsuppressive*
CKβ8-1 (splicing variant)	GRO-1α = melanoma growth-stimulating factor = KC
CKβ6/MPIF-2/Eotaxin-2	GRO-γ = MIP-2β
I-309	NAP-2 (neutrophil-activating peptide-2)
TECK	SDF-1α (stromal cell–derived factor)
LMC	SDF-1β (splicing variant)
MRP-2/MIP-1γ	
Nonsuppressive	*C Motif: suppressive*
MIP-1β = Act2	Lymphotactin
RANTES (regulated on activation of normal T-cell expressed and secreted)	
MCP-2	*CX₃C Motif: nonsuppressive*
MCP-3	Fractalkine/neurotactin
Eotaxin-1	
CKβ1/HCC-1/MCIF	
TARC	
MDC	

[a] Only those chemokines suppressive or not suppressive for inhibition of primary human bone marrow myeloid progenitor cells stimulated to proliferate by multiple cytokines are listed.

granulocyte-macrophage–colony-stimulating factor (GM-CSF) for CFU-GM and macrophage-CSF (M-CSF) for CFU-M. Murine macrophage inflammatory protein-1α (MIP-1α), MIP-1β, and MIP-2 enhanced colony formation by CFU-GM stimulated by GM-CSF and CFU-M stimulated by M-CSF. Murine MIP-2 should not be confused with members of the human MIP-2 family, which are different. The specificity of the chemokines was demonstrated by antibodies against murine MIP-1, which neutralized the enhancing activities of murine MIP-1, and antibodies against murine MIP-2, which neutralized the enhancing activity of MIP-2. These enhancing effects of murine MIP-1α, murine MIP-1β, and murine MIP-2 were apparent on both murine and human CFU-GM and were evidently limited to the GM lineage as murine MIP-1α, murine MIP-1β, and murine MIP-2 had no effect on colony formation by erythroid progenitor cells (burst-forming unit–erythroid [BFU-E]) in the presence or absence of the erythroid-specific growth factor, erythropoietin (Epo).

Progenitor cells are rare populations of cells, and unless these cells are purified, it is difficult to prove that the effects of a cytokine on the progenitor cells are direct, rather than indirect effects mediated through cytokine action on an accessory cell, which then

Table 3
Chemokine Receptors and Their Ligands[a]

Receptors	Ligand
C-C	
CCR1	MIP-1α, LKN-1/MIP-5/HCC2/NCC3, CKβ8/MPIF-1/MIP-3, CKβ8-1 (splicing variant), murine MRP-2/MIP-1γ, RANTES, MCP-3, CKβ1/HCC-1/MCIF/NCC2
CCR2a, 2b	MCP-1/murine JE, MCP-2, MCP-3, MCP-4, murine MCP-5*
CCR3	CKβ-10/MCP-4, LKN-1/MIP-5/HCC2, CKβ6/MPIF-2/Eotaxin-2, Eotaxin-1, RANTES, MCP-2, MCP-3
CCR4	TARC, MDC
CCR5	MIP-1α, MIP-1β, RANTES
CCR6	CKβ4/MIP-3α/LARC/Exodus-1
CCR7	CKβ11/MIP-3β/ELC/Exodus-3, SLC/6CKine/Exodus-2/TCA-4
CCR8	1309,** TARC, MIP-1β
CCR9	Promiscuous (nonsignaling)***
CCR?	TECK, CKβ7/MIP-4, LMC
C-X-C	
CXCR1	IL-8, GCP-2
CXCR2	IL-8, muMIP-2, GCP-2, GRO-β/MIP-2α, ENA-78, GRO-α,**** GRO-γ/MIP-2β, NAP-2
CXCR3	IP-10, MIG
CXCR4	SDF-1α, SDF-1β
CXCR5	BLC/BCA-1*
CXCR?	PF4
CX₃C	
C X₃CR1	Fractalkine/neurotactin
C	
CR?	Lymphotactin

[a]Underlined, inhibitory; nonunderlined, noninhibitory, except if noted by *, which indicates not yet tested for inhibitory activity. ** I-309 has relatively low suppressive activity compared to other chemokines. *** Chemokines binding to CCR9 include MIP-1α, MIP-1β, RANTES, MCP-1 to MCP-5, eotaxin-1, CKβ1/HCC-1; they do not cause Ca flux. **** GRO-α has no suppressive activity against CFU-GEMM, BFU-E, and CFU-GM stimulated by multiple growth factors *(36)*, but it has been reported to inhibit proliferation of the murine factor–dependent cell line 32D *(60)*. CCR? and CXCR?, Actual receptor that binds these chemokines has not yet been identified.

influences the progenitor cell *(4–6)*. Although most of the effects of murine MIP-1α, murine MIP-1β, and murine MIP-2 were assessed on relatively heterogeneous populations of mouse or human bone marrow cells, studies using very highly purified populations of murine CFU-GM and murine CFU-M, attained through separation by centrifugal elutriation, suggested that the murine MIP-1- and murine MIP-2-enhancing effects were direct acting effects on the CFU-GM and CFU-M themselves *(31)*. Since chemokines, as well as other cytokines, can have pleiotrophic effects, the demonstration of direct effects of chemokines on the progenitors does not rule out the possibility that MIP-1α, MIP-1β, and MIP-2 can also have enhancing or other effects on progenitors that are mediated indirectly on the progenitors through accessory cell action.

3.2. Suppressing Effects of MIP-1α on Proliferation
of Stem and Immature Progenitor Cells

Shortly after murine MIP-1α, murine MIP-1β, and murine MIP-2 were shown to enhance the proliferation of later subsets of CFU-GM and CFU-M, it was reported that an inhibitor of the proliferation of a myeloid stem cell compartment (CFU-S) was identified as murine MIP-1α *(33)*. During *ex vivo* treatment of mouse marrow cells, murine MIP-1α decreased the cycling status of CFU-S without influencing the frequency of CFU-S (number of CFU-S/10^5 marrow cells). The S-phase specificity of the effect was documented by a high specific activity tritiated thymidine kill technique that has been explained elsewhere *(6)*. Murine MIP-1α also decreased colony formation of CFU-A, an apparently primitive cell whose designation is not currently utilized by most laboratories. CFU-S is known not to be a competitive repopulating stem cell *(4,6)*. It is not clear whether MIP-1α can suppress the proliferation of the earliest stem cells that have long-term marrow repopulating capacity. It may be difficult to determine an effect on this earliest cell because the opinion, to date, is that this cell is essentially in a noncycling state, being in the G_1- or G_0-phase of the cell cycle *(1–6)*, and the effects of MIP-1α appear to be relatively specific for cycling cells. The high specific activity tritiated thymidine kill technique has been used here to suggest that the effects of MIP-1α are mainly in S-phase (DNA synthetic phase) of the cell cycle *(34)*. It is possible that once the early marrow repopulating stem cell enters active cell cycle, it is no longer a long-term marrow repopulating stem cell. If this is the case, then it is unlikely that MIP-1α will have an effect on this early stem cell.

Murine and human MIP-1α were determined to be non-species specific in action, and both murine and human MIP-1α were found to suppress the proliferation of the immature subsets of multipotential (CFU-granulocyte erythroid macrophage megakaryocyte [CFU-GEMM]), erythroid (BFU-E), and granulocyte-macrophage (CFU-GM) progenitors. Within the CFU-GEMM, BFU-E, and CFU-GM compartments, there are subsets of cells that are immature and respond to combinations of cytokines by forming large colonies containing many cells. The more mature subsets of cells respond to a single cytokine and form smaller-sized colonies *(3)*. MIP-1α inhibited those progenitors that responded to stimulation by the combination of multiple cytokines such as Epo, GM-CSF, or interleukin-3 (IL-3) in combination with the potent costimulating cytokines steel factor ([SLF], also known as stem cell factor [SCF]; mast cell growth factor; and the *c*-kit ligand) and/or Flt3-ligand (L) *(32,34–37)*. SLF and Flt3-L respectively bind and activate the tyrosine kinase receptors, *c*-kit and Flt3/Flk-2 *(38,39)*. The suppressive effects of murine and human MIP-1α on colony formation by human CFU-GEMM, BFU-E, and CFU-GM were determined, in large part, to be due to a direct-acting effect on these progenitors *(32,36,40)*. This was first suggested by inhibition of colony formation by highly purified populations of cells expressing a high density of CD34 antigens (CD34^{+++}) *(32,36)*, and was then more rigorously confirmed by assessing the effects of MIP-1α on the growth of single isolated CD34^{+++} human bone marrow cells stimulated by combinations of growth factors in the presence or absence of serum *(40)*.

3.3. Suppressive Effects of Other Chemokines on Proliferation
of Immature Progenitor Cells

A degree of specificity for the suppressive effects of MIP-1α on the proliferation of stem and immature progenitors was determined when MIP-1β failed to manifest suppression *(32,35)*. However, it soon became clear that MIP-1α was not the only member of the expanding family of chemokine molecules to manifest suppressive activity against the proliferation of immature progenitor cells. In short order it was found that other chemokines with suppressive activity included human forms of MIP-2α =growth-related oncogene-β (GRO-β), platelet factor 4 (PF4), IL-8, and monocyte chemoattractant protein-1 (MCP-1) (= monocyte chemoattractant and activating factor [MCAF]) *(36)*. By contrast, human forms of MIP-1β, MIP-2β (=GRO-γ), GRO-α, neutrophil-activating protein-2 (NAP-2), and RANTES were not suppressive *(36)*. Interestingly, excess MIP-1β blocked the suppressive effects of MIP-1α, and excess MIP-2β or GRO-α blocked the suppressive effects of IL-8 and PF4 *(35,36)*. These studies were reported before the specific chemokine receptors shown in Table 3 were known. The meaning of blocking remains to be determined. For example, MIP-1α and MIP-1β both bind the chemokine receptors CCR5 and CCR9 whereas MIP-1α, but not MIP-1β, also binds CCR1. Since CCR9 appears to be a nonsignaling receptor *(21)*, a simple interpretation is that the suppressive effects of MIP-1α may be mainly mediated through CCR5 and that MIP-1β cannot transmit a negative proliferative effect, but that its binding to CCR5 blocks the binding or downmodulates the suppressive action of MIP-1α. It has been suggested that MIP-1α may manifest inhibitory activity through CCR1 *(41)*; however, studies with CCR1 knockout mice suggest that CCR1 is probably not a dominant receptor for this effect *(42)*.

Why two chemokines that apparently bind the same receptor can mediate different end results is not known. Alternatively, there may be other chemokine receptors that bind MIP-1α and MIP-1β that have not yet been identified, or MIP-1β blocking may involve binding to a receptor that desensitizes the effects of another chemokine receptor that is binding and mediating the suppressive effects of MIP-1α on proliferation. That MIP-2β or GRO-α blocked the suppressive effects of IL-8 *(36)* may be explained by the binding of these three chemokines to the chemokine receptor CXCR2 (*see* Table 3), a receptor that has been demonstrated through the use of CXCR2 gene knockout mice to be involved in the negative regulation of progenitor cell proliferation *(43)*. However, the receptor for PF4 has not been identified, so unless a new signaling chemokine receptor is identified that binds MIP-2β, GRO-α, and PF4, the blocking effects of MIP-2β and GRO-α may be explained by receptor cross talk and desensitization.

Table 2 lists all the human chemokines that we have now assessed for their capacity to suppress the proliferation of human bone marrow progenitors that respond to stimulation by multiple growth factors *(32,34–37,44–51)*. Some of these chemokines have also been reported by other groups to be myelosuppressive in vitro *(52–63)*. Thus far, within the C-C chemokine family, 14 C-C chemokines have been found to be suppressive, and 8 C-C chemokines were not suppressive. Within the C-X-C chemokine family, 7 C-X-C chemokines have been found to be suppressive, and 4 C-X-C chemokines were not suppressive. The only member of the C chemokine family so far reported— lymphotactin (Ltn)—was suppressive, and the only member of the CX_3C chemokine family so far identified—fractalkine/neurotactin—was not suppressive. There is evidence, through assessment of the effects at the level of single CD34[+++] bone marrow cells, that some of these chemokines are mediating their effects directly at the level of the progenitor cell *(40)*. Not all effects may be direct and one cannot rule out both direct and indirect suppressive effects.

In an attempt to determine through which receptors the chemokines are manifesting their suppressive effects, we have listed the receptors that bind chemokines in Table 3 and underlined those chemokines that are suppressive. However, simply because we have underlined an active chemokine does not mean that it signals through that receptor to elicit a suppressive effect on proliferation. Information in Table 3 highlights the difficulty of our task in determining why some chemokines that bind a receptor elicit a negative proliferative effect, whereas others do not. Perhaps as more information on missing or orphan receptors becomes apparent, and as more biologic data are generated through the use of receptor gene knockout mice, we can begin to unravel this fascinating mystery.

3.4. Enhanced Activity of Chemokines as Suppressive Molecules for Immature Progenitor Cell Proliferation and Synergism with Other Chemokines and Members of Other Families of Cytokines

It is known that chemokines polymerize or form aggregates greater than monomers *(34,64–67)*. The active myelosuppressive form of murine MIP-1α appears to be a monomer *(34)*, suppressive effects suggested through studies that used gel filtration chromatography on a Superose-12 column and acetonitrile as a diluent. The monomeric form of MIP-1α had an approx 1000-fold higher specific activity than previously shown for the unfractionated sample. The initial sample was composed mainly of aggregated MIP-1α (>98%), and the aggregated MIP-1α was inactive as a suppressor molecule but did not block the suppressive activity of the monomer *(34)*. This study suggested, but did not prove, that the monomeric form was the active form binding to its receptor and that the monomeric form might be the physiologically relevant form. This latter possibility was, however, suggested by the enhanced specific activity of exogenously administered monomeric MIP-1α to mice in vivo *(68)*.

Additional studies with other chemokines suggest the possibility that their suppressive activities may also reside in the monomeric form *(37)*. Placing MIP-1α, PF4, IL-8, and interferon-γ-inducible protein-10 (IP-10) into an acetonitrile solution, as was done for MIP-1α, and adding low concentrations of these acetonitrile diluent-containing chemokines to phosphate-buffered saline solutions, demonstrated a large increase in specific activity of the chemokines. Of relevance, the nonsuppressive chemokines MIP-1β, MIP-2β, GRO-α, NAP-2, and RANTES were not suppressive even after pretreatment with acetonitrile. More recent studies have demonstrated that acetonitrile treatment of the chemokines CKβ7/MIP-4, CKβ4/MIP-3α/LARC/Exodus-1, monokine induced by interferon-γ (MIG), epithelial cell–derived neutrophil-activating factor-78 (ENA-78), and Ltn also greatly enhanced their specific activity as suppressor molecules of progenitor cell proliferation in vitro *(69)*. Interpretation of the previously noted evidence suggesting the activity of monomeric chemokines has been discussed in detail *(34,37,68)*.

Large increases in the specific activity of chemokines for myelosuppression have also been noted when a chemokine at very low concentration, below the level at which it is myelosuppressive, is added together with another suppressive chemokine at a very low concentration. This synergism has been noted for a large number of chemokines, including the combination of any two of the following chemokines: MIP-1α, MIP-2α, PF4, IL-8, MCP-1, and IP-10 *(36,47)*. This synergism was not apparent for the mixing of two chemokines that alone at high concentrations were not suppressive, or for the mixing of a low concentration of a suppressive chemokine with a nonsuppressive chemokine *(36)*. Whether this synergism reflects direct effects, indirect effects, or direct and indirect effects of these chemokines on the progenitor cells has not been determined. The suppressive synergism noted in vitro was even greater when low concentrations of acetonitrile-treated chemokines were tested in combination *(37)*. The actions mediating synergism may be different for different combinations of chemokines. This synergism is also seen in studies in vivo in mice *(44)*.

Chemokines have also been shown to synergize with two nonchemokine family members to suppress progenitor cell proliferation: macrophage stimulating protein, and vascular endothelial cell growth factor *(70)*.

Efforts have also been undertaken to enhance the specific suppressive activity of chemokines through the construction of chimeric molecules. A series of PF4 and IL-8 mutant molecules were analyzed *(71)*. Interestingly, a class of chimeric mutants consisting of domains of either PF4 and IL-8, GRO-α, and PF4 or GRO-β and PF4 were found to inhibit myeloid cell proliferation at concentrations between 500- and 5000-fold lower than either the IL-8 or PF4 wild-type proteins alone; these effects were comparable to or better than the activity seen when IL-8 and PF4 wild-type molecules were added together in vitro. Enhanced activity was seen with some of these mutants in mice in which exogenous administration decreased the cycling status and absolute numbers of progenitors per femur at concentrations manyfold lower than those of the IL-8 and PF4 wild-type molecules *(71)*.

3.5. Activities of Chemokines on Growth of Primary Progenitor Cells from Patients with Leukemia and Related Diseases

Although there is a report that MIP-1α suppresses in vitro growth of cells from patients with acute myelogenous leukemia (AML) *(72)*, on the whole, there appears to be heterogeneity with respect to cellular responsiveness of leukemic cells to the actions of MIP-1α *(37,73)*. In one study, none of the assessed patients with AML had progenitors responsive to inhibition by MIP-1α *(37)*. Patients with chronic myelogenous leukemia (CML) *(37,73)* and Diamond Blackfan Syndrome *(74)* also demonstrate heterogeneity in responsiveness to inhibition by MIP-1α, although at present it seems that most of the evaluated patients with CML do not have progenitors that respond to MIP-1α inhibition, even though these progenitors are in cycle at the time the MIP-1α is added with the cells (*[37]*, Broxmeyer, H. E., et al., unpublished observations). Having cells in S-phase, as assessed by high specific activity tritiated thymidine kill *(6)*, is crucial to the detection of the suppressive effects of MIP-1α, and other chemokines in vitro *(34,37)*. As an example, human cord blood myeloid progenitors, in contrast to bone marrow myeloid progenitors, are essentially in a slow or noncycling state and are insensitive to inhibition by MIP-1α and other chemokines unless the cord blood myeloid progenitors are placed into rapid cell cycle traverse in vitro by stimulation with growth-promoting cytokines *(37)*. Interestingly, if patient cells were insensitive to inhibition by MIP-1α, even though a large percentage of the cells were in active cell cycle, they were also insensitive to inhibition by MIP-2α, IL-8, PF4, MCP-1, and IP-10 *(37)*. This finding suggests multiple chemokine receptor abnormalities or a common downstream signaling effect in progenitor cells from certain patients with leukemia. By contrast, the C-C chemokine CKβ4/MIP-3α/LARC/Exodus-1 has been found to be suppressive for progenitor cell proliferation in CML, when the same cells from these patients were completely or relatively insensitive to inhibition by MIP-1α *(75)*. This suggests that the C-C chemokine receptor CCR6 (which binds CKβ4) may be a reasonable target for attempts to block the hyperproliferative state associated with CML. A screen of other chemokines may identify additional chemokines or chemokine receptors for targeting in CML.

3.6. Chemokine- and Chemokine Receptor–Like Molecules Encoded by Viruses

The recent literature has documented the presence of sequences in the genome of various viruses that encode molecules bearing a similarity to chemokines and chemokine receptors *(25–30,76)*. Examples include sequences related to CXCR1, CXCR2, and a MIP-1α/RANTES receptor in herpesvirus *(25,27)*, and sequences related to an MIP-1α/RANTES/MCP-1 receptor in human cytomegalovirus, some of which are distantly related to CCR5 and also to CXCR4 *(30)*. Moreover, Kaposi's sarcoma–associated human herpesvirus-8 encodes homologs of MIP-1α and MIP-1β *(29)*, and molluscum contagiosum virus (MCV) types 1 and 2 encode sequences similar to MIP-1α and MIP-1β *(28)*. The genes from MCV types 1 and 2 with sequence homology to MIP-1α were cloned and expressed *(28)*. Interestingly, these purified proteins suppressed colony formation by human progenitor cells stimulated to proliferate by multiple growth factors. Although these proteins did not result in chemotaxis of monocytes, as did MIP-1α, they did antagonize the chemotactic activity of MIP-1α. Most recently, it was reported that vaccinia virus and other orthopoxviruses (cowpox and camelpox) express a 35-kDa chemokine binding protein with no sequence homology to known cellular chemokine receptors *(77)*. This protein bound C-C, but not C-X-C or C, chemokines with high affinity and blocked the interactions of MCP-4 and eotaxin with their receptors. These findings suggest means by which viruses may block or circumvent the normal chemokine/chemokine receptor interactions and portions of the immune/hematopoietic regulatory responses.

3.7. Other Effects of Chemokines on Hematopoiesis

Information on the regulation of the earliest stem cell subsets is still quite limited. However, an in vitro long-term culture (LTC) system developed more than 20 yr ago allows prolonged growth of blood cells, mainly of the myeloid lineages, and a means to assess this production from a long-term culture-initiating cell (LTC-IC) *(4)*. Whether or not the LTC-IC describes a long-term marrow repopulating stem cell remains to be determined, but it is probably an early cell within the human stem cell compartment. MIP-1α was assessed for activity in the context of a human bone marrow LTC that requires a stromal cell layer for optimal output of cells, but that was modified to provide a "stroma-non-contract" system *(78)*. Under these conditions, the number of LTC-IC present after 8 wk did not change when MIP-1α was added as the only exogenous factor. However, MIP-1α did enhance output of LTC-IC when used in combination with IL-3. These results were interpreted to suggest that the effects noted depended on soluble but ill-defined stromal factors and a direct interaction of MIP-1α and other cytokines on the proliferating cells. There has not been much follow-up on these results, and it is still unclear how MIP-1α is acting under these conditions, although results suggesting that MIP-1α increases the self-renewal capacity of CFU-S after hydroxy-urea treatment in vivo *(79)* may be of relevance to the LTC-IC data.

Eotaxin-1 has recently been implicated as a growth factor during lung inflammation *(80)*. Neutralizing antibodies to eotaxin-1 administered during development of lung allergic inflammation prevented the increase in marrow myeloid progenitors, whereas in vivo administration of eotaxin-1 increased the number of marrow myeloid progenitor cells. It was suggested that eotaxin-1 acted as a CSF for granulocytes and macrophages. Eotaxin synergized with SCF, but not IL-3 or GM-CSF to stimulate growth, effects blocked by the use of pertussis toxin (PTX). Whether eotaxin is truly a CSF in the context of GM-CSF, IL-3, IL-5, or G-CSF and can directly trigger cell proliferation by itself remains to be proven and will require more rigorous studies using more purified populations of progenitors and studies at the single-cell level.

4. NEGATIVE EFFECTS OF CHEMOKINES IN VIVO ON THE PROLIFERATION OF HEMATOPOIETIC STEM AND PROGENITOR CELLS AND EVALUATION OF THEIR POSSIBLE USE AS MYELOPROTECTIVE AGENTS

4.1. MIP-1α Effects in Mice

The myelosuppressive effects of MIP-1α noted in vitro by a number of laboratories have also been confirmed through in vivo analysis of the exogenous administration of MIP-1α to mice *(22,25,81)*. The effects in vivo are believed to be S-phase specific, similar to their actions in vitro. This specificity is based on high specific activity tritiated thymidine assessment of cells from mice treated with chemokines *(33,37,68,81)*. The in vivo administration of MIP-1α to mice decreased the cycling rates of CFU-S, CFU-GEMM, BFU-E, and CFU-GM, placing them into a slow or noncycling state. Effects were noted within 3 h on cycling status of myeloid progenitors in marrow and spleen and were maintained for at least 24 h after a single injection of MIP-1α *(68,81)*. By 24 h, significant decreases were also seen in the absolute numbers of progenitors in marrow and spleen with subsequent decreases in circulating neutrophils. These effects were dose dependent, time related, and reversible. Within the framework of a few days, as long as the MIP-1α was administered, the decreases in progenitor cell cycling and numbers were apparent, but the effects were reversed within 48 h after the last injection of MIP-1α. The time sequence and reversibility were the same when a preparation of MIP-1α believed to be in monomeric form was administered to mice *(37,81)* as they were when MIP-1α in both polymerized and monomeric forms was given (the usual content of the preparation unless efforts are made to use only monomeric MIP-1α) *(34)*, except that the effects were noted at much lower concentrations when only monomeric MIP-1α was used. As an example, it took microgram quantities of MIP-1α to be suppressive when an unfractionated sample containing monomeric and polymerized MIP-1α was used (which only contains about 1% monomeric MIP-1α), yet only nanogram quantities of MIP-1α were needed when the MIP-1α was essentially in monomeric form prior to the administration of this chemokine to mice.

4.2. Preclinical and Clinical Effects of MIP-1α

Being able to place stem and progenitor cells into a slow or noncycling state offers the potential to dampen the cytotoxic effects of the chemotherapeutic drugs, by having the cells placed into a less sensitive phase of the cell cycle *(82,83)*. These possibilities were verified in mice using two S-phase-specific drugs, ara-C and hydroxyurea *(84,85)*. In both studies, CFU-Ss were apparently protected and the recovery of blood cells from cytotoxic drug treatment was accelerated when mice were pretreated with MIP-1α.

Based on the preclinical studies of MIP-1α in vitro and in vivo, and on the need to work with a molecule that did not readily aggregate into large multimeric forms, an active variant of human MIP-1α with improved pharmaceutical properties, BB10010, was developed *(86)*. BB10010 carries a single amino acid substitution of the only Asp between the third and fourth Cys to Ala and has a reduced tendency to form large polymers at physiologic pH and ionic strength. The activity of BB10010 was confirmed in receptor-binding, calcium mobilization, and biologic assays in vitro and in mice in vivo. Although BB10010 was apparently no more active on a weight-for-weight basis than MIP-1α, the fact that it aggregated to no more than tetrameric form made it more suitable for actual clinical trials, and these were performed at several clinical centers *(87,89)*. At one of the centers, BB10010 was assessed for effects on marrow and blood myeloid progenitors in patients with relapsed/refractory breast cancer *(87)*. Patients were injected subcutaneously with 5, 10, 30, or 100 µg/kg of BB10010 daily for 3 d. BB10010 significantly reduced the cycling status of marrow myeloid progenitors from pretreatment levels of 39–58% to 0–11% 1 d after the third and last injection of BB10010 *(87)*. This was associated with significant decreases in the frequency of marrow progenitors (number of colonies formed per number of cells plated) and the percentage of CD34$^+$ cells present in biopsied bone marrow. The suppressive effects were reversible in patients, but because the patients could not undergo frequent marrow aspirates, the actual speed of reversibility could not be determined *(87)*. Rather, the rapidity of reversal was documented using mice as models for the human clinical trials *(87)*.

Interestingly, even though the cycling status and actual numbers of progenitors were decreased in marrow (as assessed by calculating the reduced frequency of progenitors from the decreased percentage of marrow CD34$^+$ cells), BB10010 had no effect on nucleated cellularity or on the proliferation of the morphologically recognizable proliferating cells as assessed in marrow biopsies from the patients using immunohistochemical staining for proliferating cell nuclear antigen *(87)*. Some insight into this apparent contradiction in which decreased progenitor cell proliferation did not result in decreased nucleated cellularity was suggested by an analysis of the apoptotic rates of the nucleated cells as assessed from biopsy samples using an *in situ* DNA end-labeling technique. Decreased apoptosis of nucleated cells was seen after the administration of BB10010, suggesting a possible reason for the lack of decreased nucleated cellularity *(87)*. This finding is especially of interest, since recent studies using mice lacking the expression of the Fanconi anemia complementation C (FAC) group gene demonstrated that FAC (–/–) mouse bone marrow myeloid progenitor cells were more sensitive to inhibition by MIP-1α than were cells from marrows of wild-type littermate FAC (+/+) controls. This enhanced sensitivity to MIP-α suppression was associated with increased apoptosis of phenotypically defined stem and progenitor cells in response to the effects of MIP-1α *(90)*. Thus, it is possible that MIP-1α has different apoptotic effects on different subsets of cells: enhanced apoptosis on stem and progenitor cells and decreased apoptosis on morphologically recognizable proliferating nucleated cells.

While this possibility requires further verification and more rigorous proof, it is consistent with the biologic characteristics of MIP-1α in which it decreases proliferation of the immature progenitor cell subsets and enhances proliferation of the more mature progenitor cell subsets *(31,32)*.

Even though the stem/progenitor cell suppressive effects of MIP-1α were confirmed in a phase I clinical trial and were consistent with the preclinical mouse studies, caution in expectations of the myeloprotective effects of chemokines themselves is warranted. It is not clear yet that MIP-1α or other chemokines by themselves will be clinically myeloprotective. It did not appear that BB10010 offered myeloprotection against the effects of cyclophosphamide *(88)* or the combination of etoposide and cyclophosphamide *(89)*. This lack of protection against the toxicity of cyclophosphamide might reflect the action of the drug itself, which is known to be active in other phases of the cell cycle in addition to S-phase. A better test case would have utilized clinical myeloprotection in the context of one S-phase-specific drug, such as that used in the preclinical mouse studies *(84,85)*. However, it is rare that a single chemotherapeutic agent is used in the treatment of malignancy. In most cases, drugs with different modes of action that affect different phases of the cell cycle are combined for the greatest therapeutic effect. For ethical reasons, cyclophosphamide was the only drug that could be used as a single agent in the patients with relapsed/refractory breast cancer, since it is the only drug that when used alone has shown some clinical efficacy of action in this disease. Thus, it may not ethically be possible to use a single S-phase-specific drug in the treatment of malignancy in the context of assessing the myeloprotective effects of MIP-1α or any other chemokine. Whether a single chemokine, or even combinations of chemokines, will be myeloprotective in a clinical setting remains to be proven. It is possible that BB10010 may have to be used in combination with other cytokines or agents in order to offer the most protection in a chemotherapy setting that uses multiple drugs with different modes of action.

4.3. Preclinical and Myeloprotective Effects of Other Chemokines

A large number of chemokines (Tables 2 and 3) have myelosuppressive effects in vitro that are similar to the actions of MIP-1α. Although it is not yet clear whether all these effects are direct-acting ones on the progenitors, the final actions are apparently mediated on actively cycling progenitor cells *(34,37,44)*. Moreover, of those chemokines tested for activity in vivo in mouse models, it is clear that chemokines with suppressive activity in vitro also manifest suppressive activity in vivo, whereas chemokines that do not have suppressive activity in vitro do not manifest suppressive activity in vivo *(37,44)*. Presently, the following chemokines have been tested and found to be myelosuppressive in mouse models: MIP-2α (=GRO-β), PF4, IL-8, MCP-1, IP-10, ENA-78, Ltn, CKβ-11/MIP-3/ELC/Exodus-3, CKβ4/MIP-3α/LARC/Exodus-1, and MIG *(37,44,81)*. Those chemokines assessed in vivo and found lacking in myelosuppressive effects, consistent with their lack of suppressive activity in vitro, include MIP-1β, MIP-2β (=GRO-γ), GRO-α, and RANTES *(44,81)*.

It is also of significance that the synergism noted in myelosuppression with low concentrations of combinations of active chemokines in vitro is also apparent in vivo *(44)*. Thus, in vivo, one needs concentrations of 10 μg/mouse to see decreased cycling and absolute numbers of progenitors with either ENA-78, Ltn, CKβ-11, MIP-1α, IL-8,

PF4, MCP-1, Exodus-1, or MIG *(44)*. Inhibition is not detected with 1 µg/mouse of any of these chemokines alone. However, the addition of concentrations as low as 0.01 µg/mouse of any two of the following chemokines in combination resulted in significant myelosuppression: MIP-1α plus IL-8, MIP-1α plus PF4, IL-8 plus PF4, MCP-1 plus Exodus-1, MCP-1 plus MIG, Exodus-1 plus MIG, ENA-78 plus Ltn, ENA-78 plus CKβ11, or Ltn plus CKβ11 *(44)*. It is clear that synergism in vivo is apparent even when chemokines of different subgroups such as C-C, C-X-C, or C are mixed. We do not understand yet how suppressive synergism occurs in vitro, and it will no doubt be more complicated to dissect these effects in vivo.

In addition to MIP-1α, PF4 and IL-8 have been assessed for myeloprotective effects in the context of S-phase-specific chemotherapeutic drugs in preclinical mouse studies *(91)*. Both IL-8 and PF4 were protective for myeloid progenitor cells in mice exposed to hydroxyurea and 5-fluorouracil *(91)*. One of the IL-8/PF4 chimeric mutants was also myeloprotective, but able to manifest this effect at much lower concentrations than either wild-type IL-8 or wild-type PF4. The effects of PF4 and IL-8 in this context may reflect, in part, enhanced survival of the progenitors, an action that has been noted by one group in the absence of chemotherapeutic drugs *(92)*.

5. CHEMOKINE EFFECTS ON PROGENITOR CELL MIGRATION IN VITRO AND ON MOBILIZATION IN VIVO

5.1. Chemotactic Effects of Chemokines on Migration of Myeloid Progenitor Cells

Since chemokines were originally identified and described by their capacity to chemoattract mature leukocytes, it should not be surprising that they might also have the capacity to attract hematopoietic stem and progenitor cells. Little is known of the receptors and ligands involved in the homing and migration of stem and progenitor cells through embryonic and fetal life and in the adult. This is especially so in the context of how and why stem cells home to the marrow during transplantation with bone marrow, mobilized peripheral blood, or umbilical cord blood. At present, it is estimated that probably fewer than 10% of the cells transplanted into a conditioned host during stem cell transplantation actually home to the microenvironment in the marrow that is conducive for the self-renewal, proliferation, and differentiation of the cells, a necessity for successful long-term engraftment. If one were able to enhance the process of homing by altering/modifying the receptors and/or ligands involved in this process such that there were even a doubling in the percentage of stem/progenitor cells homing to a microenvironment conducive for growth, this would greatly increase the efficacy of stem cell transplantation. First, fewer cells would be needed for transplantation, thereby allowing transplantation with numbers of cells below those currently deemed necessary for successful engraftment. This is especially relevant for tissue sources of stem cells such as cord blood, of which there is concern that single collections of cord blood might not be of sufficient size to engraft many adult recipients *(5)*. Although engraftment rates with cord blood are high, most recipients have been children with less experience available for cord blood transplantation in adults. Second, enhancing the homing characteristics of cells might accelerate the repopulation kinetics of the engrafting cells. Third, a single collection of stem cells may be able to be used for transplantation into more than one recipient. It is obvious that an enhanced knowledge of the homing and migration of stem and progenitor cells will have important translational effects for clinical medicine.

The first chemokines implicated in the chemotaxis of hematopoietic progenitor cells were stromal cell–derived factor-1α (SDF-1α) and SDF-1β *(93–95)*. Mice null for SDF-1 died perinatally and had reduced numbers of B-lymphoid progenitors in fetal liver and fetal bone marrow *(95)*. These SDF-1 (–/–) mice also demonstrated reduced numbers of myeloid progenitor cells in bone marrow, but normal numbers of these cells in fetal liver. The results implicated SDF-1 in the migration of stem cells from fetal liver to fetal bone marrow. SDF-1 was subsequently found to attract human CD34+ progenitor cells in an in vitro system, effects that paralleled a transient elevation of cytoplasmic calcium in CD34+ cells, and the effects were PTX-sensitive *(93)*. CD34+ cells migrating toward SDF-1 included cells with a primitive phenotype (CD34+CD38– and CD34+HLA-DR–) as well as CFU-mix (=CFU-GEMM), BFU-E, and CFU-GM. Interestingly, CD34+ progenitors from mobilized peripheral blood were less sensitive than CD34+ cells in bone marrow to the chemotactic effects of SDF-1 *(93)*. The progenitor cell mobilizing effects were limited to SDF-1, because MIP-1α, MIP-1β, MCP-1, RANTES, and eotaxin-1, among C-C chemokines, and IL-8, among C-X-C chemokines, were not active *(93)*. As a matter of interest, SCF, the ligand for the tyrosine kinase receptor *c*-kit, which was previously reported to be an attractant for murine stem/progenitor cell populations *(96)*, was found to be inactive in migration induction of human CD34+ progenitor cells *(93)*. In contrast to that report, another study demonstrated the human CD34+ progenitor cell migration-inducing capacity of SCF *(94)*. The effect of SCF was mainly chemokinetic (random movement) and relatively modest compared to the chemotactic activity of SDF-1 *(94)*, and perhaps a reason that the other group *(93)* missed this activity. Interestingly, the migration-inducing effects of SCF were at least additive with those of SDF-1 for the migration of CD34+ progenitor cells *(94)*. These effects were apparent on both cord blood and bone marrow CD34+ progenitor cells, and also on the growth factor–dependent human cell line MO7e.

By use of the so-called checkerboard assay in which varying concentrations of test materials in the upper chamber, containing the cells to be assessed for migration, compete with varying concentrations of test material in the lower chamber, to which the cells are migrating, one can get a good idea of the relative chemotactic and chemokinetic potencies in a complex cytokine environment. It was in this type of culture system that plasma from bone marrow, but not from adult peripheral blood or cord blood, also showed chemotactic activity *(94)*. These results suggested that SDF-1 and SCF with other unidentified chemoattractants in the bone marrow might be involved cooperatively in the migration of stem and progenitor cells to the bone marrow and in preventing spontaneous mobilization of these primitive cells out of the bone marrow. This would include interactions with CXCR4, the receptor for SDF-1, and *c*-kit, the receptor for SCF, along with other receptor-ligand interactions.

Screening of a large number of chemokines has thus far identified only one other chemokine that attracts progenitor cells *(97)*. CKβ-11/MIP-3β/ELC/Exodus-3 is an efficacious chemoattractant for T- and B-lymphocytes *(98)*. It equally attracted naive CD45RA+ and memory type CD45RO+ T-cells, as well as CD4+ and CD8+ T-cells with a chemotactic activity comparable to that of SDF-1. It was a more efficacious chemoattractant for B-cells than MIP-1α. CKβ-11 induced calcium mobilization in lymphocytes, which could be desensitized by SDF-1, suggesting possible cross regulation in their signaling since the receptor for CKβ-11 is CCR7. In addition to its potential importance in the trafficking of T-cells in thymus, and T- and B-cell migration to secondary lymphoid organs, CKβ-11 also attracted a subset of myeloid progenitor cells from human bone marrow and cord blood *(97)*. In contrast to SDF-1, which attracted multiple types of progenitors (CFU-GEMM, BFU-E, CFU-GM) *(93,94)*, CKβ-11 attracted progenitors that were mainly responsive to stimulation by M-CSF and that produced macrophages *(97)*. The expression of CCR7, the receptor for CKβ-11, was detected at an mRNA level in the attracted as well as the input human CD34$^+$ progenitors. The expression of CKβ-11 mRNA was not constitutive, but was inducible in bone marrow stromal cells by inflammatory agents such as bacterial lipopolysaccharide (LPS), interferon-γ and tumor necrosis factor-α *(97)*. Taken together, the results suggested that CKβ-11 is expressed in the bone marrow microenvironment after induction with certain inflammatory cytokines and LPS and might play a role in the trafficking of macrophage progenitors into and out of the bone marrow in inflammatory conditions. It has recently been reported that CCR7 also binds the chemokine secondary lymphoid-tissue chemokine (SLC)/6Ckine/Exodus-2 *(99)*. SLC has many of the same activities as CKβ-11, including induction of the migration of CFU-GM type progenitors *(100)*.

In addition to the inactivity of MIP-1α, MIP-1β, IL-8, MCP-1, RANTES, and eotaxin-1 in the migration of progenitor cells *(93)*, it was found that CKβ-1/HCC-1/MCIF, CKβ4/MIP-3α/LARC/Exodus-1, CKβ-6/MPIF2/Eotaxin-2, CKβ-7/MIP-4, CKβ-8/MPIF-1, CKβ-10/MCP-4, and CKβ-12/IL-1α-inducible chemokine were also inactive in the chemotaxis of progenitor cells *(97)*. Thus, it appears that chemokine-induced migration of progenitor cells is not a characteristic of most chemokines. It is, however, likely that other chemokines will be effective in inducing the movement of progenitors. If SDF-1 is active for CFU-GEMM, BFU-E, and CFU-GM *(93,94)* and CKβ-11 and SLC are effective for macrophage progenitors *(97,100)*, it is possible that other chemokines might be found that are selective for granulocyte progenitors, or for only one of a group of other progenitors. Of course, it would be of great help, in a clinical sense, to find a chemoattractant for stem cells, especially those with long-term marrow repopulating capacity.

The interplay of chemotactic chemokines is highlighted by the combined roles of SDF-1 and CKβ-11. SDF-1 shows chemotactic preference for immature thymocytes (subsets of triple-negative thymocytes and double-positive subsets) over mature single positive thymocytes, whereas CKβ-11 shows low chemotactic activity on the immature thymocytes, but strongly attracts mature single-positive thymocytes *(101)*. Thus, from the effects on progenitors and thymocytes, it is apparent that SDF-1 acts on more immature cells than does CKβ-11. Interactions such as these are of probable significance in developmental hematopoiesis, and may be influenced by other chemokines and cytokines.

5.2. Mobilizing Effects of Chemokines on Stem and Progenitor Cells

Stem and progenitor cells mobilized from the marrow to the blood in response to growth factors such as G-CSF, GM-CSF, Epo, or SCF have been used for autologous and allogeneic transplantation and have increased the use of peripheral blood cells for such purposes *(5)*. In attempts to enhance stem/progenitor cell mobilization, chemokines have been assessed in this context. IL-8 has been shown to induce the rapid mobilization in mice of hematopoietic stem cells that have radioprotective capacity and long-term myeloid and lymphoid cell repopulating ability *(102)*. IL-8 also induced rapid mobilization of progenitor cells in rhesus monkeys *(103)*. Although the stem/progenitor cell mobilizing effects of G-CSF, GM-CSF, and other growth factors are usually enhanced over time after injection of these cytokines, and peak within days, the effects of IL-8 were very rapid (within minutes) and were quickly reversible to background levels (within 1 or 2 h). Murine MIP-2 also induced this rapid mobilization *(104)*. Interestingly, the progenitor cell mobilization with murine MIP-2 was enhanced by pretreatment of mice with G-CSF *(104)*, an effect very similar to that noted for the MIP-1α analog BB10010 in mice; BB10010 and MIP-1α synergized to induce mobilization of CFU-S and marrow repopulating cells *(105)*. The mobilizing effects of BB10010 and G-CSF were even more apparent in splenectomized mice.

Based on its mobilizing effects in mice *(105)*, BB10010 was also evaluated for mobilizing effects in patients with relapsed/refractory breast cancer as part of a phase I clinical trial *(87)*. In the clinical trial, B10010 demonstrated significant myeloid progenitor cell mobilizing capacity. These effects, however, were rather modest 3.4- to 5.6-fold average enhancements with a wide range within each progenitor cell category (0.9- to 1.2-fold to 11.4- to 26.0-fold). Although there was a large variability in the pretreatment progenitor cell numbers between patients, there was no correlation between the starting progenitor cell numbers and the degree of induced mobilization by BB10010 *(87)*. A significant difference was noted between the mobilizing effect of BB10010 in mice and in humans. The effects in mice, which occur within 1 h, were much quicker than in humans. In the majority of patients, the largest-fold increases were noted by d 3, and in some cases, the maximal increases were detected by 24 h after the first dose *(87)*. No significant increases were seen in the numbers of circulating progenitors at the 1- and 4-h time points after the first injection of BB10010. The modest increases in mobilization of progenitors in humans in response to BB10010 is consistent with the effects seen when BB10010 was used alone in mice for these purposes *(105)*. It is likely that in order for chemokines to be efficacious in humans for stem/progenitor cell mobilization, they will have to be used in combination with other cytokines in a way noted for murine MIP-2 *(104)* or BB10010 *(105)* in mice.

Understanding what keeps stem/progenitors in the marrow, and how these cells are mechanistically released into the blood, should help in the rational design of clinically effective mobilization procedures. It is likely that chemokines and chemokine receptors will play an important role, as evidenced by the information obtained from chemokine receptor gene knockout mice, as described in the following section.

6. MECHANISMS OF ACTION OF CHEMOKINES AND UNRAVELING THE POTENTIAL REDUNDANCY IN CHEMOKINE/CHEMOKINE RECEPTOR INTERACTIONS

6.1. Signal Transduction by Chemokines

Little is known regarding the intracellular signal transduction events mediating the effects of chemokines on the proliferation or movement of hematopoietic stem and progenitor cells.

Since chemokine receptors are G protein–linked receptors whose effects can be downmodulated by PTX, it is clear that many of the effects of chemokines are probably mediated through some of the G proteins. Using the human growth factor–dependent cell line MO7e *(106)*, which has been a useful model for assessing intracellular effects in progenitor cells *(107,108)*, it has been determined that some of the effects of MIP-1α and IP-10 are mediated through cyclic AMP (cAMP) *(109,110)*, involve the phosphorylation and activation of Raf kinase *(109)*, and may involve phosphatidyl-choline (PC) metabolism *(110)*. Treatment of MO7e cells with MIP-1α increased PC and phosphocholine turnover rates in cells that were synergistically stimulated to proliferate by the combination of GM-CSF and SCF but not by those factors acting alone *(110)*. The proliferation-suppressing effects of MIP-1α and other chemokines on primary progenitor cells and on MO7e cells are seen only when cells are synergistically stimulated to proliferate by combinations of cytokines *(37)*. MIP-1α and IP-10 induced a dose- and time-dependent increase in intracellular cAMP in MO7e cells *(109)*, and exogenous PC and dibutyryl cAMP were found to suppress the proliferation of MO7e colony-forming cells to a level similar to that of MIP-1α *(110)*. These findings suggested that a human MIP-1α receptor is coupled to phospholipid and cAMP metabolism in a manner similar to that of other seven-transmembrane, G protein–linked receptors and that a PC hydrolytic cycle and increased cAMP are part of the mechanisms of action of MIP-1α.

It is highly probable that although several different chemokines can mediate the suppression of progenitor cell proliferation, probably through a number of different receptors, the intracellular signals triggered by these chemokine–chemokine receptor interactions may be different in some of these cases. MIP-1α-mediated growth inhibition of a murine growth factor–dependent cell line, FDCP-Mix, was found to be associated with inositol 1,4,5 triphosphate generation *(111)*. Using nonstem, nonprogenitor cell systems, others have demonstrated that MIP-1α can activate Stats in T-lymphocytes *(112)*. Moreover, others have linked MIP-1β binding to CCR5 with activation of the related adhesion focal tyrosine kinase (RAFTK), with subsequent activation of the cytoskeletal protein, paxillin, and the downstream transcriptual activator, *c*-Jun N-terminal kinase (JNK)/stress-activated protein (mitogen-activated protein) kinase *(SAPK)* *(113)*. It was noted that inhibition of RAFTK by a dominant-negative kinase mutant markedly attenuated JNK/SAPK activity. These intracellular signals may be involved in chemotaxis of mature cells, but since MIP-1β has not been shown to be active as an inhibitor of progenitor cell proliferation or as an inducer of migration of progenitor cells, it is not yet clear whether this pathway *(113)* is mechanistically involved in the chemokine effects on progenitor cells.

6.2. Use of Chemokine Receptor Gene Knockout Mice to Evaluate Dominant Effects of This Receptor

Because of the potential redundancy in chemokine effects, especially for negative regulation of progenitor cell proliferation (*see* Tables 2 and 3), it is difficult to determine which effects are physiologically relevant. The use of gene knockout mice offers the possibility of determining which chemokine receptors might play a dominant role in these effects. To this end, many chemokine receptor gene knockout mice have been evaluated for proliferation of progenitor cells and for movement of these cells.

The expansion of neutrophils and B-lymphocytes had been seen in mice lacking expression of the murine IL-8 receptor homolog, CXCR2 (–/–) *(114)*. It was further determined that bone marrow cells from these CXCR2 (–/–), but not from wild-type littermate control CXCR2 (+/+), mice were insensitive to inhibition by human IL-8 and murine MIP-2, but not to inhibition by a number of other chemokines that do not utilize CXCR2 as their receptor *(43)*. Under normal environmental conditions, the CXCR2 (–/–) mice had a hyperproliferation of myeloid progenitor cells in the bone marrow, spleen, and blood, suggesting that CXCR2 serves as a dominant negative regulatory receptor for progenitor cell proliferation, and also possibly for progenitor cell migration. Interestingly, when CXCR2 (–/–) and (+/+) mice were bred and raised under germ-free conditions, the numbers of marrow, spleen, and blood progenitors were much lower than in these same mice raised under normal environmental conditions. However, differences in progenitors per organ between mice bred under germ-free and normal environmental conditions were greater for the CXCR2 (–/–) than (+/+) mice *(43)*. These studies provided evidence for a large expansion of myeloid progenitors in CXCR2, with this effect being environmentally inducible.

Studies of CCR2 (–/–) mice demonstrated that the CCR2 (–/–), but not (+/+), bone marrow cells were insensitive to inhibition by human MCP-1 and murine JE, but not to inhibition by other chemokines that utilize receptors other than CCR2 *(115)*. Evaluation of the cycling status of CCR2 (–/–) bone marrow cells demonstrated that they were in a much higher proliferative state than marrow from CCR2 (+/+) mice *(116)*. However, in contrast to the CXCR2 (–/–) mice, there was no increase in absolute numbers of progenitor cells. Further analysis of phenotypically defined stem/progenitor cells (*c*-kit⁺/Lin⁻) demonstrated that although these progenitors were in a higher proliferative state in CCR2 (–/–) than in CCR2 (+/+) marrow, they were also undergoing apoptosis at a significantly higher rate *(116)*, which was apparently counterbalancing the enhanced proliferative state. These results implicated CCR2 also as a negative regulatory chemokine receptor.

Evaluation of cells from CCR1 (–/–) mice did not point to CCR1 as a dominant receptor for negative regulation *(42)*. Although it has been suggested that human CCR1 may mediate the suppressive effects of MIP-1α on the proliferation of erythroid progenitors, based on the use of antibodies to CCR1 to block MIP-1α inhibition *(84)*, this effect is probably not a dominant one *(42)*. Bone marrow cells from CCR1 (–/–) mice were as sensitive as cells from CCR1 (+/+) mice to inhibition by both human and murine MIP-1α *(42)*. Additionally, no significant differences were apparent in the cycling rates or absolute numbers of myeloid progenitors in the marrow, spleen, and blood of CCR1 (–/–) compared with CCR1 (+/+) mice.

Whereas CCR1 was not implicated as a dominant receptor for negative regulation of proliferation, it was implicated as a receptor involved in other aspects of chemokine actions on progenitor cells *(117)*. Although the distribution of mature leukocytes was normal in CCR1 (–/–) mice, steady-state and LPS-induced trafficking of myeloid progenitor cells was disordered in CCR1 (–/–) mice *(117)*. LPS induced a similar migration of myeloid progenitor cells out of the marrows of CCR1 (–/–) and (+/+) mice. However, the usual LPS-induced increase in myeloid progenitor cell movement to the spleen, noted in the CCR1 (+/+) mice, was not seen in the spleens of CCR1 (–/–) mice. In fact, after LPS induction, progenitors in the spleens of CCR1 (–/–) mice were, in some cases, lower than the numbers in noninduced CCR1 (–/–) spleens. These changes were associated with increased numbers of progenitors in the blood of CCR1 (–/–) compared with (+/+) mice *(117)*. Additionally, the MIP-1α progenitor cell mobilizing effects noted in normal mice of several different strains *(105)*, including CCR1 (+/+) mice, were not detected in CCR1 (–/–) mice *(42)*. Interestingly, myeloid progenitors in the CCR1 (–/–) mice could be more actively mobilized to the blood in response to G-CSF than those in CCR1 (+/+) mice *(42)*. This totally unexpected finding adds another level of complexity to growth factor–induced mobilization of progenitor cells and suggests that CCR1 may be acting somehow, in a negative sense, to limit G-CSF-induced mobilization.

Although CCR1 was not implicated in negative regulation of the proliferation of myeloid progenitor cells, it was found to be involved in the MIP-1α enhancement of the proliferation of the more mature progenitor cells *(42)*. Both human and murine MIP-1α enhanced colony formation by CFU-GM stimulated by GM-CSF and by CFU-M stimulated by M-CSF in marrow cells from the CCR1 (+/+) mice, but this enhancement was not seen in marrow cells from the CCR1 (–/–) mice *(42)*.

It is probable that further useful information will come from evaluation of the proliferation and movement of stem and progenitor cells in other chemokine receptor knockout mice, or in mice in which the expression of the chemokines themselves are deleted or enhanced. A further level of detail will most likely result from the use of dual chemokine receptor or chemokine knockout mice.

An unexpected effect of knocking out the u-opioid receptor was an increased proliferation of myeloid progenitor cells in the marrow and spleen, which established a link between hematopoiesis and the opioid system *(118)*. Since the u-opioid receptor is a G protein–coupled receptor, it makes one wonder if there is a link between the u-opioid system and the chemokine/chemokine receptor system.

7. CONCLUSION

The chemokine/chemokine receptor system is evolving into a complicated but perhaps not so redundant system that has regulatory networks for several different functional activities. In terms of hematopoiesis and regulation of the proliferation and movement of hematopoietic stem and progenitor cells, the major questions are as follows: Which chemokines and chemokine receptors are dominant for which effects? Exactly how are they working alone and in the context of other chemokines and cytokines and their receptors? Is there a way to take advantage of this information in the design of relevant clinical trials for the treatment of hematopoietic disorders?

ACKNOWLEDGMENTS

The authors thank Becki Miller for typing the manuscript. Some of the more recent studies from the authors that were cited in this review were supported by U.S. Public Health Grants R01 HL56416, R01 DK53674, R01 HL54037, P01 HL53586, and T32 DK07519 (H.E.B.).

REFERENCES

1. Broxmeyer, H. E. 1982. Granulopoiesis, in *The Human Bone Marrow* (Trubowitz, S., and S. Davis, eds.), CRC, Boca Raton, FL, pp. 145–208.

 2. Broxmeyer, H. E. 1982. Hematopoietic stem cells, in *The Human Bone Marrow* (Trubowitz, S., and S. Davis, eds.), CRC, Boca Raton, FL, pp. 77–123.

 3. Broxmeyer, H. E. 1992. Update: Biomolecule-cell interactions and the regulation of myelopoiesis, in *Concise Reviews in Clinical and Experimental Hematology* (Murphy, M. J., Jr., ed.), Alpha Med, Dayton, OH, pp. 119–149.

 4. Broxmeyer, H. E. 1993. Role of cytokines in hematopoiesis, in *Clinical Aspects of Cytokines: Role in Pathogenesis, Diagnosis and Therapy* (Oppenheim, J. J., J. L. Rossio, and A. J. H. Gearing, eds.), Oxford University Press, New York, pp. 201–206.

 5. Broxmeyer, H. E., and F. O. Smith. 1998. Cord blood stem cell transplantation, in *Stem Cell Transplantation* (Forman, S. I., K. G., Blume, and E. D. Thomas, eds.), Blackwell Scientific, Cambridge, MA, Chapter 41, pp. 431–443.

 6. Cooper, S., and H. E. Broxmeyer. 1996. Measurement of interleukin-3 and other hematopoietic growth factors, such as GM-CSF, G-CSF, M-CSF, erythropoietin and the potent co-stimulating cytokines steel factor and Flt-3 ligand, in *Current Protocols in Immunology* (Coligan, J. E., A. M. Kruisbeek, D. H. Margulies, E. M. Shevach, W. Strober, and R. Coico, eds.), John Wiley & Sons, New York, Suppl. 18, pp. 6.4.1–6.4.12.

 7. Broxmeyer, H. E., G. W. Douglas, G. Hangoc, S. Cooper, J. Bard, D. English, M. Arny, L. Thomas, and E. A. Boyse. 1989. Human umbilical cord blood as a potential source of transplantable hematopoietic stem/progenitor cells. *Proc. Natl. Acad. Sci. USA* **86:** 3828–3832.

 8. Broxmeyer, H. E., G. Hangoc, S. Cooper, R. C. Ribeiro, V. Graves, M. Yoder, J. Wagner, S. Vadhan-Raj, P. Rubinstein, and E. R. Broun. 1992. Growth characteristics and expansion of human umbilical cord blood and estimation of its potential source for transplantation of adults. *Proc. Natl. Acad. Sci. USA* **89:** 4109–4113.

 9. Broxmeyer, H. E. 1991. Commentary: self-renewal and migration of stem cells during embryonic and fetal hematopoiesis: important, but poorly understood events. *Blood Cells* **17:** 282–286.

10. Cumano, A., F. Dieterlen-Lievre, and I. Godin. 1996. Lymphoid potential, probed before circulation in mouse, is restricted to caudal intraembryonic splanchnopleura. *Cell* **86:** 907–916.

11. Medvisnky, A., and E. Dzierzak. 1996. Definitive hematopoiesis is autonomously initiated by the AGM region. *Cell* **86:** 897–906.

12. Sanchez, M., A. Holmes, C. Miles, and E. Dzierzak.1996. Characterization of the first definitive hematopoietic stem cells in the AGM and liver of the mouser embryo. *Immunity* **5:** 513–525.

13. Turpen, J. B., C. M. Kelley, P. E. Mead, and L. I. Zon. 1997. Bipotential primitive-definitive hematopoietic progenitors in the vertebrate embryo. *Immunity* **7:** 325–334.

14. Yoder, M. C., K. Hiatt, P. Dutt, P. Mukherjee, D. M. Bodine, and D. Orlic. 1997. Characterization of definitive lymphohematopoietic stem cells in the day 9 murine yolk sac. *Immunity* **7:** 335–344.

15. Adams, D. H., and A. R. Lloyd. 1997. Chemokines: leucocyte recruitment and activation cytokines. *Lancet* **349:** 490–495.

16. Baggiolini, M., B. Dewald, and B. Moser. 1994. Interleukin-8 and related chemotactic cytokines—CXC and CC chemokimes. *Adv. Immunol.* **55:** 97–179.

17. Baggiolini, M. 1998. Chemokines and leukocyte traffic. *Nature* **392:** 565–568.

18. Murphy, P. M. 1996. Chemokine receptors: structure, function and role in microbial pathogenesis. *Cytokine & Growth Factor Rev.* **7:** 47–64.

19. Rollins, B. J. 1997. Chemokines. *Blood* **90:** 909–928.

20. Baggiolini, M., B. Dewald, and B. Moser. 1997. Human chemokines: an update. *Annu. Rev. Immunol.* **15:** 675–705.

21. Nibbs, R. J. B., S. M. Wylie, J. Yang, N. R. Landau, and G. J. Graham. 1997. Cloning and characterization of a novel promiscuous human β-chemokine receptor D6. *J. Biol. Chem.* **272:** 32,078–32,083.

22. Darbonne, W. C., G. C. Rice, M. A. Mohler, T. Apple, C. A. Hegert, A. J. Valente, and J. B. Baker. 1991. Red blood cells are a sink for interleukin 8, a leukocyte chemotaxin. *J. Clin. Invest.* **88:** 1362.

23. Hadley, T. J., and S. C. Peiper. 1997. From Malaria to chemokine receptor: the emerging physiologic role of the duffy blood group antigen. *Blood* **89:** 3077–3091.

24. Neote, K., W. Darbonne, J. Ogez, R. Horuk, and T. J. Schall. 1993. Identification of a promiscuous inflammatory peptide receptor on the surface of red blood cells. *J. Biol. Chem.* **268:** 12,247.

25. Ahuja, S. K., J. L. Gao, and P. M. Murphy. 1994. Chemokine receptors and molecular mimicry. *Immunol. Today* **15:** 281–287.

26. Arvanitakis, L., E. Geras-Raaka, A. Varma, M. C. Gershengorn, and E. Cesarman. 1997. Human herpesvirus KSHV encodes a constitutively active G-protein-coupled receptor linked to cell proliferation. *Nature* **385:** 347–350.

27. Gao, J. L., and P. M. Murphy. 1994. Human cytomegalovirus open reading frame US28 encodes a functional β chemokine receptor. *J. Biol. Chem.* **269:** 28,539–28,542.

28. Krathwohl, M. D., R. Hromas, D. R. Brown, H. E. Broxmeyer, and K. H. Fife. 1997. Functional characterization of the c-c chemokine-like molecules encoded by molluscum contagiosum virus types 1 and 2. *Proc. Natl. Acad. Sci. USA* **94:** 9875–9880.

29. Nicholas, J., V. R. Ruvilo, W. H. Burnes, G. Sandford, X. Wan, D. Ciufo, S. B. Hendrickson, H. G. Guo, G. S. Hayward, and M. S. Reitz. 1997. Kaposi's sarcoma-associated human herpesvirus-8 encodes homologues of macrophage inflammatory protein-1 and interleukin-6. *Nat. Med.* **3:** 287–292.

30. Pleskoff, O., C. Treboute, A. Brelot, N. Heveker, M. Seman, and M. Alizon. 1997. Identification of a chemokine receptor encoded by human cytomegalovirus as a cofactor for HIV-1 entry. *Science* **272:** 1874–1878.

31. Broxmeyer, H. E., B. Sherry, L. Lu, S. Cooper, C. Carow, S. D. Wolpe, and A. Cerami. 1989. Myelopoietic enhancing effects of murine macrophage inflammatory proteins 1 and 2 *in vitro* on colony formation by murine and human bone marrow granulocyte-macrophage progenitor cells. *J. Exp. Med.* **170:** 1583–1594.

32. Broxmeyer, H. E., B. Sherry, L. Lu, S. Cooper, K.-O. Oh, P. Tekamp-Olson, B. S. Kwon, and A. Cerami. 1990. Enhancing and suppressing effects of recombinant murine macrophage inflammatory proteins on colony formation *in vitro* by bone marrow myeloid progenitor cells. *Blood* **76:** 1110–1116.

33. Graham, G. J., E. G. Wright, R. Hewick, S. D. Wolpe, N. M. Wilkie, D. Donaldson, S. Lorimore, and I. B. Pragnell. 1990. Identification and characterization of an inhibitor of haemopoietic stem cell proliferation. *Nature* **344:** 442–444.

34. Mantel, C., Y.-J. Kim, S. Cooper, B. Kwon, and H. E. Broxmeyer. 1993. Polymerization of murine macrophage inflammatory protein-1α inactivates its myelosuppressive effects *in vitro*. The active form is monomer. *Proc. Natl. Acad. Sci. USA* **90:** 2232–2236.

35. Broxmeyer, H. E., B. Sherry, S. Cooper, F. W. Ruscetti, D. E. Williams, P. Arosio, B. S. Kwon, and A. Cerami.1991. Macrophage inflammatory protein (MIP)-1β abrogates the capacity of MIP-1α to suppress myeloid progenitor cell growth. *J. Immunol.* **147:** 2586–2594.

36. Broxmeyer, H. E., B. Sherry, S. Cooper, L. Lu, R. Maze, M. P. Beckmann, A. Cerami, and P. Ralph.1993. Comparative analysis of the suppressive effects of the human macrophage inflammatory protein family of cytokines (chemokines) on proliferation of human myeloid progenitor cells. *J. Immunol.* **150:** 3448–3458.

37. Broxmeyer, H. E., S. Cooper, N. Hague, L. Benninger, A. Sarris, K. Cornetta, S. Vadhan-Raj, P. Hendrie, and C. Mantel.1995. Human chemokines: enhancement of specific activity and effects *in vitro* on normal and leukemic progenitors and a factor dependent cell line and *in vivo* in mice. *Ann. Hematol.* **71:** 235–246.

38. Broxmeyer, H. E., R. Maze, K. Miyazawa, C. Carow, P. C. Hendrie, S. Cooper, G. Hangoc,

S. Vadhan-Raj, and L. Lu. 1991. The Kit receptor and its ligand, steel factor, as regulators of hematopoiesis. *Cancer Cells* **3**: 480–487.

39. Lyman, S. D., S. E. W. Jacobsen. 1998. C-kit ligand and Flt3 ligand: stem/progenitor cell factors with overlapping yet distinct activities. *Blood* **91**: 1104–1134.

40. Lu, L., M. Xiao, S. Grigsby, W. X. Wang, B. Wu, R.-N. Shen, and H. E. Broxmeyer. 1993. Comparative effects of suppressive cytokines on isolated single CD34^{+++} stem/progenitor cells from human bone marrow and umbilical cord blood plated with and without stem. *Exp. Hematol.* **21**: 1442–1446.

41. Su. S. B., N. Mukaida, J. B. Wang, Y. Zhang, A. Takami, S. Nakao, and K. Matsushima. 1997. Inhibition of immature-erythroid progenitor cell proliferations by macrophage inflammatory protein-1α by interacting mainly with a C-C chemokine receptor. CCR1. *Blood* **90**: 605–611.

42. Broxmeyer, H. E., S. Cooper, G. Hangoc, J. L. Gao, and P. M. Murphy. 1997. Chemokine receptor CCR1 acts as a dominant receptor for MIP-1α enhancement of proliferation of mature progenitors *in vitro*, MIP-1α mobilization of progenitors *in vivo*, and MIP-1α enhancement of G-CSF induced mobilization, but not for MIP-1α suppression of immature progenitors *in vitro*: effects elucidated using CCR1 knock-out mice. *Blood* **90(Suppl. 1, Pt. 1):** 571a (abstract).

43. Broxmeyer, H. E., S. Cooper, G. Cacalano, N. L. Hague, E. Bailish, and M. W. Moore. 1996. Interleukin-8 receptor is involved in negative regulation of myeloid progenitor cells *in vivo*: evidence from mice lacking the murine IL-8 receptor homolog. *J. Exp. Med.* **184:** 1825–1832.

44. Broxmeyer, H. E., L. M. Pelus, R. Hromas, B. Kwon, B. Youn, K. Fife, M. D. Krathwohl, C. Kim, J. R. White, G. Hangoc, and S. Cooper. 1997. Myelosuppression *in vitro* and *in vivo* by newly identified members of the cysteine cysteine (CC), CXC and C chemokine family and synergistic suppression *in vivo* by combinations of these chemokines. *Blood* **90(Suppl. 1, Pt. 1):** 475a (abstract).

45. Hromas, R., P. W. Gray, D. Chantry, M. Krathwohl, K. Fife, G. I. Bell, J. Takeda, S. Aronica, M. Gordon, S. Cooper, H. E. Broxmeyer, and M. Klemsz. 1997. Cloning and characterization of exodus, a novel β-chemokine. *Blood* **89**: 3315–3322.

46. Hromas, R., M. Klemsz, M. Krathwohl, K. Fife, S. Cooper, C. Schnizlein-Bick, and H. E. Broxmeyer. 1997. Isolation and characterization of exodus-2, a novel c-c chemokine with a unique 37 amino acid carboxy terminal extension. *J. Immunol.* **159(Cutting Edge):** 2554–2558.

47. Sarris, A. H., H. E. Broxmeyer, U. Wirthmueller, N. Karasavvas, J. Krueger, and J. V. Ravetch. 1993. Human interferon inducible protein 10: expression and purification of recombinant protein demonstrate inhibition of early human hematopoietic progenitors. *J. Exp. Med.* **178:** 1127–1132.

48. Youn, B. S., I.-K. Jang, H. E. Broxmeyer, S. Cooper, N. A. Jenkins, D. J. Gilbert, N. G. Copeland, T. A. Elick, M. J. Fraser, Jr., and B. S. Kwon. 1995. A novel chemokine, macrophage inflammatory protein-related protein-2, inhibits colony formation of bone marrow myeloid progenitors. *J. Immunol.* **155:** 2661–2667.

49. Youn, B. S., S. M. Zhang, E. K. Lee, D. H. Park, H. E. Broxmeyer, P. M. Murphy, M. Locati, J. E. Pease, K. K. Kim, K. Antol, and B. S. Kwon. 1997. Molecular cloning of leukotactin-1: a novel human β-chemokine, a chemoattractant for neutrophils, monocytes and lymphocytes, and a potent agonist at CC chemokine receptors 1 and 3. *J. Immunol.* **159(Cutting Edge):** 5201–5205.

50. Youn, B. S., S. M. Zhang, H. E. Broxmeyer, S. Cooper, K. Antol, M. Fraser, and B. S. Kwon. 1998. Characterization of CKβ8 and CKβ8-1: two alternatively spliced forms of human β-chemokine, chemoattractants for neutrophils, monocytes and lymphocytes, and potent agonists at CC chemokine receptor 1. *Blood* **91**: 3118–3126.

51. Youn, B. S., S. Zhang, H. E. Broxmeyer, K. Antol, M. J. Fraser, Jr., G. Hangoc, and B. S.

Kwon. 1998. Isolation and characterization of LMC, a novel lymphocyte and monocyte chemoattractant human CC chemokine with myelosuppressive activity. *Biochem. Biophys. Res. Commun.* **247:** 217–222.

52. Clements, J. M., S. Craig, A. J. H. Gearing, M. G. Hunter, C. M. Heyworth, T. M. Dexter, and B. I. Lord. 1992. Biological and structural properties of MIP-1α expressed in yeast. *Cytokine* **4:** 76–82.

53. Gewirtz, A. M., B. Calabretta, B. Rucinski, S. Niewiarowski, and W. Y. Xu. 1988. Inhibition of human megakaryocytopoiesis *in vitro* by platelet factor 4 (PF4) and a synthetic COOH-terminal PF4 peptide. *J. Clin. Invest.* **83:** 1477–1486.

54. Gewirtz, A. M., J. Zhang, J. Ratajczak, M. Ratajczak, K. S. Part, C. Li, Z. Yan, and M. Poncz. 1995. Chemokine regulation of human megakaryocytopoiesis. *Blood* **86:** 2559–2567.

55. Graham, G. J., M. G. Freshney, D. Donaldson, and I. B. Pragnell. 1992. Purification and biochemical characterisation of human and murine stem cell inhibitors (SCI). *Growth Factors* **7:** 151–160.

56. Han, Z. C., L. Sensebe, J. F. Abgrall, and J. Briere. 1990. Platelet factor 4 inhibits human megakaryocytopoiesis *in vitro*. *Blood* **75:** 1234.

57. Keller, J. R., S. H. Bartelmez, E. Sitnicka, F. W. Ruscetti, M. Ortiz, J. M. Gooya, and S. E. W. Jacobsen. 1994. Distinct and overlapping direct effects of macrophage inflammatory protein-1α and transforming growth factor β on hematopoietic progenitor/stem cell growth. *Blood* **84:** 2175–2181.

58. Maltman, J., I. B. Pragnell, and G. J. Graham. 1993. Transforming growth factor β: is it a downregulator of stem cell inhibition by macrophage inflammatory protein 1α? *J. Exp. Med.* **178:** 925–932.

59. Mayani, H., M. T. Little, W. Dragowska, G. Thornbury, and P. M. Lansdrop. 1995. Differential effects of the hematopoietic inhibitors MIP-1α, TGF-β, and TNF-α on cytokine-induced proliferation of subpopulations of CD34[+] cells purified from cord blood and fetal liver. *Exp. Hematol.* **23:** 422–427.

60. Patel, V. P., B. L. Kreider, Y. Li, H. Li, K. Leung, T. Salcedo, B. Nardelli, V. Pippalla, S. Gentz, R. Thotakura, D. Parmelee, R. Gentz, and G. Garotta. 1997. Molecular and functional characterization of two novel human CC chemokines as inhibitors of two distinct classes of myeloid progenitors. *J. Exp. Med.* **185:** 1163–1172.

61. Sanchez, X., K. Suetomi, B. Cousins-Hodges, J. K. Horton, and J. Navarro. 1998. CXC chemokines suppress proliferation of myeloid progenitor cells by activation of the CXC chemokine receptor 2. *J. Immunol.* **160:** 906–910.

62. Schwartz, G. N., F. Liao, R. E. Gress, and J. M. Farber. 1997. Suppressive effects of recombinant human monokine induced by IFN-γ (rHuMig) chemokine on the number of committed and primitive hematopoietic progenitors in liquid cultures of CD34[+] human bone marrow cells. *J. Immunol.* **159:** 895–904.

63. VanRanst, P. C. F., H. W. Snoeck, F. Lardon, M. Lenjou, G. Nijs, S. F. A. Weekx, I. Rodrigus, Z. N. Berneman, and D. R. Van Bockstaele. 1996. TGF-β and MIP-1α exert their main inhibitory activity on very primitive CD34[++]CD38[−] cells but show opposite effects on more mature CD34[+]CD38[+] human hematopoietic progenitors. *Exp. Hematol.* **24:** 1509–1515.

64. Graham, G. J., J. Mackenzie, S. Lowe, M. L. S. Tsang, J. A. Weatherbee, A. Issacson, J. Medicherla, F. Fang, P. C. Wilkinson, and I. B. Pragnell. 1994. Aggregation of the chemokine MIP-1α is a dynamic and reversible phenomenon. *J. Biol. Chem.* **269:** 4974–4978.

65. Paolini, J. F., D. Willard, T. Consler, M. Luther, and M. S. Krangel. 1994. The chemokines IL-8, monocyte chemoattractant protein-1, and I-309 are monomers at physiologically relevant concentrations. *J. Immunol.* **153:** 2704–2717.

66. Patel, S. R., S. Evans, K. Dunne, G. C. Knight, P. J. Morgan, P. G. Varley, and S. Craig.

1993. Characterization of the quaternary structure and conformational properties of the human stem cell inhibitor protein LD78 in solution. *Biochemistry* **32:** 5466–5471.

67. Rajarathnam, K., B. D. Sykes, C. M. Kay, B. Dewald, T. Geiser, M. Baggiolini, and I. Clark-Lewis. 1994. Neutrophil activation by monomeric interleukin-8. *Science* **264:** 90–92.

68. Cooper, S., C. Mantel, and H. E. Broxmeyer. 1994. Myelosuppressive effects *in vivo* with very low dosage of monomeric recombinant murine macrophage inflammatory protein-1α. *Exp. Hematol.* **22:** 186–193.

69. Broxmeyer, H. E., C. H. Kim, S. H. Cooper, G. Hangoc, R. Hromas, and L. M. Pelus. 1999. Effects of CC, CXC, C, and CX₃C chemokines on proliferation of myeloid progenitor cells, and insights into SDF-1 induced chemotaxis of progenitors. *N.Y. Acad. Sci.,* in press.

70. Broxmeyer, H. E., S. Cooper, Z.-H. Li, L. Lu, A. Sarris, M.-H. Wang, C. Metz, M.-S. Chang, D. B. Donner, and E. J. Leonard. 1996. Macrophage-stimulating protein, a ligand for the *RON* receptor protein tyrosine kinase, suppresses myeloid progenitor cell proliferation and synergizes with vascular endothelial cell growth factor and members of the chemokine family. *Ann. Hematol.* **73:** 1–9.

71. Daly, T. J., G. J. LaRosa, S. Dolich, T. E. Maione, S. Cooper, and H. E. Broxmeyer. 1995. High activity suppression of myeloid progenitor proliferation by chimeric mutants of interleukin 8 and platelet factor 4. *J. Biol. Chem.* **270:** 23,282–23,292.

72. Ferrajoli, A., M. Talpaz, T. F. Zipf, C. Hirsch-Ginsberg, E. Estey, S. D. Wolpe, and Z. Estrov. 1994. Inhibition of acute myelogenous leukemia progenitor proliferation by macrophage inflammatory protein-1α. *Leukemia* **8:** 798–805.

73. Eaves, C. J., J. D. Cashman, S. D. Wolpe, and A. C. Eaves. 1993. Unresponsiveness of primitive chronic myeloid leukemia cells to macrophage inflammatory protein 1α, an inhibitor of primitive normal hematopoietic cells. *Proc. Natl. Acad. Sci. USA* **90:** 12,015–12,019.

74. McGuckin, C. P., W. M. Liu, S. E. Ball, E. C. Gordon-Smith, and M. R. Uhr. 1996. Diamond Blackfan anaemia: differential pattern of *in vitro* progenitor response to macrophage inflammatory protein 1-alpha. *Br. J. Haematol.* **92:** 280–286.

75. Broxmeyer, H. E., S. Cooper, G. Hangoc, and R. Hromas. 1997. Unpublished observations.

76. Senkevich, T. G., J. J. Bugert, J. R. Sisler, E. V. Koonin, G. Darai, and B. Moss. 1996. Genome sequence of a human tumorigenic poxvirus: prediction of specific host response-evasion genes. *Science* **273:** 813–816.

77. Alcami, A., J. A. Symons, P. D. Collins, T. J. Williams, and G. L. Smith. 1998. Blockage of chemokine activity by a soluble chemokine binding protein from vaccinia virus. *J. Immunol.* **160:** 624–633.

78. Verfaillie, C. M., P. M. Catanzarro, and W. N. Li. 1994. Macrophage inflammatory protein-1α, interleukin 3 and diffusible marrow stromal factors maintain human hematopoietic stem cells for at least eight weeks *in vitro. J. Exp. Med.* **179:** 643–649.

79. Lord, B. I. 1995. MIP-1α increases the self-renewal capacity of the hemopoietic spleen-colony-forming cells following hydroxyurea treatment *in vivo. Growth Factors* **12:** 145–149.

80. Peled, A., J. A. Gonzalo, C. Lloyd, and J. C. Gutierrez-Ramos. 1998. The chemotactic cytokine eotaxin acts as a granulocyte-macrophage colony-stimulating factor during lung inflammation. *Blood* **91:** 1909–1916.

81. Maze, R., B. Sherry, B. S. Kwon, A. Cerami, and H. E. Broxmeyer. 1992. Myelosuppressive effects *in vivo* of purified recombinant murine macrophage inflammatory protein-1 alpha. *J. Immunol.* **149:** 1004–1009.

82. Broxmeyer, H. E. 1995. The cell cycle as therapeutic target. *Cancer Invest.* **13:** 617–624.

83. Broxmeyer, H. E., and S. Vadhan-Raj. 1996. Hemopoietic stem and progenitor cell protection, in *Manual of GM-CSF* (Marty, M., ed.), Blackwell Science, Oxford, UK, pp. 197–207.

84. Dunlop, D. J., E. G. Wright, S. Lorimore, G. J. Graham, T. Tolyoake, D. J. Kerr, S. D. Wolpe, and I. B. Pragnell. 1992. Demonstration of stem cell inhibition and myeloprotective effects of SCI/rhMIP-1α *in vivo. Blood* **79:** 2221–2225.

85. Lord, B. I., T. M. Dexter, J. M. Clements, A. A. Hunter, and A. J. H. Gearing. 1992. Macrophage-inflammatory protein protects multipotent hematopoietic cells from the cytotoxic effects of hydroxyurea *in vivo. Blood* **79:** 2605–2609.

86. Hunter, M. G., L. Bawden, D. Brotherton, S. Craig, S. Cribbes, L. G. Czaplewski, T. M. Dexter, A. H. Drummond, A. H. Gearing, C. M. Heyworth, B. I. Lord, M. McCourt, P. G. Varley, L. M. Wood, R. M. Edwards, and P. J. Lewis. 1995. BB-10010: an active variant of human macrophage inflammatory protein-1α with improved pharmaceutical properties. *Blood* **86:** 4400–4408.

87. Broxmeyer, H. E., A. Orazi, N. L. Hague, G. W. Sledge, Jr., H. Rasmussen, and M. S. Gordon. 1998. Myeloid progenitor cell proliferation and mobilization effects of BB10010, a genetically engineered variant of human macrophage inflammatory protein-1α, in a phase I clinical trial in patients with relapsed/refractory breast cancer. *Blood Cells, Molecules Dis.* **24:** 14–30.

88. Gordon, M. S., W. J. McCaskill-Stevens, and H. E. Broxmeyer. 1996. A phase I trial of subcutaneous (sc) BB-10010 in breast cancer patients (pts) receiving high-dose cyclophosphamide (C). *Exp. Hematol.* **24:** 1104 (abstract).

89. Bernstein, S. H., C. J. Eaves, R. Herzig, J. Fay, J. Lynch, G. L. Phillips, N. Christiansen, D. Reece, S. Ericson, M. Stephan, M. Kovalsky, K. Hawkins, H. Rasmussen, A. Devos, and G. P. Herzig. 1997. A randomized phase II study of BB-10010: a variant of human macrophage inflammatory protein-1α for patients receiving high-dose etoposide and cyclophosphamide for malignant lymphoma and breast cancer. *Br. J. Haematol.* **99:** 888–895.

90. Haneline, L., H. E. Broxmeyer, S. Cooper, G. Hangoc, M. Carreau, M. Buchwald, and D. W. Clapp. 1998. Altered proliferation kinetics, deregulated responsiveness to multiple inhibitory cytokines and enhanced tumor necrosis factor-α mediated apoptosis in hematopoietic cells from fac –/– mice. *Blood* **91:** 4092–4098.

91. Broxmeyer, H. E., S. Cooper, T. Maione, M. Gordon, and T. Daly. 1995. Myeloprotective effects of the chemokines interleukin-8 and platelet factor 4 in a mouse model of cytosine arabinoside (ARA-C) chemotherapy. *Exp. Hematol.* **23:** 900.

92. Han, Z. C., M. Lu, J. Li, M. Defard, B. Boval, N. Schlegel, and J. P. Caen. 1997. Platelet-factor 4 and other CXC chemokines support the survival of normal hematopoietic cells and reduce the chemosensitivity of cells to cytotoxic agents. *Blood* **89:** 2328–2335.

93. Aiuti, A., I. J. Webb, T. Springer, and J. C. Gutierrez-Ramos. 1997. The chemokine SDF-1 is a chemoattractant for human CD34⁺ hematopoietic progenitor cells and provides a new mechanism to explain the mobilization of CD34⁺ progenitors to peripheral blood. *J. Exp. Med.* **185:** 111–120.

94. Kim, C. H., and H. E. Broxmeyer. 1998. In vitro behavior of hematopoietic progenitor cells under the influence of chemoattractants: stromal cell-derived factor-1, steel factor and the bone marrow environment. *Blood* **91:** 100–110.

95. Nagasawa, T., S. Hirota, K. Tachibana, N. Takakura, S. Nishikawa, Y. Kitamura, N. Yoshida, H. Kikutani, and T. Kishimoto. 1996. Defects of B-cell lymphopoiesis and bone-marrow myelopoiesis in mice lacking CXC chemokine PBSF/SDF-1. *Nature (Lond.)* **382:** 635–638.

96. Okumura, N., K. Tsuki, Y. Ebihara, I. Tanaka, N. Sawai, K. Koike, A. Komiyama, and T. Nakahata. 1996. Chemotactic and chemokinetic activities of stem cell factor on murine hematopoietic progenitor cells. *Blood* **87:** 4100.

97. Kim, C. H., L. M. Pelus, J. R. White, and H. E. Broxmeyer. 1998. CKβ-11/MIP-3β/ELC, a CC chemokine, is a chemoattractant with a specificity for macrophage progenitors amongst myeloid progenitor cells. *J. Immunol.* **161:** 2580–2585.

98. Kim, C. H., L. M. Pelus, J. R. White, E. Appelbaum, K. Johanson, and H. E. Broxmeyer. 1998. CKβ-11/MIP-3β/EB-11-ligand chemokine (ELC) is an efficacious chemoattractant for T- and B-cells. *J. Immunol.* **160:** 2418–2424.

99. Yoshida, R., M. Nagira, M. Kitaura, N. Imagawa, T. Imai, and O. Yoshie. 1998. Secondary lymphoid-tissue chemokine is a functional ligand for CC chemokine receptor CCR7. *J. Biol. Chem.* **273:** 7118–7122.

100. Kim, C. H, L. M. Pelus, and H. E. Broxmeyer. 1998. Regulation of trafficking and proliferation of myeloid progenitors by CCR7 ligands: SLC/6 Ckine/Exodus 2 and CKβ-11/MIP-3/ELC. *Blood* **92(Suppl 1, Part 1):** 370a (abstract).

101. Kim, C. H., L. M. Pelus, J. R. White, and H. E. Broxmeyer. 1998. Differential chemotactic behavior of developing T cells in response to thymic chemokines. *Blood* **91:** 4434–4443.

102. Laterveer, L., I. J. D. Lindley, M. S. Hamilton, R. Willemze, and W. E. Fibbe. 1995. Interleukin-8 induces rapid mobilization of hematopoietic stem cells with radioprotective capacity and long-term myelolymphoid repopulating ability. *Blood* **85:** 2269–2275.

103. Laterveer, L., I. J. D. Lindley, D. P. M. Heemskerk, J. A. J. Camps, E. K. J. Pauwels, R. Willemsz, and W. E. Fibbe. 1996. Rapid mobilization of hematopoietic progenitor cells in rhesus monkeys by a single intravenous injection of interleukin-8. *Blood* **87:** 781–788.

104. Wang, J. B., N. Mukaida, Y. Zhang, T. Ito, S. Nakao, and K. Matsushima. 1997. Enhanced mobilization of hematopoietic progenitor cells by mouse MIP-2 and granulocyte colony-stimulating factor in mice. *J. Leuk. Biol.* **62:** 503–509.

105. Hendrie, P. C., K. Miyazawa, Y.-C. Yang, C. D. Langefeld, and H. E. Broxmeyer. 1991. Mast cell growth factor (c-kit ligand) enhances cytokine stimulation of proliferation of human factor dependent cell line. M07e. *Exp. Hematol.* **19:** 1031–1037.

106. Lord, B. I., L. B. Woolford, L. M. Wood, L. G. Czaplewski, M. McCourt, M. G. Hunter, and R. M. Edwards. 1995. Mobilization of early hematopoietic progenitor cells with BB-10010: a genetically engineered variant of human macrophage inflammatory protein-1α. *Blood* **85:** 3412–3415.

107. Miyazawa, K., P. C. Hendrie, C. Mantel, K. Wood, L. K. Ashman, and H. E. Broxmeyer. 1991. Comparative analysis of signaling pathways between mast cell growth factor (c-kit ligand) and granulocyte-macrophage colony stimulating factor in a human factor-dependent myeloid cell line involves phosphorylation of Raf-1, GTPase-activating protein and mitogen-activated protein kinase. *Exp. Hematol.* **19:** 1110–1123.

108. Tauchi, T., G. S. Feng, R. Shen, M. Hoatlin, G. C. Bagby, L. Lu, and H. E. Broxmeyer. 1995. Involvement of SH2-containing phosphotyrosine phosphatase Syp in erythropoietin receptor signal transduction pathways. *J. Biol. Chem.* **270:** 5631–5635.

109. Aronica, S. M., C. Mantel, R. Gonin, M. S. Marshall, A. Sarris, S. Cooper, N. Hague, X. F. Zhang, and H. E. Broxmeyer. 1995. Interferon-inducible protein 10 and macrophage inflammatory protein-1α inhibit growth factor stimulation of Raf-1 kinase activity and protein synthesis in a human growth factor-dependent hematopoietic cell line. *J. Biol. Chem.* **270:** 21,998–22,007.

110. Mantel, C., S. Aronica, Z. Luo, M. S. Marshall, Y.-J. Kim, and H. E. Broxmeyer. 1995. Macrophage inflammatory protein 1α enhances growth-factor stimulated phospholipid turnover and increases cAMP levels in the human factor-dependent cell line. M07e. *J. Immunol.* **154:** 2342–2350.

111. Heyworth, C. M., M. A. Pearson, T. M. Dexter, G. Wark, P. J. Owen-Lynch, and A. D. Whetton. 1995. Macrophage inflammatory protein-1α mediated growth inhibition in a haemopoietic stem cell line is associated with inositol 1,4,5 trisphosphate generation. *Growth Factors* **12:** 165–172.

112. Wong, M., and E. N. Fish. 1998. RANTES and MIP-1α activate STATs in T cells. *J. Biol. Chem.* **273:** 309–314.

113. Ganju, R. K., P. Dutt, L. Wu, W. Newman, H. Avraham, S. Avraham, and J. E. Groopman. 1998. β-chemokine receptor CCR5 signals via the novel tyrosine kinase RAFTK. *Blood* **91:** 791–797.

114. Cacalano, G., J. Lee, K. Kikly, A. M. Ryan, S. Pitts-Meek, B. Hultgren, W. I. Wood, and M. W. Moore. 1994. Neutrophil and B cell expansion in mice that lack the murine IL-8 receptor homolog. *Science* **265:** 682–684.

115. Boring, L., J. Gosling, S. W. Chensue, S. L. Kunkel, R. V. Farese, Jr., H. E. Broxmeyer, and I. F. Charo. 1997. Impaired monocyte migration and reduced type 1 (Th1) cytokine responses in C-C chemokine receptor 2 knockout mice. *J. Clin. Invest.* **100:** 2552–2561.

116. Reid, S., A. Ritchie, L. Boring, S. Cooper, G. Hangoc, I. F. Charo, and H. E. Broxmeyer. 1999. Enhanced myeloid progenitor cell cycling and apoptosis in mice lacking the chemokine receptor, CCR2. *Blood*, in press.

117. Gao, J. L., T. A. Wynn, Y. Chang, E. Lee, B. E. Broxmeyer, E. Cooper, H. L. Tiffany, H. Westphal, J. Kwon-Chung, and P. M. Murphy. 1997. Impaired host defense, hematopoiesis, granulomatous inflammation and type 1/type 2 cytokine balance in mice lacking cc chemokine receptor 1. *J. Exp. Med.* **185:** 1959–1968.

118. Tian, M., H. E. Broxmeyer, Y. Fan, Z. Lai, S. Zhang, S. Aronica, S. Cooper, R. M. Bisby, R. Steinmetz, S. J. Engle, A. Mestek, J. Gong, J. D. Pollock, M. R. Vasko, M. N. Lehman, H. T. Jansen, M. Ying, P. J. Stambrook, J. A. Tischfield, and L. Yu. 1997. Altered hematopoiesis, behavior, and sexual function in μ opioid receptor-deficient mice. *J. Exp. Med.* **185:** 1517–1522.

16

Macrophage Inflammatory Protein-1α
and Stem Cell Inhibition

Gerard J. Graham and Robert J. B. Nibbs

1. INTRODUCTION

Much interest has recently focused on the regulation of hemopoietic stem cell (HSC) proliferation as such studies are of fundamental importance in a range of therapeutic contexts. For example, both inhibitors and stimulators of stem cell proliferation have potential roles to play in alleviating myelosuppression following chemotherapeutic cancer treatments. In addition, the ability to manipulate the proliferative status of the HSC may be crucial in assuring the efficacy of gene therapeutic regimes. This chapter outlines the biology of the hemopoietic system and sets out to define the role of macrophage inflammatory protein-1α (MIP-1α) as an inhibitor of HSC proliferation.

2. HSC BIOLOGY

2.1. HSC Compartment and Bioassays

The earliest assay for the HSC was developed in the early 1960s by Till and McCulloch *(87)*. This assay involves subjecting mice to a lethal dose of irradiation, of which they would normally die owing to bone marrow failure. If following the irradiation a source of syngeneic murine bone marrow is transplanted into the mouse, stem cells in the transplanted marrow serve to replenish the damaged system, and during the process of hemopoietic regeneration, some of the stem cells seed onto the surface of the spleen and form colonies. These colonies, which are referred to as colony forming unit–spleen (CFU-S) colonies, are multilineage and clonal and, in addition, demonstrate a limited ability to self-renew. These characteristics prompted researchers, at the time, to claim that the CFU-S cell was the HSC.

A number of difficulties have arisen over the definition of the CFU-S cell as the HSC; e.g., CFU-S are unable to generate lymphoid progeny, and, in addition, in murine bone marrow transplantation experiments, it has been noted that there is little correlation between CFU-S numbers in the transplanted marrow and the success of long-term hemopoietic reconstitution *(27)*. These and other observations have led stem cell biologists to propose the existence of more primitive stem cells that have a more direct relationship with long-term repopulation. Indeed, evidence for such pre-CFU-S cells has been put forward, and there is now an emerging hierarchy of stem cells that appear

From: *Chemokines and Cancer*
Edited by: B. J. Rollins © Humana Press Inc., Totowa, NJ

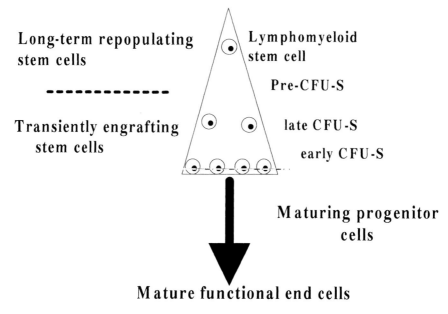

Fig. 1. The HSC compartment.

to be more primitive than the CFU-S cell *(36,75,76)*. It is clear, however, that pre-CFU-S cells and CFU-S cells all fulfill the basic criteria required of a stem cell, i.e., self-renewal and differentiation capacity. Thus, although the pre-CFU-S stem cells are clearly more primitive than the CFU-S cells, both populations must be regarded as being stem cell–like, therefore, we now talk not of a stem cell *per se* but of a stem cell compartment sitting at the more primitive end of the hemopoietic system and comprising these overlapping stem cell populations (*see* Fig. 1).

Although the stem cell compartment is complicated, it has recently been able to be functionally subdivided into two major compartments on the basis of reconstitution ability *(42,43)*. Thus, the population of cells, including the CFU-S cells and the other more mature components of the stem cell compartment, when transplanted into a lethally irradiated recipient mouse, will allow recovery of the mouse, which survives for about 4–6 wk after transplant and then dies as a result of bone marrow failure. By contrast, the more primitive elements of the stem cell compartment have no independent ability to rescue a lethally irradiated mouse. What is required for full and long-term reconstitution of the irradiated murine hemopoietic system is a combination of these two cell types, with the CFU-S and other less primitive stem cells acting as transiently engrafting stem cells, bolstering the system for the first few weeks posttransplant and the very primitive stem cell components acting to mediate longer-term reconstitution. The marked inability of these cells to repopulate in the absence of transient engrafting stem cells suggests that they may need to be seeded into a supportive and regulatory niche before they can contribute to the reconstitution process. Therefore, the role of the CFU-S and other transiently engrafting cells is to maintain the system long enough for the very primitive cells to find such supportive niches. Hence, the simple functional distinction is between long-term repopulating stem cells and transiently engrafting stem cells.

Typically the long-term repopulating or primitive hemopoietic cells are detected by in vivo long-term repopulating assays using marked transplanted bone marrow. In addition to this cumbersome in vivo assay are several in vitro assays, such as the long-term culture-initiating cell assay and the pre-CFU-S assay. While such cells are primitive in nature, their precise relationship with the long-term repopulating stem cells has yet to be defined. The transiently engrafting stem cells are routinely detected using the CFU-S assay and a range of in vitro assays such as the colony forming unit–agar (CFU-A), the high proliferative potential–colony forming cell (HPP-CFC) assays, and the colony forming unit–granulocyte, erythroid, macrophage, megakaryocyte (CFU-GEMM) and CFCmix assays (*see* ref. *86* for reviews of hemopoietic stem/progenitor cell asays).

2.2. Control of HSC Proliferation

As shown in Figure 1, the HSC compartment sits at the heart of the hemopoietic system, and it is at this cellular level that all hemopoietic function can ultimately be regulated. In particular, regulation of the proliferation of this pivotal cell will have profound implications for the functioning of the entire system. For this and other reasons, a full understanding of the nature of the factors acting to control stem cell proliferation is central to our overall appreciation of the hemopoietic system.

Most studies on the proliferative status of HSC suggest that these cells are largely quiescent with as few as 4–6% being in active cell cycle at any one time. Following radiation or chemotherapeutic insult to the hemopoietic system, these quiescent HSCs rapidly enter cell cycle and, through processes of self-renewal and differentiation, serve to replenish the damaged system. Having achieved this, the HSCs then reenter the quiescent state. It has therefore been inferred from these observations that the HSC must be under both positive and negative proliferative regulation and that the overall proliferative status of the HSC is regulated by the relative levels of these two opposing activities.

2.2.1. Stimulatory Factors

An almost bewildering array of factors capable of stimulating HSC proliferation has now been identified. However, in general, stimulatory factors do not work in isolation and require the synergy of partners for effective stimulation *(3)*. Thus, factors such as stem cell factor (SCF) and Flt3 ligand can induce synergy with a range of other peptide growth factors to stimulate HSC proliferation *(4,38,88)*. In this context, it has been demonstrated that factors such as SCF act to maintain the viability of the quiescent progenitors and that the factor of synergy such as interleukin-6 (IL-6) induces the proliferation of these viable quiescent HSCs *(40,44,46,51,52)*. It is currently unclear whether such synergy of HSC proliferative factors induces self-renewal in the stem cell population or whether the proliferation induced is accompanied by differentiation or phenotypic alterations. Clearly, HSCs express telomerase, suggesting an extended life span, but HSCs are known to age following either stimulation by growth factors or serial transplantation *(62,63)*. The role of stimulatory factors in vivo and also in therapeutic contexts needs to be more accurately defined.

2.2.2. Inhibitory Factors

Several inhibitors of HSC proliferation that show overlapping biologic effects have been identified and characterized *(25)*. As well as being of importance to our understanding of the regulation of HSC proliferation, stem cell inhibitory factors may have a therapeutic role as myeloprotective agents for use during chemotherapeutic treatments for cancer *(25)*. The major inhibitory molecules identified to date include the following:

2.2.2.1. THE TETRAPEPTIDE

The tetrapeptide, a small peptide inhibitor, was first identified by Frindel and Guigon *(21)* as a low mol wt dialyzable inhibitory molecule present in fetal calf bone marrow *(19)*. The peptide has now been purified and sequenced, indicating it to be a tetrapeptide with the sequence AcSDKP *(53)*. It is suggested that this peptide is derived from Thymosin-β4, which carries the AcSDKP sequence at its amino terminus *(34)*.

The tetrapeptide is active in inhibiting CFU-S cells and appears to act by blocking the reentry of quiescent stem cells into the cell cycle *(61,81)*. A physiologic role for the tetrapeptide has been inferred from studies with antibodies that trigger CFU-S into the cell cycle *(20)*, and, in addition, a role in regulating regenerative hemopoiesis has been suggested by studies on cytotoxic drug–treated mice *(21)*.

2.2.2.2. THE PENTAPEPTIDE

The pentapeptide, a peptide that is present in rodent bone marrow and is produced by human leukocytes, has been purified and sequenced revealing the sequence pEEDCK *(48,74)*. This peptide is active in inhibiting murine and human granulocyte macrophage–colony forming cell (GM-CFC) and murine CFU-S cells *(49,71,72,73)*. The inhibitory activity is optimal at 10^{-13}M, but the dose response is "bell-shaped" and inhibition is lost at higher concentrations, owing, in large part, to the ability of this peptide to dimerize using the cysteine residues on opposing monomers. Intriguingly, this dimeric variant is active as a stimulator of GM-CFC proliferation and shows no inhibitory activities *(22,50)*. Again, the stimulatory variant displays a biphasic dose-response curve with optimal activity at 10^{-9}M.

2.2.2.3. TRANSFORMING GROWTH FACTOR-β (TGF-β)

There are five TGF-β isoforms identified to date, three of which are expressed in mammalian cells. The TGF-βs are members of a large family of related peptides that include activin, inhibin, and the product of DECAPENTAPLEGIC. Members of this family play diverse roles in embryonic development and adult cell function *(64,84,85)*. TGF-β is secreted from cells in an inactive latent form that requires activation. This is likely to be achieved in vivo using the protease plasmin; however, other nonphysiologic activation mechanisms have been identified *(6,33)*.

TGF-β appears to be able to inhibit the proliferation of cells throughout the stem cell compartment; however, this is dependent on the precise cell type being examined and on the relative growth factor environment in which the cell is being cultured *(41,45)*. TGF-β is constitutively expressed in bone marrow *(11)* and in long-term bone marrow cultures *(16)*, and data from antisense and antibody studies suggest that it may be able to function as an autocrine or paracrine inhibitor of HSC proliferation *(35,54,83)*.

3. MIP-1α AS A STEM CELL INHIBITOR

Our preliminary studies into the characterization of novel stem cell inhibitors involved the identification of a stem cell inhibitory activity in the conditioned medium of the murine macrophage cell line J774.2. The peptide responsible for this activity was purified to homogeneity, and sequencing showed it to be identical to MIP-1α *(28)*.

The human homolog of MIP-1α is also active in inhibiting stem cell proliferation *(29)*, as are the murine and human MIP-1β peptides *(30)*. We have been unable to demonstrate the effects of other chemokines in our stem cell inhibitory assays; however, a number of other chemokines with stem cell inhibitory properties have been identified *(1,82,94)*.

3.1. MIP-1α Stem Cell Inhibition In Vitro

It appears from several studies that the inhibitory properties of MIP-1α are restricted to the transiently engrafting stem cell compartment *(5,7,28,45,59)* and that this peptide has little detectable inhibitory effects on very primitive elements of the stem cell compartment, such as the long-term repopulating stem cells or various primitive cell types detected by the HPP-CFC assays *(78,83)*.

Within the context of transiently engrafting stem cells, a range of assays has been used to demonstrate MIP-1α inhibitory effects. For example, this peptide appears capable of inhibiting primitive cells detected in the CFU-GEMM and burst-forming unit–erythroid assays as well as the classical CFU-S and CFU-A stem cell assays. Our own analysis using the CFU-S assay has demonstrated that human MIP-1α preferentially inhibits the proliferation of more primitive CFU-S cells (d12 CFU-S), and has a relatively weaker effect on more mature members of the CFU-S stem cell pool *(15)*. This work is confirmed by studies on sorted components of the stem cell compartment indicating that whereas transiently engrafting stem cells sorted on the basis of the absence of lineage markers and the presence of low levels of Thy1 (lin-Thy1 lo) are inhibitable by MIP-1α, the more mature lin-/Thy1 cells are resistant to the inhibitory effects of this peptide *(45)*. Indeed, there maybe some stimulation of the more mature components of the stem cell compartment, and this is confirmed by a number of studies suggesting MIP-1α to be active as a stimulator of progenitor cell proliferation under appropriate circumstances *(7,10,89)*.

In addition to the direct effects of MIP-1α in inhibiting primitive hemopoietic cells, there is evidence implicating MIP-1α or related chemokines in the inhibitory properties of other agents. Thus, the neuropeptide Neurokinin A has been shown to be capable of inhibiting GM-CFC and, in addition, to induce the expression of both MIP-1α and TGF-β in bone marrow stroma *(80)*. Neutralizing antibody studies have suggested that both TGF-β and MIP-1α conspire to bring about the inhibitory effects seen with this peptide. As described previously, the tetrapeptide inhibitor is also active in inhibiting a range of transiently engrafting stem cells, and evidence has been presented from long-term bone marrow cultures suggesting that this inhibition is not direct but that it may be achieved using an MIP-1α-like intermediate *(8)*.

The relatively restricted theater of influence of MIP-1α within the stem cell compartment is in contrast to the effects of TGF-β, which are seen throughout the stem cell compartment *(45)*. Although the relevance of this observation remains to be determined, it may suggest relatively different physiologic or pathologic roles for these two inhibitors. Under steady-state conditions, it is likely that the majority of hemopoietic function is regulated at the level of the transiently engrafting stem cells with little input from the more primitive long-term repopulating stem cells. Thus, although the inhibition of long-term repopulating stem cells may be desirable under certain conditions of regeneration, it is likely that the transiently engrafting stem cells, the target of MIP-1α inhibition, may be more in need of active and frequent proliferative regulation. This may partially explain the relatively restricted pattern of MIP-1α function within the stem cell compartment. Note, however, that data from studies on MIP-1α null mice (*[12]* and unpublished observations) have failed to demonstrate any abnormalities of transiently engrafting stem cells in these animals. These data therefore suggest that MIP-1α is not an indispensable requirement for stem cell regulation in vivo and that there may be some level of redundancy built into this important control system.

In addition to HSCs, data from our laboratory have demonstrated MIP-1α to be active as an inhibitor of in vitro keratinocyte growth *(70)*. Our results suggest that murine MIP-1α is a reversible inhibitor of clonogenic epidermal cell proliferation and that the likely intradermal source of this chemokine is the population of epidermal Langerhans cells. One complicating feature of this relationship between MIP-1α and the control of keratinocyte proliferation is that whereas MIP-1α generated by transient transfection of the mammalian COS cell line is active on both HSCs and keratinocytes, the bacterially generated form of the protein is active only on HSCs. We have hypothesized that this discrepancy relates to the requirement by MIP-1α for an accessory factor to allow it to function as a keratinocyte inhibitor. Thus, it is possible that traces of such a factor may be generated by the COS cells but not by the bacterial cells. A second possibility is that the keratinocyte inhibitory activity of MIP-1α requires that the protein be structurally altered; hence, this alteration would be conferred on the protein during expression in COS cells but not during expression by the bacterial system. We have now looked exhaustively for evidence of an accessory factor and have found none. In fact, we have purified the COS cell MIP-1α to essentially complete homogeneity and it retains its kerato-inhibitory activity. We are therefore currently investigating the possibility that subtle structural alterations are required to "unleash" the kerato-inhibitory effects of MIP-1α. However, we still have no clear thoughts on what these alterations may be.

3.2. MIP-1α Stem Cell Inhibition In Vivo and Potential Clinical Usefulness

The potential clinical roles of stem cell inhibitory factors are well documented *(26)*. Briefly, during most chemotherapeutic regimes, the dose of chemotherapeutic agents used is limited, to a large extent, by the damage that these agents do to uninvolved normal tissues. The most fragile tissue in the body in this respect is the hemopoietic system, and thus hemopoietic damage is frequently the primary dose-limiting factor in cytotoxic drug therapies. If it were possible to protect the stem cell compartment from therapeutic damage, it might be possible to increase the dosage of cytotoxic drug used and also, perhaps, its efficacy. Following treatment the patient could then repopulate the damaged elements of his or her hemopoietic system from the protected stem cell population.

To date several studies from our own and other laboratories have demonstrated the ability of MIP-1α to function as a stem cell inhibitor in vivo following exogenous administration *(15,55,60)*. In addition, administered MIP-1α has been demonstrated to be active in protecting the transiently engrafting stem cell population from chemotherapeutic damage using the drugs 5-fluorouracil and cytosine arabinoside. Typically, 10–20 μg of protein is required per mouse for effective inhibition and protection of the stem cells; however, one study suggests that using appropriately prepared MIP-1α, very small amounts of MIP-1α, can achieve the same end point *(14)*.

MIP-1α, therefore, can clearly function in vivo and appears to have no detectable associated toxicity. One problem, however, is that the cytotoxic agents that have been used in these studies have been single agents and have been cycle specific in that they will kill only cycling cells. In routine chemotherapy, it is more common to use combinations of cytotoxic agents, one or more of which are likely to be non–cell cycle–specific drugs. Thus, protection against such agents may not be achievable using cell cycle blockers such as MIP-1α. Although few data are available on this topic, studies from our own and other laboratories (*[24]* and Parker, A., et al., unpublished data) imply that MIP-1α can protect against the cytotoxic effects of the non–cell cycle–specific drug cyclophosphamide, suggesting that indeed this peptide may be useful as a hemoprotective agent in combination therapy without the requirement for cycle specificity of the drugs used.

One additional therapeutic use lies in the treatment of some leukemias. It has been demonstrated, in a number of studies, that transiently engrafting stem cells from chronic myelogenous leukemia (CML) patients are insensitive to the inhibitory effects of MIP-1α *(17,37)*. However, the reasons for this resistance are not currently known, but it has been demonstrated that CML stem cells express MIP-1α receptors although the precise receptors expressed on these cells have not yet been identified *(9)*. In addition, a subset of acute myelogenous leukemia patients demonstrate a sensitivity of their transiently engrafting stem cells to MIP-1α but other subtypes do not *(18,68)*. It is therefore possible to envisage a therapeutic approach to leukemia in which the wild-type stem cells are rendered quiescent using MIP-1α, while the non-MIP-1α -responsive leukemic cells are killed by cytotoxic drug therapy. Such a kill could be achieved either in vivo or ex vivo with subsequent administration of the treated bone marrow.

3.3. Structure Function Studies on MIP-1α

Despite having a peptide mol wt of about 8 kDa, MIP-1α, in common with several other C-C chemokines, has the ability to form large noncovalent self-aggregates *(29)*. These aggregates appear to be held together by electrostatic forces, and their size is dictated by the concentration of the monomeric chemokine. Typically, MIP-1α at a concentration of 0.1 mg/mL in physiologic buffers has a native mol wt of about 100 kDa, and thus appears to be an aggregated dodecamer. There are a number of practical consequences of this self-aggregation, one being that depending on the precise chemical environment, it is very difficult to derive meaningful receptor-binding data for MIP-1α. We believe that this aggregation is a consequence of the aggregation tendency such that when all cell surface binding sites are occupied by monomeric MIP-1α, this receptor-bound MIP-1α acts as a nucleating center for further self-aggregation. This ensures aggregation that the receptor binding neither saturates nor competes with cold ligand. A further consequence of the self-aggregation is that crystals of MIP-1α are difficult to grow precluding X-ray crystallographic structural analysis.

As mentioned previously, it is hoped that MIP-1α will have a therapeutic role as a myeloprotective agent, and it is in this context that other practical consequences of the self-aggregation tendency become apparent. Thus, if aggregated MIP-1α is administered to a patient, it will be wasteful and unnecessarily expensive and may indeed have a very low specific activity.

For these reasons, we and others have attempted to understand the biochemical basis for the self-aggregation process in the hope that this understanding would allow a rational design of MIP-1α variants with reduced self-aggregation potential *(31,39)*. It became apparent from these studies that a feature common to the aggregating chemokines was an acidic carboxyl terminal tail, and thus a simple model of self-aggregation involving electrostatic interactions between this tail and internal basic residues in apposing monomers was proposed. We have subsequently gone on to demonstrate that this is indeed the case and that neutralization of the carboxy terminal acidic amino acids progressively reduces the aggregated state of MIP-1α. Intriguingly, the differentially aggregated mutants generated (tetramers, dimers, and monomers), all are active in stem cell inhibitory and monocyte migratory assays, although none is more active than the wild-type protein. In fact, these three mutants and the wild-type protein have essentially identical and superimposable bioactivity profiles in the two test assays, suggesting that ultimately all of these mutants must disaggregate in the solutions used in the assays and must therefore ultimately interact with their receptors in the monomeric form. We have now confirmed that this is the case, and the conclusion that chemokines interact with their receptors in the monomeric form is now a generally held view for both C-C and C-X-C chemokines *(69,79)*.

A further property of MIP-1α that we have investigated using mutagenesis has been the tendency for this and other chemokines to bind to proteoglycans. It is known from studies on basic fibroblast growth factor that proteoglycans may modulate function *(93)*, and, indeed, IL-8 has been shown to have enhanced activity on neutrophils when presented along with heparin and heparan sulfate *(91)*. However, little is known regarding the role of proteoglycan binding in MIP-1α function. Typically, proteoglycan binding sites in peptides comprise clusters of basic amino acid residues, and we have identified the likely binding site in MIP-1α. Mutagenesis of this site resulting in neutralization of two of the basic charges has resulted in the generation of a MIP-1α variant that has no apparent ability to bind to proteoglycan affinity columns *(32)*. Intriguingly, this peptide has a native mol wt of 16 kDa and thus appears to be a dimer at a concentration at which the wild-type protein is dodecameric. This reinforces the notion that self-aggregation is a consequence of interaction between carboxy terminal acidic residues and internal basic residues.

Bioactivity analysis of the nonheparin-binding variant of MIP-1α revealed that it retained essentially wild-type activity in the stem cell inhibitory assay, suggesting that in this context, proteoglycan binding is not a prerequisite for function. By contrast, this mutant appeared to be completely inactive on monocytes. Further analysis has revealed that this functional uncoupling of stem cell inhibition from monocyte chemoattraction in MIP-1α is a consequence of altered binding to the CCR1 receptor. This appears to be the result of the fact that the proteoglycan binding site that is mutated in this variant is also a site that is involved either directly or indirectly in the binding of this mutant to CCR1.

More recently, studies on human MIP-1α have identified the same site as being of importance in proteoglycan binding *(47)*. Intriguingly, mutagenesis of this site in human MIP-1α does not abrogate CCR1 binding. The basis for the discrepancy between these two studies is currently unclear but may relate either to species difference or, more likely, to the nature of the mutagenesis performed. Koopman and Krangel *(80)* used an alanine replacement strategy for mutagenesis whereas we have replaced the lysine and arginine residues, within the heparin-binding domain, with asparagine and serine residues, respectively. Preliminary studies on RANTES mutants at this site suggest that the nature of the amino acid replacement used is important in defining subsequent interaction of mutants with CCR1 (Pakianathan, D., and Graham, G.J., unpublished data).

3.4. Interaction of MIP-1α with Other Stem Cell Inhibitory Molecules

Throughout our studies on MIP-1α, we have been struck by the broad range of biologic similarities among this peptide and other inhibitory proteins, most notably members of the TGF-β family of peptides. Thus, both MIP-1α and TGF-β will inhibit proliferation of HSCs and will, under appropriate circumstances, stimulate the proliferation of more mature progenitor cells. In addition, and as outlined in more detail subsequently, both are also active in inhibiting the proliferation of clonogenic epidermal cells. This finding has prompted us to investigate the possibility that this apparent functional redundancy may be accounted for on the basis of one of these regulators acting through induction of the other.

Our analysis to date has suggested that a complex and dynamic relationship exists between MIP-1α and TFG-β *(56,57)*. For example, TGF-β is active in potently suppressing MIP-1α transcript levels in murine bone marrow macrophages. Activity is seen with subpicomolar levels of TGF-β and is shared by the three TGF-β isoforms, TGF-β1, -β2, and -β3. In addition, this decrease in transcript level is reflected in a reduction in the levels of MIP-1α protein in TGF-β-treated macrophage cell lines, suggesting a functional consequence of this downregulation. This effect is not restricted to MIP-1α, and other chemokines are also suppressed by this regulator. In addition to the effects on the chemokines, it also appears that TGF-β is active in suppressing MIP-1α receptor levels. In particular, TGF-1β can suppress CCR1 levels in both human and murine monocytes/macrophages. This suggests that in an inflammatory context in which CCR1 is likely to be important, the presence of TGF-β may act to suppress both ligand production and receptor generation, thus acting to suppress both arms of the MIP-1α inflammatory machinery. The presence of an endogenous TGF-β-mediated suppression of MIP-1α expression in bone marrow macrophages is demonstrable using the pan TGF-β neutralizing agent latency associated peptide (LAP) *(23)*. Treatment of macrophages with this agent induces the expression of MIP-1α, suggesting the levels to be actively and endogenously suppressed by TGF-β.

In looking at the reciprocal relationship between TGF-β and MIP-1α, it has become apparent that MIP-1α induces TGF-β expression in bone marrow macrophages and thus serves to ensure its own suppression. It appears, therefore, that in all interactions between TGF-β and MIP-1α, whether they be pertinent to inflammatory or stem cell inhibitory contexts, the system tends toward suppression of the levels of MIP-1α and at least one of its receptors.

These data therefore suggest that in terms of stem cell inhibition, TGF-β may be a more dominant regulatory molecule, given its widespread expression in vivo. It is possible, however, that MIP-1α is more active as a stem cell inhibitor under conditions in which its expression is actively induced over the TGF-β-mediated transcriptional block. Such circumstances may include the return of proliferating stem cells to quiescence following proliferation induced during an inflammatory response. Indeed, a number of regulators have recently been identified, most notable IL-3 and granulocyte-macro-phage colony-stimulating factor (GM-CSF), that can induce MIP-1α expression in bone marrow macrophages even in the presence of TGF-β (Jarmin and Graham, unpublished data). In addition, it is clear that MIP-1α can be detected in normal human and murine bone marrow and peripheral blood *(11)*, and therefore the restricted relationship between TGF-β and MIP-1α demonstrated in vitro may be confounded in vivo, a set-ting in which the MIP-1α producer cells will be open to a wide range of complex and interacting regulatory factors.

4. MIP-1α RECEPTOR BIOLOGY AND SIGNAL TRANSDUCTION OF RELEVANCE TO STEM CELL INHIBITION

Identification of the receptor molecules responsible for MIP-1α-mediated stem cell inhibition has been hampered by technical problems. First, it is difficult to separate those cells inhibited by MIP-1α in sufficient purity to allow in-depth molecular analy-sis. Second, cell lines established from immature hemopoietic cell types are generally insensitive to the inhibitory effects of MIP-1α (Graham, G., and Nibbs, R., unpub-lished observations), although the MO7e cell line may be an exception (see below).

However, some studies do provide clues to the properties of the stem cell inhibitory receptor. First, of the chemokines tested, only MIP-1α and, to a lesser extent, MIP-1β appear to be active on the cell detected in a CFU-A/S assay, implying that the receptor on these cells shows relative specificity for these two chemokines. However, this may not be an accurate assumption since other chemokines may be able to bind to the CFU-A/S receptor without necessarily eliciting an inhibitory response. Second, we have generated a murine MIP-1α mutant, HepMut (*see* Subheading 3.3.), that is equipotent to wild-type MIP-1α in CFU-A assays but that has lost its monocyte chemotactic func-tion owing to abrogation of CCR1 binding activity *(32)*. The stem cell inhibitory recep-tor should therefore be able to interact with HepMut. Finally, Avalos and colleagues *(2)* attempted to calculate the affinity of receptors on purified stem cells for iodinated MIP-1α and arrived at a figure for the dissociation constant of approx 300 p*M*, sugges-tive of a relatively high affinity interaction. Thus, we can tentatively hypothesize that the CFU-A/S stem cell inhibitory receptor is specific for MIP-1α and MIP-1β, exhibit-ing high affinity for MIP-1α, and retains interaction with HepMut.

Currently, 10 genes have been cloned from humans and mice that are able to interact with β-chemokines, namely CCR1–CCR8, D6, and Duffy *(66,67,77)*. These are all members of the heptahelical G protein–coupled receptor superfamily, and show vary-ing degrees of sequence homology. Using cell sorting, we have been able to show mRNA for D6 and, to a lesser extent, CCR3 and CCR5, in cell populations enriched for MIP-1α-responsive stem cells *(66)*. When expressed in heterologous cell types, such as Chinese hamster ovary or 293 cells, four of the receptors—CCR1, CCR3, CCR5, and D6—bound MIP-1α and MIP-1β. Of these receptors, CCR5 and D6 bound MIP-1α and MIP-1β with high affinity (subnanomolar) whereas CCR1 and CCR3 bound these ligands with lower affinity (nanomolar). In each case, the receptors bound MIP-1α with a higher affinity than MIP-1β. In addition to MIP-1α and MIP-1β, all four of these receptors bind other members of the extensive β-chemokine family: CCR1 and CCR5 bind RANTES, CCR3 binds eotaxin, and D6 binds RANTES and MCP-1 and MCP-3. Moreover, CCR1 is completely unable to bind to HepMut, and CCR3, CCR5, and D6 each shows a significantly lower affinity interaction with this mutant compared to wild-type MIP-1α (Graham, G., and Nibbs, R., unpublished observations). Although this may not necessarily reflect the ability of HepMut to signal through these proteins, it provides further circumstantial evidence to support the unlikely involvement of these known receptors in stem cell inhibition.

However, with the possible exceptions of CCR1 and D6, which appears to be nonsignaling chemokine receptor *(67)*, none of the known MIP-1α receptors can be confidently excluded until further interventionist approaches have been taken, such as homologous recombination to generate receptor null stem cells. It is possible, e.g., that MIP-1α and MIP-1β may elicit ligand-specific signals on interaction with CFU-A/S cell receptors, despite these same receptors displaying more promiscuous β-chemokine binding in in vitro models. Alternatively, it may be necessary to engage two distinct receptor types on stem cells to inhibit proliferation, which may have only MIP-1α and MIP-1β as common ligands.

Very little is known about the signaling pathways utilized by the activated MIP-1α receptor on stem cells to bring about proliferative inhibition. The growth factor–dependent cell line MO7e, derived from a patient with an acute megakaryocytic leukemia, has been used as a model system to study signaling in vitro *(1,58)*. These cells are routinely grown in serum-containing medium supplemented with GM-CSF. To observe proliferative inhibition by MIP-1α, it is necessary first to starve the cells of serum and cytokines, then pulse for 1 h in medium containing serum, GM-CSF, and MIP-1α. The cells in S-phase are then killed by incubation with tritiated thymidine and the surviving cells scored in a colony-forming assay containing GM-CSF and SCF. It is feasible that this cell line may not accurately reflect CFU-A/S inhibition, but it is currently the only system amenable for signaling studies in vitro. Moreover, it is possible that these cells may express MIP-1α receptors not involved in inhibition that could also be signaling into the cell to confuse results. Nonetheless, Mantel and colleagues *(58)* were able to show dose- and time-dependent increases in phosphatidylcholine (PC) turnover and cAMP levels on treatment of the cells with MIP-1α. They concluded that the rise in cAMP may be important in proliferative inhibition because (1) exogenous dibutyryl cAMP also inhibited MO7e proliferation in the previously cited colony-forming assay, and (2) no change in cAMP levels was seen on RANTES treatment, which does not inhibit proliferation but does stimulate PC turnover.

A subsequent publication showed that MIP-1α was able to inhibit GM-CSF/SCF-stimulated Raf-1 phosphorylation in MO7e cells, hence reducing the activity of this central signaling kinase, and it has been postulated that this may be owing to the increase in cAMP *(1)*. Indeed, it has been shown in several other cell types that cAMP can prevent Raf-1 activation, thereby blocking mitogenic stimuli working through the mitogen-activated protein (MAP) kinase cascade *(13,92)*. A recent publication suggests that this is mediated by cAMP-dependent protein kinase A (PKA) activation of Rap-1, a small G protein related to the Ras superfamily, which in turn inhibits Raf-1 *(90)*. Treatment of MO73 cells with an inhibitor of PKA prevents MIP-1α-mediated inhibition of cell proliferation as measured by the colony-forming assay *(1)*.

Increases in cAMP are induced by activation of adenylate cyclase, and this enzyme can be controlled by components of the $G_{\alpha\beta\gamma}$ heterotrimer involved in signaling through heptahelical receptors of the type known to bind MIP-1α (see above) *(65)*. Different

G_α-subunits exert different effects on adenylate cyclase: $G_{\alpha s}$ stimulates whereas $G_{\alpha i}$ inhibits. The effect of the $G_{\beta\gamma}$ heterodimer depends on the isoform of adenylate cyclase that is involved: it can activate or inhibit. Thus, cAMP levels may either increase or decrease depending on the available G proteins the receptor can be coupled to, and the adenylate cyclase isoforms present in the cell. To further complicate the matter, an increase in cAMP can *stimulate* the MAP kinase cascade in some cell types, e.g., PC12 cells. This seems to also be mediated through PKA activation of Rap-1, though this time resulting in activation of B-raf with subsequent activation of the MAP kinases *(90)*. Bearing all this in mind, it is possible that the same receptor may induce cAMP to rise or fall depending on the cell type it is expressed in, and that this change in cAMP can either inhibit nor activate the MAP kinase pathway depending on the relative abundance of Raf-1 and B-raf. Thus, in summary, the ability of MIP-1α to inhibit stem cells may not necessarily be a consequence of expression of a stem cell–specific inhibitory receptor, but rather be caused by the cellular environment in which the receptor is activated.

5. CONCLUSION

Clearly much needs to be done to define in more detail the mode of action of MIP-1α as an inhibitor of stem cell proliferation. In particular, identification of the receptor responsible for articulating the stem cell inhibitory properties of MIP-1α will be invaluable in facilitating studies into the mechanisms of inhibition by this chemokine. In addition, identification of the receptor may shed light on the pathogenesis of a number of leukemias and may indeed suggest novel therapeutic approaches to treatment of these malignancies.

It is our hope that in the near future, judicious use of MIP-1α and other inhibitory regulators will improve current therapeutic treatments for cancer, and we and others are actively engaged in wide-ranging biochemical and clinical studies with a view to achieving this goal.

ACKNOWLEDGMENTS

The authors were supported by grants from the Cancer Research Campaign.

REFERENCES

1. Aronica, S. M., C. Mantel, R. Gonin, M. S. Marshall, A. Sarris, S. Cooper, N. Hague, X.-F. Zhang, and H. E. Broxmeyer. 1995. Interferon-inducible protein 10 and macrophage inflammatory protein-1a inhibit growth factor stimulation of Raf-1 kinase activity and protein synthesis in a human growth factor-dependent hematopoietic cell line. *J. Biol. Chem.* **270:** 21,988–22,007.
2. Avalos, B. R., K. J. Bartynski, P. J. Elder, M. S. Kotur, W. G. Burton, and N. M. Wilkie. 1994. The active monomeric form of macrophage inflammatory protein-1a interacts with high- and low-affinity classes of receptors on human hematopoietic cells. *Blood* **84:** 1790–1801.
3. Bodine, D. M., P. S. Crosier, and S. C. Clark. 1991. Effects of hematopoietic growth factors on the survival of primitive stem cells in liquid suspension. *Blood* **78:** 914–920.
4. Bodine, D. M., D. Orlic, N. C. Birkett, N. E. Seidel, and K. M. Zsebo. 1992. Stem cell factor increases colony-forming unit-spleen number *in vitro* in synergy with interleukin-6 and *in vivo* in Sl/Sl^d mice as a single factor. *Blood* **79:** 913–919.

5. Bonnet, D., F. M. Lemoine, A. Najman, and M. Guigon. 1995. Comparison of the inhibitory effect of AcSDKP, TNF-α, TGF-β, and MIP-1α on marrow-purified CD34$^+$ progenitors. *Exp. Hematol.* **23:** 551–556.

6. Brown, P. D., L. M. Waterfield, A. D. Levinson, and M. Sporn. 1990. Physicochemical activation of recombinant latent transforming growth factor-betas 1, 2 and 3. *Growth Factors* **3:** 35–43.

7. Broxmeyer, H. E., B. Sherry, L. Lu, S. Cooper, K.-O. Oh, P. Tekamp-Olson, B. S. Kwon, and A. Cerami. 1990. Enhancing and suppressing effects of recombinant murine macrophage inflammatory proteins on colony formation *in vitro* by bone marrow myeloid progenitor cells. *Blood* **76:** 1110–1116.

8. Cashman, J. D., A. C. Eaves, and C. J. Eaves. 1994. The tetrapeptide AcSDKP specifically blocks the cycling of primitive normal but not leukemic progenitors in long-term culture: evidence for an indirect mechanism. *Blood* **84:** 1534–1542.

9. Chasty, R. C., G. S. Lucas, and J. Owen-Lynch. 1995. Macrophage inflammatory protein-1a receptors are present on cells enriched for CD34 expression from patients with chronic myeloid leukemia. *Blood* **86:** 4270–4277.

10. Clements, J. M., S. Craig, A. J. H. Gearing, M. G. Hunter, C. M. Heyworth, T. M. Dexter, and B. I. Lord. 1992. Biological and structural properties of MIP-1a expressed in yeast. *Cytokine* **4:** 76–82.

11. Cluitmans, F. H. M., B. H. J. Essendam, J. E. Landegent, R. Willemze, and J. H. F. Falkenberg. 1995. Constitutive *in vivo* cytokine and haemopoietic growth factor gene expression in the bone marrow and peripheral blood of healthy individuals. *Blood* **85:** 2038–2044.

12. Cook, D. N., M. A. Beck, T. M. Coffman, S. L. Kirby, J. F. Sheridan, I. B. Pragnell, and O. Smithies. 1995. Requirement of MIP-1α for inflammatory response to viral infection. *Science* **269:** 1583–1586.

13. Cook, S. J., and F. McCormick. 1993. Inhibition by cyclic AMP of Ras-dependent activation of Raf. *Science* **262:** 1069–1072.

14. Cooper, S., C. Mantel, and H. E. Broxmeyer. 1994. Myelosuppressive effects *in vivo* with very low dosages of monomeric recombinant murine macrophage inflammatory protein-1a. *Exp. Hematol.* **22:** 186–193.

15. Dunlop, D. J., E. G. Wright, S. Lorimore, G. J. Graham, T. Holyoake, D. J. Kerr, S. D. Wolpe, and I. B. Pragnell. 1992. Demonstration of stem cell inhibition and myeloprotective effects of SCI/rhMIP-1α *in vivo*. *Blood* **79:** 2221–2225.

16. Eaves, C. J., J. D. Cashman, R. J. Kay, G. J. Dougherty, T. Otsuka, L. A. Gaboury, D. E. Hogge, P. M. Landsdorp, A. C. Eaves, and R. K. Humphries. 1991. Mechanisms that regulate the cell cycle status of very primitive hematopoietic cells in long-term human marrow cultures. II. Analysis of positive and negative regulators produced by stromal cells within the adherent layer. *Blood* **78:** 110–117.

17. Eaves, C. J., J. D. Cashman, S. D. Wolpe, and A. C. Eaves. 1993. Unresponsiveness of primitive chronic myeloid leukemia cells to macrophage inflammatory protein 1a, an inhibitor of primitive normal hematopoietic cells. *Proc. Natl. Acad. Sci. USA* **20:** 12,015–12,019.

18. Ferrajoli, A., M. Talpaz, and T. F. Zipf. 1994. Inhibition of acute myelogenous leukemia progenitor proliferation by macrophage inflammatory protein 1-α. *Leukemia* **8:** 798–805.

19. Frindel, E., and M. Guigon. 1977. Inhibition of CFU entry into cycle by a bone marrow extract. *Exp. Hematol.* **5:** 74–76.

20. Frindel, E., and J.-P. Monpezat. 1989. The physiological role of the endogenous colony forming unit spleen (CFU-S) inhibitor acetyl-N-ser-asp-lys-pro (AcSDKP). *Leukaemia* **3:** 753, 754.

21. Frindel, E., A. Masse, Ph. Pradelles, L. Volkov, and M. Rigaud. 1992. Correlation of endogenous acetyl-Ser-Asp-Lys-Pro plasma levels in mice and the kinetics of the pluripo-

tent hemopoietic stem cells entry into the cycle after cytosine arabinoside treatment: fundamental and clinical aspects. *Leukemia* **6**: 599–601.

22. Frostad, S., T. Kalland, A. Aakvaag, and O. D. Laerum. 1993. Hemoregulatory peptide (HP5b) dimer effects on normal and malignant cells in culture. *Stem Cells* **11**: 303–311.

23. Gentry, L. E., and B. W. Nash. 1990. The pro domain of pre-pro-Transforming Growth Factor-beta 1 when independently expressed is a functional binding protein for the mature Growth-Factor. *Biochemistry* **29**: 6851–6857.

24. Gilmore, G. L., D. K. DePasquale, and R. K. Shadduck. 1996. BB10010, a synthetic variant of MIP-1a, reduces neutropenic interval in cyclophosphamide treated mice. *Blood* **88**: 3270.

25. Graham, G. J., and I. B. Pragnell. 1990. Negative regulators of haemopoiesis—current advances. *Prog. Growth Factor Res.* **2**: 181–191.

26. Graham, G. J., and I. B. Pragnell. 1991. Treating cancer: the potential role of stem cell inhibitors. *Eur. J. Cancer* **27**: 952, 953.

27. Graham, G. J., and I. B. Pragnell. 1992. The haemopoietic stem cell: properties and control mechanisms. *Semin. Cell Biol.* **3**: 423–434.

28. Graham, G. J., E. G. Wright, R. Hewick, S. D. Wolpe, N. M. Wilkie, D. Donaldson, S. Lorimore, and I. B. Pragnell. 1990. Identification and characterisation of an inhibitor of haemopoietic stem cell proliferation. *Nature* **344**: 442–444.

29. Graham, G. J., M. F. Freshney, D. Donaldson, and I. B. Pragnell. 1992. Purification and biochemical characterisation of human and murine stem cell inhibitors (SCI). *Growth Factors* **7**: 151–160.

30. Graham, G. J., L. Zhou, J. A. Weatherbee, M. L.-S. Tsang, M. Napolitano, W. J. Leonard, and I. B. Pragnell. 1993. Characterisation of a receptor for MIP-1α and related proteins on human and murine cells. *Cell Growth Differ.* **4**: 137–146.

31. Graham, G. J., J. Mackenzie, S. Lowe, M. L.-S. Tsang, J. A. Weatherbee, A. Issacson, J. Medicherla, F. Fang, P. C. Wilkinson, and I. B. Pragnell. 1994. Aggregation of the chemokine MIP-1α is a dynamic and reversible phenomenon: biochemical and biological analyses. *J. Biol. Chem.* **269**: 4974–4978.

32. Graham, G. J., P. C. Wilkinson, R. J. B. Nibbs, S. Lowe, S. O. Kolset, A. Parker, M. G. Freshney, M. L.-S. Tsang, and I. B. Pragnell. 1996. Uncoupling of stem cell inhibition from monocyte chemoattraction in MIP-1α by mutagenesis of the proteoglycan binding site. *EMBO J.* **15**: 6506–6515.

33. Grainger, D. J., P. R. Kemp, A. C. Liu, R. M. Lawn, and J. C. Metcalfe. 1994. Activation of transforming growth factor-β is inhibited in transgenic apolipoprotein(a) mice. *Nature* **370**: 460–462.

34. Grillon, C., K. Rieger, J. Bakala, D. Schott, J.-L. Morgat, E. Hannapel, W. Voelter, and M. Lenfant. 1990. Involvement of thymosin β4 and endoproteinase Asp-N in the biosynthesis of the tetrapeptide Ac.Ser.Asp.Lys.Pro a regulator of the haematopoietic system. *FEBS Lett.* **274**: 30–34.

35. Hatzfeld, J., M.-L. Li, E. L. Brown. 1991. Release of early human hematopoietic progenitors from quiescence by antisense transforming growth factor β1 or Rb oligonucleotides. *J. Exp. Med.* **174**: 925–929.

36. Hodgson, G. S., and T. R. Bradley. 1979. Properties of haematopoietic stem cells surviving 5-fluorouracil treatment: evidence for a pre-CFU-S cell? *Nature* **281**: 383, 384.

37. Holyoake, T. L., M. G. Freshney, and A. M. Sproul. 1993. Contrasting effects of rh-MIP-1α and TGF-β1 on Chronic Myeloid Leukaemia progenitors *in vitro*. *Stem Cells* **11(Suppl. 3)**: 122–128.

38. Holyoake, T. L., M. G. Freshney, L. McNair, A. N. Parker, P. J. McKay, W. P. Stewart, E. Fitzsimmons, G. J. Graham, and I. B. Pragnell. 1996. *Ex vivo* expansion with stem cell factor and Interleukin-11 augments both short-term recovery posttransplant and the ability to serially transplant marrow. *Blood* **87**: 4589–4595.

39. Hunter, M. G., L. Bawden, D. Brotherton, S. Craig, S. Cribbes, L. G. Czaplewski, T. M. Dexter, A. H. Drummond, A. H. Gearing, C. M. Heyworth, B. I. Lord, M. McCourt, P. G. Varley, L. M. Wood, R. M. Edwards, and P. J. Lewis. 1995. BB-10010: an active variant of human macrophage inflammatory protein-1α with improved pharmaceutical properties. *Blood* **86:** 4400–4408.

40. Ikebuchi, K., J. N. Ihle, Y. Hirai, G. G. Wong, S. C. Clark, and M. Ogawa. 1988. Synergistic factors for stem cell proliferation: further studies of the Target stem cells and the mechanism of stimulation by interleukin-1, interleukin-6, and granulocyte colony-stimulating factor. *Blood* **72:** 2007–2014.

41. Jacobsen, S. E. W., J. R. Keller, and F. W. Ruscetti. 1991. Bidirectional effects of transforming growth factor β (TGF-β) on colony-stimulating factor-induced human myelopoiesis *in vitro*: differential effects of distinct TGF-β isoforms. *Blood* **78:** 2239–2247.

42. Jones, R. J., P. Celano, S. J. Sharkis, and L. L. Sensenbrenner. 1989. Two phases of engraftment established by serial bone marrow transplantation in mice. *Blood* **73:** 397–401.

43. Jones, R. J., J. E. Wagner, P. Celano, M. S. Zicha, and S. J. Sharkis,. 1990. Separation of pluripotent haematopoietic stem cells from spleen colony forming cells. *Nature* **347:** 188, 189.

44. Katayama, N., S. C. Clark, and M. Ogawa. 1993. Growth factor requirement for survival in cell-cell dormancy of primitive murine lymphohematopoietic progenitors. *Blood* **81:** 610–616.

45. Keller, J. R., S. H. Barteimez, E. Sitnicka, F. W. Ruscetti, M. Ortiz, J. M. Gooya, and S. E. W. Jacobsen. 1994. Distinct and overlapping direct effects of macrophage inflammatory protein-1α and transforming growth factor β on hematopoietic progenitor/stem cell growth. *Blood* **84:** 2175–2181.

46. Keller, J. R., M. Ortiz, and F. W. Ruscetti. 1995. Steel factor (c-kit ligand) promotes the survival of hematopoietic stem/progenitor cells in the absence of cell division. *Blood* **85:** 1757–1764.

47. Koopman, W., and M. S. Krangel. 1997. Identification of a glycosaminoglycan-binding site in chemokine macrophage inflammatory protein-1α. *J. Biol. Chem.* **272:** 10,103–10,109.

48. Laerum O. D., and H. R. Maurer. 1973. Proliferation kinetics of myelopoietic cells and macrophages in diffusion chambers after treatment with granulocyte extracts (chalones). *Virchows Arch. B. Cell Pathol.* **14:** 293–305.

49. Laerum, O. D., and W. R. Paukovits. 1984. Inhibitory effects of a synthetic pentapeptide on haemopoietic stem cells *in vitro* and *in vivo*. *Exp. Hematol.* **12:** 7–17.

50. Laerum, O. D., O. Sletvold, R. Bjerknes, J. A. Eriksen, J. H. Johansen, J.-S. Schanche, T. Tveteras, and W. R. Paukovits. 1988. The dimer of hemoregulatory peptide (HP5B) stimulates mouse and human myelopoiesis in vitro. *Exp. Hematol.* **16:** 274–280.

51. Leary, A. G., Y. Hirai, T. Kishimoto, S. C. Clark, and M. Ogawa. 1989. Survival of hemopoietic progenitors in the G_0 period of the cell cycle does not require early hemopoietic regulators. *Proc. Natl. Acad. Sci. USA* **86:** 4335–4338.

52. Leary, A. G., H. Q. Zeng, S. C. Clark, and M. Ogawa. 1992. Growth factor requirements for survival in G_0 and entry into the cell cycle of primitive human hemopoietic progenitors. *Proc. Natl. Acad. Sci. USA* **89:** 4013–4017.

53. Lenfant, M., J. Wdzieczak-Bakala, E. Guittet, J.-C. Prome, D. Sotty, and E. Frindel. 1989. Inhibitor of hematopoietic pluripotent stem cell proliferation: purification and determination of its structure. *Proc. Natl. Acad. Sci. USA* **86:** 779–782.

54. Li, M.-L., A. A. Cardoso, P. Sansilvestri, A. Hatzfeld, E. L. Brown, H. Sookdeo, J.-P. Levesque, S. C. Clark, and J. Hatzfeld. 1994. Additive effects of steel factor and antisense TGF-β1 oligodeoxynucleotide in CD34+ hematopoietic progenitor cells. *Leukaemia* **8:** 441–445.

55. Lord, B. I., T. M. Dexter, J. M. Clements, M. A. Hunter, and A. J. H. Gearing. 1992.

Macrophage inflammatory protein protects multipotent haemopoietic cells from the cyto-toxic effects of hydroxyurea *in vivo. Blood* **79**: 2605–2609.

56. Maltman, J., I. B. Pragnell, and G. J. Graham. 1993. Transforming growth factor β: is it a downregulator of stem cell inhibition by macrophage Inflammatory protein-1α? *J. Exp. Med.* **178**: 925–932.

57. Maltman, J., I. B. Pragnell, and G. J. Graham. 1996. Specificity and reciprocity in the interactions between TGF-β: and macrophage inflammatory protein-1α. *J. Immunol.* **156**: 1566–1571.

58. Mantel, C., S. Aronica, Z. Luo, M. S. Marshall, Y. J. Kim, S. Cooper, N. Hague, and H. E. Broxmeyer. 1995. Macrophage inflammatory protein-1α enhances growth factor-stimu-lated phosphatidylcholine metabolism and increases cAMP levels in the human growth factor-dependent cell line MO7e, events associated with growth suppression. *J. Immunol.* **154**: 2342–2350.

59. Mayani, H., M.-T. Little, W. Dragowska, G. Thornbury, and P. M. Lansdorp. 1995. Differ-ential effects of the hematopoietic inhibitors MIP-1α, TGF-β, and TNF-α on cytokine-induced proliferation of subpopulations of CD34+ cells purified from cord blood and fetal liver. *Exp. Hematol.* **23**: 422–427.

60. Maze, R., B. Sherry, B. S. Kwon, A. Cerami, and H. E. Broxmeyer. 1992. Myelo-suppressive effects *in vivo* of purified recombinant murine macrophage inflammatory pro-tein-1α. *J. Immunol.* **149**: 1004–1009.

61. Monpezat, J.-P., and E. Frindel. 1989. Further studies on the biological activities of the CFU-S inhibitory tetrapeptide AcSDKP. II. The precise point of the cell cycle sensitive to AcSDKP: studies on the effect of AcSDKP on GM-CFC and on the possible involvement of T-lymphocytes in the AcSDKP response. *Exp. Hamatol.* **17**: 1077–1080.

62. Morrison, S. J., K. R. Prowse, P. Ho, and I. L. Weissman. 1996. Telomerase activity in hematopoietic cells is associated with self-renewal potential. *Immunity* **5**: 207–216.

63. Morrison, S. J., A. N. Wandycz, K. Akashi, A. Globerson, and I. L. Weissman. 1996. The aging of hematopoietic stem cells. *Nat. Med.* **2**: 1011–1017.

64. Mummery, C. L., and A. J. M. Van Den Eijnden-Van Raaij. 1993. Type β transforming growth factors and activins in differentiating embryonal carcinoma cells, embryonic stem cells and early embryonic development. *Int. J. Dev. Biol.* **37**: 169–182.

65. Neer, E. J. 1995. Heterotrimeric G proteins: organizers of transmembrane signals. *Cell* **80**: 249–257.

66. Nibbs, R. J. B., S. M. Wylie, I. B. Pragnell, and G. J. Graham. 1997. Cloning and characterisation of a novel murine β-chemokine receptor D6: comparison to three other related macrophage inflammatory protein-1α receptors CCR-1, CCR-3 and CCR-5. *J. Biol. Chem.* **272**: 12495–12504.

67. Nibbs, R. J. B., S. M. Wylie, J. Yang, N. R. Landau, and G. J. Graham. 1997. Cloning and characterisation of a novel promiscuous human β-chemokine receptor D6. *J. Biol. Chem.* **272**: 32078–32083.

68. Owen-Lynch, P. J., J. A. Adams, and M. L. Brereton. 1996. The effect of the chemokine rhMIP-1α, and a non-aggregating variant BB-10010, on blast cells from patients with acute myeloid leukaemia. *Br. J. Haematol.* **95**: 77–84.

69. Paolini, J. F., D. Willard, T. Consler, M. Luther, and M. S. Krangel. 1994. The chemokines IL-8, monocyte chemoattractant protein-1 and I-309 are monomers at physiologically rel-evant concentrations. *J. Immunol.* **153**: 2704–2717.

70. Parkinson, E. K., G. J. Graham, P. Daubersies, J. E. Burns, C. Heufler, M. Plumb, G. Schuler, and I. B. Pragnell. 1993. Hemopoietic stem cell inhibitor (SCI/MIP-1α) also inhib-its clonogenic epidermal keratinocyte proliferation. *J. Invest. Dermatol.* **101**: 113–117.

71. Paukovits, W. R., A. Hergl, and R. Schulte-Hermann. 1990. Hemoregulatory peptide pGlu-Flu-Asp-Cys-Lys: a new synthetic derivative for avoiding dimerization and loss of inhibi-tory activity. *Mol. Pharmacol.* **38**: 401–409.

72. Paukovits, W. R., M.-H. Moser, K. A. Binder, and J. B. Paukovits. 1991. Protection from arabinofuranosylcytosine and *n*-mustard-induced myelotoxicity using hemoregulatory peptide pGlu-Glu-Asp-Cys-Lys monomer and dimer. *Blood* **77**: 1313–1319.

73. Paukovits, W. R., M.-H. Moser, and J. B. Paukovits. 1993. Pre-CFU-S quiescence and stem cell exhaustion after cytostatic drug treatment: protective effects of the inhibitory peptide pGlu-Glu-Asp-Cys-Lys (pEEDCK). *Blood* **81**: 1755–1761.

74. Paukovits, W. R., and O. D. Laerum. 1982. Isolation and synthesis of a hemoregulatory peptide. *Z. Naturforsch.* **37c**: 1279.

75. Ploemacher, R. E., and N. H. C. Brons. 1988. Isolation of hemopoietic stem cell subsets from murine bone marrow. II. Evidence for an early precursor of day 12 CFU-S and cells associated with radioprotective ability. *Exp. Hematol.* **16**: 27–30.

76. Ploemacher, R. E., and R. H. C. Brons. 1989. Separation of CFU-S from primitive cells responsible for reconstitution of the bone marrow hemopoietic stem cell compartment following irradiation: evidence for a pre-CFU-S cell. *Exp. Hematol.* **17**: 263–270.

77. Premak, B. A., and T. J. Schall. 1996. Chemokine receptors: gateways to inflammation and infection. *Nat. Med.* **2**: 1174–1178.

78. Quesniaux, F. J., G. J. Graham, I. Pragnell, D. Donaldson, S. D. Wolpe, N. N. Iscove, and B. Fagg. 1993. Use of 5-fluorouracil to analyze the effect of macrophage inflammatory protein-1α on long-term reconstituting stem cells *in vivo*. *Blood* **81**: 1497–1504.

79. Rajarathnam, K., B. D. Sykes, C. M. Kay, B. Dewald, T. Geiser, M. Baggiolini, and I. Clark-Lewis. 1994. Neutrophil activation by monomeric interleukin-8. *Science* **264**: 90–92.

80. Rameshwar, P. and P. Gascon. 1996. Induction of negative hematopoietic regulators by neurokinin-A in bone marrow stroma. *Blood* **88**: 98–106.

81. Robinson, S., M. Lenfant, J. Wdzieczak-Bakala, and A. Riches. 1993. The molecular specificity of action of the tetrapeptide acetyl-N-ser-asp-lys-pro (AcSDKP) in the control of haemopoietic stem cell proliferation. *Stem Cells* **11**: 422–427.

82. Sarris, A. H., H. E. Broxmeyer, U. Wirthmueller, N. Karasavvas, S. Cooper, L. Lu, J. Krueger, and J. V. Ravetch. 1993. Human interferon-inducible protein 10: expression and purification of recombinant protein demonstrate inhibition of early human hematopoietic progenitors. *J. Exp. Med.* **178**: 1127–1132.

83. Soma, T., J. M. Yu, and C. E. Dunbar. 1996. Maintenance of murine long-term repopulating stem cells in *ex vivo* culture is affected by modulation of transforming growth factor-β but not macrophage inflammatory protein-1α activities. *Blood* **87**: 4561–4567.

84. Sporn, M. B., A. B. Roberts, L. M. Wakefield, and B. de Crombrugghe. 1987. Some recent advances in the chemistry and biology of transforming growth factor-beta. *J. Cell Biol.* **105**: 1039–1045.

85. Sporn, M. B., and A. B. Roberts. 1992. Transforming growth factor-beta: recent progress and new challenges. *J. Cell Biol.* **119**: 1017–1021.

86. Testa, N. G., and G. Molineux. 1993. *Haemopoiesis: A Practical Approach*. IRL, Oxford, England.

87. Till, J. E., and E. A. McCulloch. 1961. A direct measurement of the radiosensitivity of normal mouse bone marrow cells. *Radiat. Res.* **14**: 213–219.

88. Tsuji, K., S. D. Lyman, T. Sudo, S. C. Clark, and M. Ogawa. 1992. Enhancement of murine hematopoiesis by synergistic interactions between steel factor (ligand for *c-kit*, interleukin-11, and other early acting factors in culture. *Blood* **79**: 2855–2860.

89. Van Ranst, P. C. F., H.-W. Snoeck, F. Lardon, M. Lenjou, G. Nijs, S. F. Weekx, I. Rodrigus, Z. N. Berneman, and D. R. Van Bockstaele. 1996. TGF-β and MIP-1α exert their main inhibitory activity on very primitive CD34++CD38− cells but show opposite effects on more mature CD34+CD38+ human hematopoietic progenitors. *Exp. Hematol.* **4**: 1509–1515.

90. Vossler, M. R., H. Yao, R. D. York, M.-G. Pan, C. S. Rim, and P. J. S. Stork. 1997. cAMP activates MAP Kinase and Elk-1 through a B-Raf- and Rap1-dependent pathway. *Cell* **89**: 73–82.

91. Webb, L. M. C., M. U. Ehrengruber, I. Clark-Lewis, M. Baggiolini, and A. Rot. 1993. Binding to heparin sulphate or heparin enhances neutrophil responses to interleukin 8. *Proc. Natl. Acad. Sci. USA* **90:** 7158–7162.

92. Wu, J., P. Dent, T. Jelinek, A. Wolfman, M. J. Weber, and T. W. Sturgill. 1993. Inhibition of the EGF activated MAP Kinase signalling pathway by Adenosine 3′, 5′-monophosphate. *Science* **262:** 1065–1069.

93. Yayon, A., M. Klagsbrun, J. D. Esko, P. Leder, and D. M. Ornitz. 1991. Cell surface, heparin-like molecules are required for binding of basic fibroblast growth factor to its high affinity receptor. *Cell* **64:** 841–848.

94. Youn, B.-S., I.-K. Jang, H. E. Broxmeyer, S. Cooper, N. A. Jenkins, D. J. Gilbert, N. G. Copeland, T. A. Elick, M. J. Fraser, Jr., and B. S. Kwon. 1995. A novel chemokine, macrophage inflammatory protein-related protein-2, inhibits colony formation of bone marrow myeloid progenitors. *J. Immunol.* **155:** 2661–2667.

Index

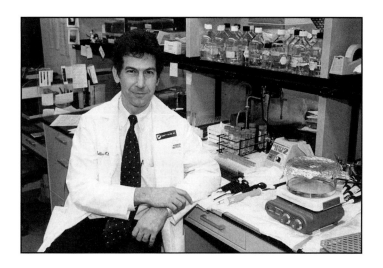

Dr. Barrett J. Rollins received his MD and PhD degrees from Case Western Reserve University. He performed a residency in Internal Medicine at Boston's Beth Israel Hospital, and then a fellowship in Medical Oncology at Dana-Farber Cancer Institute. He is currently on the staff at that institution as well as being a member of the faculty at Harvard Medical School.